Controlled Release of
**Pesticides and
Pharmaceuticals**

Controlled Release of
Pesticides and Pharmaceuticals

Edited by
Danny H. Lewis

Southern Research Institute
Birmingham, Alabama

SPRINGER SCIENCE+BUSINESS MEDIA, LLC

Library of Congress Cataloging in Publication Data

International Symposium on Controlled Release of Bioactive Materials (7th: 1980: Ft. Lauderdale, Fla.)
   Controlled release of pesticides and pharmaceuticals.
   "Proceedings of the Seventh International Symposium on Controlled Release of Bioactive Materials, held July 27-30, 1980, in Ft. Lauderdale, Florida"—T.p. verso.
   Includes bibliographies and index.
   1. Delayed-action preparations—Congresses. 2. Pesticides, Controlled release—Congresses. I. Lewis, Danny H. II. Title.
RS201.D4I57 1980   615'.191   81-7336
ISBN 978-1-4757-0739-7   ISBN 978-1-4757-0737-3 (eBook)   AACR2
DOI 10.1007/978-1-4757-0737-3

Proceedings of the Seventh International Symposium on
Controlled Release of Bioactive Materials, held July 27 – 30,
1980, in Ft. Lauderdale, Florida

©1981 Springer Science+Business Media New York
Originally published by Plenum Press, New York in 1981

PREFACE

        This volume is a result of the 7th International Symposium
on Controlled Release of Bioactive Materials held in Ft. Lauderdale,
Florida, on July 27-30, 1980. Controlled-release technology has
rapidly emerged over the past decade as a new science offering novel
approaches to a variety of practical problems in health care, food
production, and ecology. These symposia, organized and held annually
by the Controlled Release Society, Inc., provide an opportunity
for exchange of information among research scientists, regulatory
agencies, and consumers. The symposia are unique in the diverse
disciplines represented among the participants. Included among
the 186 attendees representing more than a dozen countries at the
1980 meeting were chemists, engineers, biologists, entomologists,
botanists, pharmacologists, physicians, and many others representing
the pharmaceutical, veterinary, and agrochemical areas.

        Each paper contained in this volume was reviewed and refereed
by experts in the field of controlled-release technology. The
assistance of the approximately 30 referees involved in that task
is greatly appreciated.

        The efforts of the many people involved in organizing the
meeting and preparing the manuscripts are appreciated. Particularly
helpful were Mr. Don Davis and his staff at Southern Research
Institute who did the graphic arts and layout. Special thanks are
due to Dr. Howard Creed for his editorial assistance and to Mrs.
Doris Thrower, who typed the complete volume in final form.

        The administrative and technical assistance provided by Southern
Research Institute in the preparation of this volume is appreciated.

                                          D.H. Lewis

                                          March, 1981

CONTENTS

CONTENTS

CONTROLLED RELEASE: BENEFITS VS. RISKS

Donald R. Cowsar

Southern Research Institute
2000 Ninth Avenue South
Birmingham, Alabama 35255

During the decade of the 1970s, new controlled-release technology continued to emerge from research laboratories around the
world. A few controlled-release formulations and devices have
already reached the market place, and many others are currently
undergoing premarketing trials. One might say that controlled
release has transgressed from its infancy through its childhood,
and it is rapidly maturing to occupy a vital position in many important industries. The future of controlled release appears bright
indeed.

The science and technology of controlled release is clearly
multidiciplinary. The non-routine interactions among polymer
chemists, biologists, biochemists, agrochemists, etomologists,
physical pharmacists, physicians, dentists, veterinarians, engineers,
and others have provided the synergism required for major technical
innovations. In 1855, when E. Fick stated in his emprical First
Law of Diffusion that "the flow is proportional to the gradient
in concentration", I am certain he never dreamed that Folkman and
Long[1] would apply the law to formulate a zero-order delivery system
for cardiac drugs or that Baker and Lonsdale[2] would derive fifty-
two ancillary equations quantifying controlled release by diffusion
from devices of many different geometries. Today, at least 1000
controlled-release scientists throughout the world publish their
work each year in journals ranging from Mosquito News to the Proceedings of the National Academy of Sciences.

When contrasted to conventional drug and pesticide formulary,
controlled release offers many benefits, some small and some very
large. To obtain benefits of large magnitude, one sometimes has
to take substantial risk. Fortunately, with nearly all of the

1

controlled release formulations developed so far, the risk to indivi-
duals and the environment appears minimized while the benefits appear
maximized. Indeed, a significant benefit of many agrochemical controlled-release formulations is that they minimize environmental
risks. Some of the major benefits of controlled release are summarized below.

A fundamental limitation of conventional formulations is that
they give up their agent to the surrounding medium at time-varying
rates that are highest initially and decline continually thereafter.
The rate of decline (duration of action) usually depends not upon
the dose but upon the host, and much more of the agent is required
to prolong the action than one might anticipate. Controlled-release
technologists, on the other hand, have developed a new arsenal of
"smart" systems which deliver agents with precision at predetermined, low rates. In many instances the agents are delivered
directly to the target organ or organism with only minimal intervention, and hence, only minimal therapeutic or environmental risk.
At least one order of magnitude less agent is usually required when
the delivery system provides a constant (zero-order) release rate.

Given that agents are efficacious, i.e., that they are effective
for the purpose intended, conventional formulations have failed
because of faulty compliance by the user with the prescribed regimen.
Since most controlled-release formulations are designed to function
for prolonged periods after a single administration, user compliance
rarely compromises their efficacy. In fact, some agents which were
only marginally efficacious when formulated conventionally, have
become highly effective in controlled-release formulations. If,
however, unexpected side effects occur with agents administered
via controlled release, many controlled-release formulations are
not reversible, and the side effects persist until the dose regimen
is complete. The more severe are the side effects, the greater
the risk.

As mentioned earlier, Fickian diffusion is often the mechanism
by which agents are released from controlled-release formulations.
Similarly, diffusion through cell walls is usually the mechanism
by which agents are taken up by the target organisms. For poorly
diffusing agents, uptake can only be increased by increasing the
extracellular concentration, i.e., the amount of agent administered
in each dose. Thus, agent uptake rather than agent release becomes
the controlling factor. By entrapping poorly diffusing agents in
tiny lipid spherules (i.e., liposomes), controlled-release technologists have produced formulations of conventional agents with
greatly enhanced potency. The liposomes are transported intact
through cell walls, and the entrapped agents are released slowly
within the cells as lipase enzymes attack the lipid materials.
The potential benefits of liposomes appear large indeed, while the

risks appear minimal. Current risk-vs.-benefit assessments of
liposome formulations are focused on potential side effects. Since
the lipid membrane of the liposomes disguises the encapsulated
agent, the distribution of the agent among body organs can be vastly
different for liposomal vs. conventional doses.

During the past few years, considerable research emphasis has
been given to targeted controlled-release systems which seek out
receptor sites and deliver their payloads as a "silver bullet" only
to the target organ or organism. This approach could significantly
augment the therapeutic index of many agents, especially those
highly toxic drugs used for cancer chemotherapy. Smart formulations
or devices which can respond to physiological rhythms or dynamic
cycles may be in the future of controlled-release technology. Currently, it is a major challenge to life scientists to determine
the extent to which the temporal patterning of agent delivery may
influence the balance of desired and undesired effects. If a significant benefit can be postulated, the polymer chemists, engineers,
and other designers of controlled-release systems can likely meet
the challenge with "smarter", more sophisticated systems.

REFERENCES

1.   J. Folkman and D.M. Long, Jr., J. Surg. Res. 4:139 (1964).
2.   R.W. Baker and H.K. Lonsdale, in: "Controlled Release of Bio-
      logically Active Agents," A.C. Tanquary and R.E. Lacey, eds.,
      Plenum Press, New York (1974). pp. 195-224.

EXPERIMENTAL APPROACHES FOR ACHIEVING BOTH ZERO-ORDER AND MODULATED CONTROLLED RELEASE FROM POLYMER MATRIX SYSTEMS

Dean S.T. Hsieh and Robert Langer

Department of Nutrition and Food Science, M.I.T.,
Cambridge, Massachusetts 02139 and the Department
of Surgery, Children's Hospital Medical Center,
Boston, Massachusetts 02115

INTRODUCTION

One of the major drawbacks of all practical approaches thus far developed for fabricating diffusion-controlled matrices for drug delivery is that the release rates decrease with time. From a pharmaceutical standpoint, it would be desirable for many such systems to display zero-order release kinetics. Furthermore, in some circumstances (e.g., insulin delivery in diabetics) it would be useful to be able to achieve increased dosages on demand. In the present study, we present experimental approaches for achieving both of these objectives.

ZERO-ORDER MATRIX SYSTEMS

In an earlier study, we used the Higuchi model to analyze a variety of matrix shapes in order to achieve zero-order kinetics. It was found that optimal results were achieved with a hemisphere that was laminated with an impermeable coating except for a small concavity in the center face.[1] All drug was therefore forced to be released through this concavity. With this geometry, an increasing area of drug became available as the distance from the releasing surface increased. This effect compensated for the decreasing release rates normally seen in matrix systems caused by time-dependent increases in drug-diffusion distance from the matrix surface; near-constant release was predicted. We have now developed experimental approaches to test the prediction. In the model system described below, sodium salicylate is used as the drug and polyethylene as the polymer.

5

Preparation of Zero-Order Hemispheres

Sodium salicylate (Fisher Scientific) and polyethylene (PEP-315, Union Carbide) were initially passed through a 60-mesh screen (Dual Mfg. Co.) separately. These ingredients were then mixed together in a cube blender (Type UG No. 16643, Erweka - G.M.B.H.) for five minutes in batches of different weight ratios or loadings. The brass molds, shown in Figure 1, had two halves fastened together with wing nuts. The molds had six hollow cylinders (3/8" diameter, 4.5" long) that were round-bottomed (with a 3/16" radius).

To fabricate hemispheres, each hollow cylinder was loaded with 220 mg of sodium salicylate-polyethylene blend and placed into a 150°C oven for 30 minutes. After this heating, a brass plunger (3/8" diameter) was inserted into each cylinder as hard as manually possible. This plunger was flat-bottomed except for a central depression into which one half of a 2-mm steel bead (Type 440C Ultraspheric, Inc.) was glued.

After compression of the drug-polymer blend, the plunger was removed. To maintain the small concavity during cooling and coating, a 2-mm steel bead was then inserted into the depression of each hemisphere with the aid of forceps. The mold was allowed to cool at room temperature and was then disassembled. The hemispheres were removed from the mold and then trimmed with a scalpel (No. 10 Blade, Bard-Parker) to remove any irregular edges. The average weight of a hemisphere after trimming was 210 ± 5 mg. The average diameter was 9.10 ± 0.01 mm.

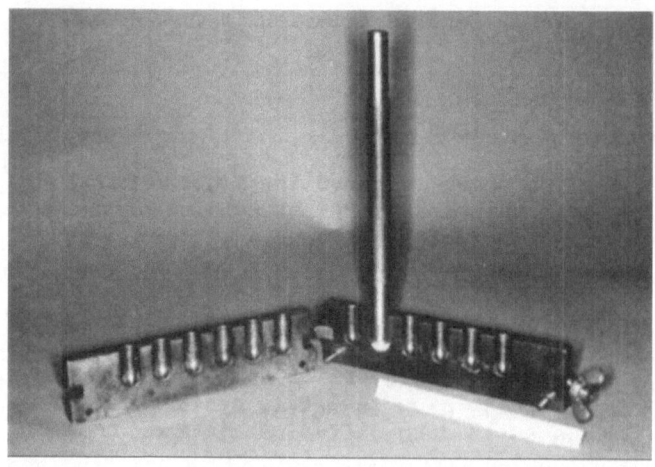

Figure 1. Mold for making hemisphere pellets.

Each hemisphere was coated with five applications of paraffin (Paraplast tissue embedding medium). For this process 30 gm of paraffin was placed in a 150-ml Pyrex beaker and heated to 85 ± 2°C on a hot plate. The hemisphere was held with a forceps and dipped briefly (2-3 seconds) into the molten paraffin. Each coating was allowed to harden for at least one minute with exposure to air. For each subsequent coating, the hemisphere was held at a different position and then dipped into the paraffin again. After five coatings, the steel bead was removed with forceps. The only uncoated space was the center concavity where the bead had been.

Kinetic Studies

Studies were conducted to measure the release of salicylate into saline from these hemispheres. For these studies, each matrix was immersed in a scintillation vial (No. 986548, Wheaton Scientific) with 10 ml of saline solution (0.9% NaCl). Each matrix was weighted down with a small piece of stainless-steel wire wrapped around it. Any bubbles present on the uncoated releasing surface were removed by aspiration with a pasteur pipette. The vials were placed on a Thomas Rotating Apparatus at speed 4. (Preliminary experiments showed no significant difference in release with this shaking versus more vigorous stirring.) Each matrix was transferred into a new vial with fresh saline at periodic intervals. The released sodium salicylate concentrations were determined spectrophotometrically by measuring absorbance at 294 nm.

As controls, hemispheres of pure polyethylene were prepared both uncoated and completely coated (including the concavity). Similarly, completely coated hemispheres with the 30% salicylate-polyethylene blend were prepared. All of these controls were tested for release kinetics.

Results and Discussion

Figure 2 shows photographs of a hemisphere, prepared from a blend comprising 10% sodium salicylate and 90% polyethylene. The left one (a) is the view of the flat surface of the hemisphere; note the central depression via which drug diffuses. The right one (b) is the view of the round bottom of the hemisphere.

An example of the release rates obtained from these hemispheres is shown in Figure 3. As noted, zero-order release was demonstrated. Further studies have verified that zero-order release is obtained by this technique with different loadings and that release from the hemisphere more closely approximated linearity than with other shapes (e.g., a wedge[2,3]) previously proposed as zero-order release systems. All controls showed no salicylate absorbance.

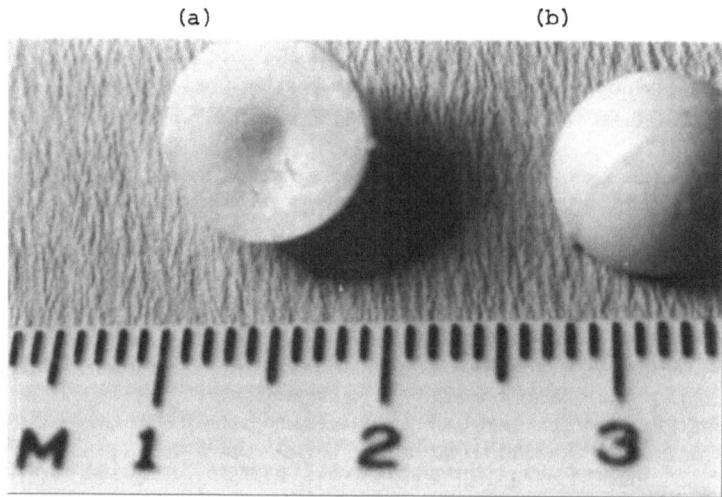

Figure 2. Hemisphere pellets. (a) top; (b) bottom.

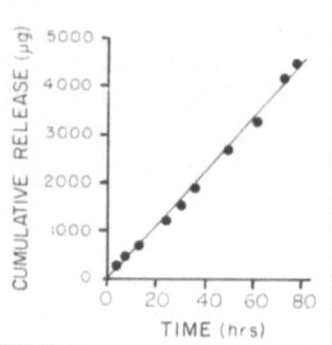

Figure 3. Release of sodium salicylate 30% (w/w) from
           polyethylene.

It should be noted that the geometry suggested relies on the fact that diffusion of the drug through the polymer is the rate-limiting step.[4] If, for example, surface erosion was rate limiting, then a geometry whose surface area did not change as a function of time (e.g., a long thin slab) would be required to obtain zero-order release kinetics.[5]

MAGNETICALLY MODULATED SUSTAINED-RELEASE SYSTEMS

One problem central to the field of sustained-release technology is that all vehicles so far developed display drug-release rates that are either constant or decay with time. There has been no way to change or modulate the release rate on demand, once release has commenced.

Here we report the development of a polymeric system capable of delivering molecules at increased rates on demand. By the simple technique of embedding small magnetic steel beads in the polymer along with the drug, release rates can be increased when desired by an oscillating external bar magnet. The procedures used and the initial results obtained are described below.

Preparation of Magnetic Sustained-Release Polymers

The procedure for preparing magnetic sustained-release systems was modified from our earlier methods of preparing non-magnetic sustained-release implants;[6] it is shown in Figure 4. Polymer casting solution was made by dissolving ethylene-vinyl acetate copolymer[6,7] in methylene chloride to achieve a 10% (w/v) solution. One-half gram of powdered simulating drug (bovine serum albumin; (BSA) Sigma Chemical Co., St. Louis, MO), which had been sieved to contain particles between 149 and 210 μm, was mixed with 10 ml of casting solution. The suspension was poured quickly onto a leveled glass mold (7 x 7 x 0.5 cm) which had been previously cooled by placing it on dry ice for five minutes. The mold remained on the dry ice throughout the procedure. Immediately following the pouring of the polymer-drug-mixture, magnetic steel beads (79.17% iron, 17% chromium, 1% carbon, 1% magnanese, 1% silicone, 0.05% phosphorus, 0.05% sulfur, and 0.75% molybdenum; 1.4 mm diameter; from Ultra-spherics, Inc., Marie, MI) were placed onto the mixture with a loading device.

The loading device was made of one bacterial culture petri-dish (Falcon 1001, Oxnard, CA) with the bottom sitting inside the inverted lid (Figure 5a) Both the bottom and the lid had an identical arrangement of 263 holes (1.8 mm diameter) with 3-mm spacing. While the plates were shifted with respect to each other so that

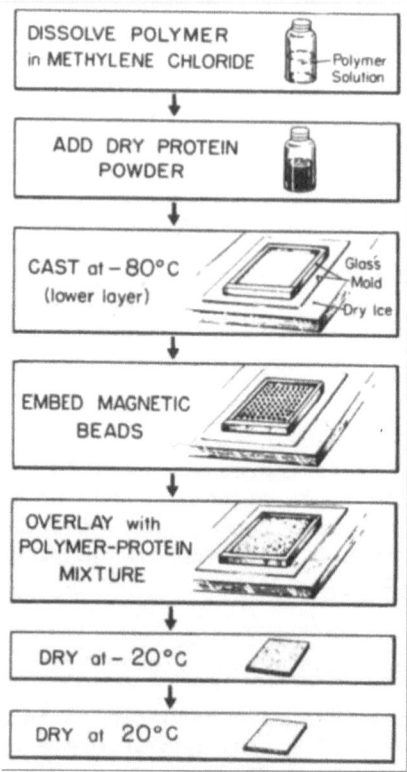

Figure 4. Flow diagram of the procedure for preparing magnetic
         sustained-release polymers.

the upper and lower holes were offset, the upper holes were filled
with magnetic steel beads (Figure 5b). The plates with magnetic
beads were positioned over the polymer slab in the mold. When the
plates were shifted back so that all the holes were aligned, the
magnetic steel beads dropped onto the polymer in a uniform array
(Figure 5c).

    Two minutes after the magnetic beads were added, a top layer
of BSA-polymer mixture identical to the bottom layer was cast over
the beads. After the entire mixture had solidified (approximately
ten minutes), the slab was transferred to a -20°C freezer for 48
hours followed by further drying at 20°C under a houseline vacuum
(600 millitorrs) for an additional 24 hours.

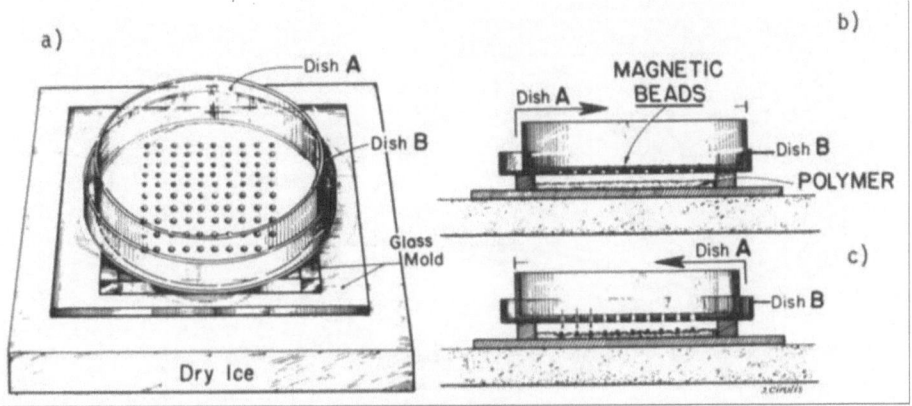

Figure 5.   Diagram of a loading device and the procedures of load-
            ing magnetic beads. (a) Assembly of the petri-dish (top
            and bottom) loading device, the glass mold, and dry ice;
            (b) To load beads onto the device, the top lid and bot-
            tom lid are offset with respect to each other. The
            holes are filled with magnetic beads. As long as the
            lids are offset, the beads will remain in the loading
            device; (c) To place beads onto the polymer, the holes
            of the top lid and bottom lid are aligned; the magnetic
            beads now drop onto the polymer slab.

     The use of low-temperature casting and drying prevents migra-
tion of the drug powder.[6] The use of a three-step procedure to
embed the beads between two layers of partially fluid polymer-BSA
mixture provides vertical homogeneity of the beads; the device used
to place the beads between polymer layers provides horizontal uniformity.

Kinetic Studies

     First, sixteen 1 cm^2 squares were excised from the central
portion of the dried slab. Each square contained approximately
14 beads/cm^2. Each square was placed in a glass scintillation vial
(Wheaton Scientific Co., Millville, NJ) containing 10 ml of physiological saline (0.9% w/v). Then the vials containing polymer squares
were placed onto a plastic tray above a triggering device (Figure 6).

     The triggering device was modified from a commercial speed-
controlled rocker (Minarik Electric Co., Los Angeles, CA) by simply
placing a permanent magnet bar (Crucore Magnet Bar, No. RE80108,
Permag Northeast Co., Billerica, MA) on one end of the rocker and

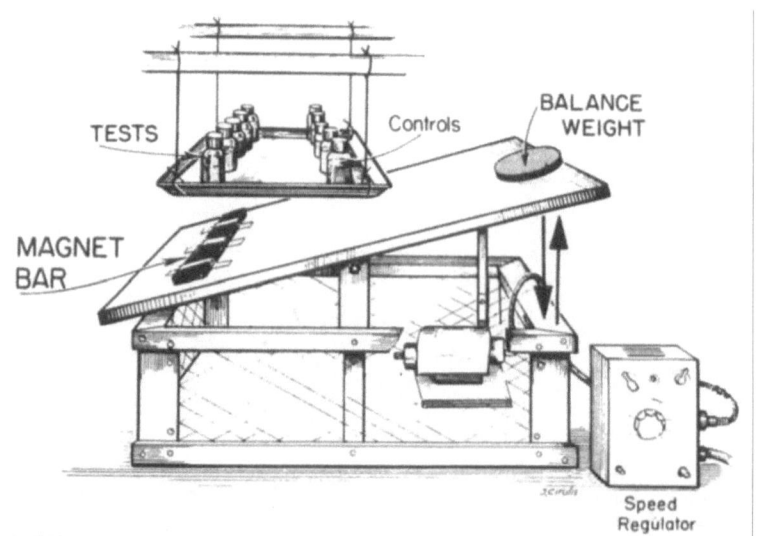

Figure 6.   Diagram of a motor driven see-saw rocker used as a
             triggering device.

a balanced weight on the other end (Figure 6). The frequency of
motion was 18 cycles/minutes. Thus an oscillating magnetic field
ranging from 1/2 gauss (the magnetic field strength on the surface
of the earth) to approximately 1,000 gauss on the surface of the
magnetic bar was created for triggering.

The vials (n=8) containing polymeric squares made as described
in Figure 4 were exposed to the oscillating magnetic field for six-
hour periods followed by six hours of non-exposure. Cyclic shift-
ing between triggering and non-triggering was conducted for five
days.

Four different control experiments were conducted:

(1)   Polymeric squares excised from the same slab as those
       used in the triggering experiment were subjected to the
       same manipulations except that the bar magnet was absent.

(2)   Polymeric squares were made without magnetic steel beads.
       These polymer squares were exposed to the oscillating
       magnetic field.

(3) Polymeric squares containing BSA and steel beads were exposed to intervals of shaking in the absence of the bar magnet. The shaking was done by placing the polymeric squares on a Thomas Clinical Rotator at speed 3.

(4) Polymeric squares containing BSA and steel beads were exposed to a stationary magnetic field in which the bar magnet was maintained in apposition to the polymer throughout alternating six-hour periods.

Results and Discussion

When exposed to the oscillating magnetic field, the polymeric squares released up to 100% more BSA than when the magnetic field was discontinued (Figure 7). For example, the first six-hour exposure period showed an average release rate of 125 µg/hour compared to the 40 µg/hour in the following six hours of no exposure. The differential decreased with increasing time, but was still significant at the end of the experiment (37 µg/hour versus 25 µg/hour). Increased rates of release upon exposure to the oscillating magnetic field were repeatedly observed in the course of this test. Furthermore, in none of the four control experiments were modulated release rates observed.[8]

We have also tested the biocompatibility of the polymers containing steel beads by implanting them into the rabbit cornea using previously described techniques.[9] No inflammation was detected.

The mechanism by which the magnetic field is able to induce a modulated sustained-release pattern is currently under investigation. In an earlier study, we identified small channels in ethylene-vinyl acetate copolymer-drug matrices through which the drugs can migrate.[10] It is possible that the oscillating magnetic field causes alternating compression and expansion of these channels, thereby facilitating drug movement out of the matrix. Regardless of the mechanism, the further development of systems with modulated release patterns induced by magnetism or other means (e.g., enzymatic[11]) may prove useful in the delivery of various hormones such as insulin in vivo.

CONCLUSIONS

These studies demonstrate that matrix systems can be modified to produce either zero-order or modulated sustained-release devices. Work is underway to develop improved designs for both systems and to test them in animals. The studies reported have, we hope, extended the capability of polymer matrix systems to produce desired release-kinetic patterns.

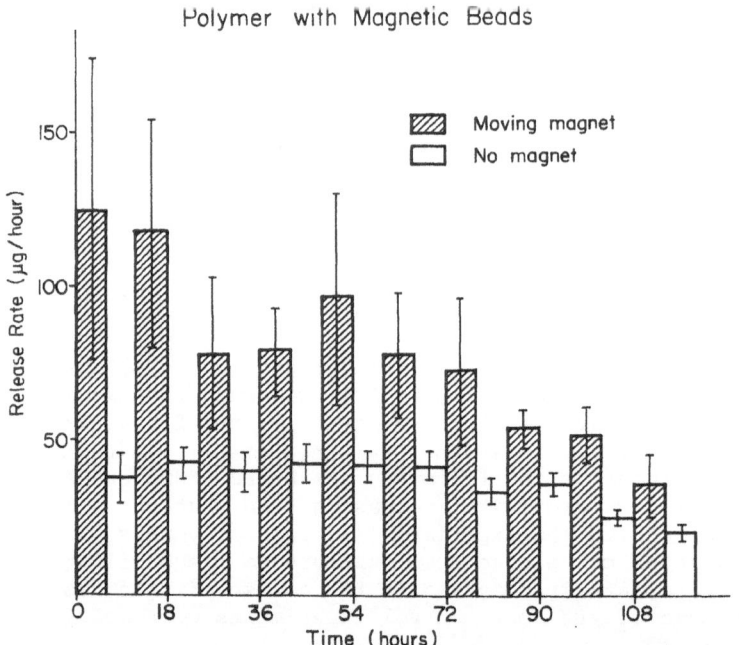

Figure 7. Modulated sustained release of bovine serum albumin from
           polymeric vehicles by magnetism. Each histogram repre-
           sents the average release rate of BSA from polymer
           squares (1 cm x 1 cm).

ACKNOWLEDGEMENTS

     This study was supported by NIH grant GM 26698. We would like
to thank Annette LaRocca for typing the manuscript.

REFERENCES

1. W. Rhine, V. Sukhatme, D. Hsieh, and R. Langer, in: "Controlled
    Release of Bioactive Materials," R.W. Baker, ed., Academic
    Press, New York (1980). p. 177.
2. B Brooke, and R. Washkuhn, J. Pharm. Sci 66:159 (1977).
3. R.A. Lipper, and W.I. Higuchi, J. Pharm. Sci. 66:163 (1977).
4. R. Langer, Chem. Eng. Commun. 6:1 (1980).
5. H. Hopfenberg, in: "Controlled Release Polymeric Formulations,"
    D.R. Paul and F.W. Harris, eds., American Chemical Society,
    Washington (1976). p. 26.
6. W.D. Rhine, D.S.T. Hsieh, and R. Langer, J. Pharm. Sci. 69:265
    (1980).

7. R. Langer, and J. Folkman, Nature 263:797 (1976).
8. D. Hsieh, R. Langer, and J. Folkman, Proc. Natl. Acad. Sci. in press.
9. R. Langer, H. Brem, and D. Tapper, J. Biomed. Mat. Res., in press.
10. R. Langer, W. Rhine, D. Hsieh, and R. Bawa, in: "Controlled Release of Bioactive Materials," R.W. Baker, ed., Academic Press, New York (1980). p. 83.
11. J. Heller, and P. Trescony, J. Pharm. Sci. 68:919 (1979).

PHARMACOKINETIC MODELING OF GENTAMICIN RELEASE

FROM A PROSTHETIC HEART VALVE

L.S. Olanoff, J.M. Anderson, and R.D. Jones

Departments of Pathology and Macromolecular
Science, Case Western Reserve University,
Cleveland, Ohio 44106, and Division of
Surgical Research, St. Luke's Hospital,
Cleveland, Ohio 44104

INTRODUCTION

Sustained release of biological agents is a concept that has
received increased attention over the past decade. The primary
goal of sustained drug release is the prolonged delivery of a drug
to a particular body compartment or anatomical target site. This
goal is accomplished by the application of a therapeutic drug
delivery system designed to control both temporal and spatial aspects
of drug disposition.

Previous investigations in the field of controlled drug delivery
have centered on the design and in vitro testing of the device.
Animal experimentation has been largely limited to reports on the
temporal pharmacodynamic performance of the drugs released from
the implanted, inserted, or surface-applied polymer vehicles. Few
studies have attempted to provide details of the kinetic behavior
of these release systems throughout the period of in vivo evaluation. These data are essential to exploring the pharmacokinetic
characteristics of such systems and providing for the development
of predictive models. These models also increase experimental efficiency by allowing the use of preliminary measurements and analyses
to optimize the further design of the controlled drug-release
systems, conserving time and animal resources.

The project to be discussed in this report concerns the release
of gentamicin from a drug vehicle fabricated within a prosthetic
heart valve. In brief, the system consists of a dispersion of gentamicin sulfate in a silicone rubber polymer molded to serve as a

17

sewing rim insert within the replacement heart valve. The ability
of the system to provide local sustained release of the antibiotic
in vitro and in vivo, for the prevention of prosthetic valve endocarditis, has been detailed in previous publications.[1,2] This paper
will report on efforts to formulate diffusion models to describe
the in vitro release of gentamicin from the silicone rubber sewing
rim insert, and the correlation of in vitro drug release with in
vivo drug delivery through the incorporation of the above drug diffusion models in a simple pharmacokinetic simulation.

METHODS

     The construction and in vitro and in vivo evaluation of the
gentamicin releasing prosthetic heart valve has been previously
detailed.[2] In brief, prosthetic mitral valves were constructed
by substituting the drug-release system in place of the standard-
valve sewing rim. The drug-release system was fabricated by milling
together 0.52 gm of crystalline gentamicin sulfate, 57-58% potency
(Schering Corp., Bloomfield, NJ), and 0.78 gm silicone rubber stock
(Grade MDX-44515, Dow Corning Medical Products, Midland, MI) until
a uniform dispersion of the drug in the unpolymerized rubber was
obtained. The silicone rubber loaded at 40% by weight with gentamicin sulfate was then compression molded and allowed to cure in
a steam autoclave at 220°F for five mins. In those experiments
involving drug concentration analysis, 0.35 to 0.5 mg of the drug
was added in the form of ^{3}H-gentamicin sulfate (Amersham-Searle
Corp.). Some of the drug-loaded valve rim inserts were coated after
cure with an additional layer of drug-free silicone rubber by dip-
ping the insert once in a solution of 10% silicone rubber (Product
Q7-2213, Dow Corning Medical Products, Midland, MI) in 1,1,1-tri-
chloroethane. The coating thickness was 72 ± 16 µ (mean ± SD) as
measured by a microscope equipped with a calibrated micrometer
attachment. These samples were designated as the "coated valve
inserts".

     In vitro release of gentamicin was determined with the use of
flow cells in which the valve rim inserts were mounted in a configuration similar to that used in the prosthetic valve. Small teflon
stirring bars within each cell were rotated continuously to minimize boundary layer effects at the diffusional surfaces. The total
effluent was collected daily, and the drug release was determined
by liquid scintillation analysis of the ^{3}H-gentamicin.

     Prosthetic valves were implanted in the mitral position in
dogs by standard techniques of cardiopulmonary bypass with a modified rotating disc oxygenator. Following anesthesia with sodium
pentobarbital, 30 mg/kg, heparin was administered, 3,000 U/kg, and,
after institution of full cardiopulmonary support, the normal mitral

valve leaflets were excised, and the valve prosthesis was fixed
in place with 12 to 14 atraumatic polyester sutures. No protamine
was given postoperatively, and the dog was not given anticoagulants
other than the intraoperative heparin, which was metabolized over
the next four to five hrs as determined by in vitro titration.
In the in vivo experiments, prosthetic valves containing silicone-
rubber rim inserts loaded with 40% gentamicin sulfate (by weight),
both coated and uncoated forms, were evaluated. In five of each
of the uncoated and coated gentamicin-loaded prosthetic valves,
[3]H-gentamicin sulfate was added during fabrication for radioassay
measurements of serum gentamicin concentrations postimplantation
in dogs. Following contact of the prosthetic valve with the heart
tissue surface, blood samples for gentamicin measurement were obtained at 5 min intervals throughout the cardiopulmonary bypass
procedure, and at 30 mins, 1 hr, and 5 hrs after its termination.
In addition, blood gentamicin levels were monitored daily for the
first three to four days postimplantation and one to two times
weekly until blood levels fell below measurable limits (<0.1 µg/ml).

The equations of the in vitro diffusion models and the in vivo
pharmacokinetic simulation were solved numerically by an iterative
technique[3] with the use of a PDP-12 computer (Digital Electronics
Corporation, Maynard, MA).

Gentamicin elimination constants and volume of distribution
values, employed in the in vivo pharmacokinetic model, were determined by injecting the dogs with a small intravenous bolus of the
antibiotic at least one week prior to surgery and observing the
fall in serum values for 20 hours immediately following the injection. The analysis of the data used to derive the above constants
is reported elsewhere.[3]

THEORETICAL BACKGROUND

A widely used mathematical diffusion model for the release
of drugs from monolithic matrix devices, where the drug consists
of a combination of dissolved and solid dispersed forms within a
polymer slab, is the set of equations derived by T. Higuchi.[4] The
same simulation has also been extended to approximate in vitro drug
release from polymer matrix devices of cylindrical configurations
(Chien et al,[5] Chien and Lambert,[6] Roseman[7]).

A far better conceptual model for drug release from cylindrical
matrices is provided by Roseman and W. Higuchi.[8] Expressed in terms
of the physical dimensions of a cylindrical rod where at time, t,
solid drug is considered dispersed from the rod center to some distance, a', to where the eluting front has progressed from the surface (Figure 1), Roseman and Higuchi's equation takes the following
form:

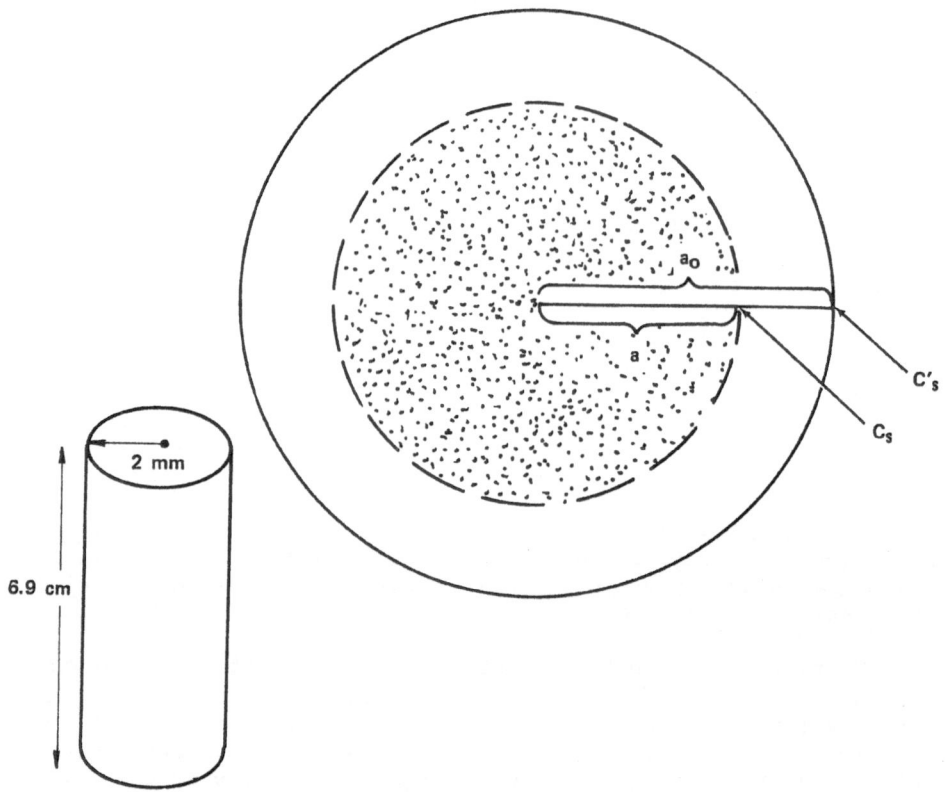

Figure 1. Above: diagram of cut edge of uncoated valve rim insert
           (see text for definition of symbols). Below: measured
           dimensions of cylindrical approximation of valve rim
           insert. Release from cylinder end surfaces not included
           in the approximation.

$$\frac{a'^2}{2} \ln \frac{a'}{a_o} + \frac{a_o^2 - a'^2}{4} = \frac{D_e \cdot C_s \cdot t}{A} \tag{1}$$

where a_o = radial distance from center of the rod to its surface

         D_e = diffusion coefficient of the drug in the polymer

         C_s = drug solubility constant in the polymer

         A = initial drug concentration (dispersed + dissolved
              forms) in the polymer

At the distance, a', the effective drug concentration driving the diffusion process is the drug solubility constant, C_s. Alternatively, in terms of cumulative amount of drug released, Q, and initial amount of drug, M_o, where Q/M_o equals the fraction of drug released at time, t, equation (1) becomes,

$$(1 - Q/M_o) \cdot \ln (1 - Q/M_o) + \frac{Q}{M_o} = \frac{4 \cdot C_s \cdot D_e \cdot t}{A \cdot a_o^2} \tag{2}$$

Equation (2) was used to describe gentamicin release from the ring-shaped uncoated rim-insert device incorporated in the prosthetic valve design.[3] In this example the ring configuration was approximated as a bent cylinder without ends, which was appropriate since equation (2) does not account for release of the drug from the ends of a cylindrical device. For the valve rim insert M_o, A and a_o^2 were known quantities, and Q and t were measured during the in vitro gentamicin release experiments. The quantity $D_e \cdot C_s$ was calculated by transforming equation (2) to the point in time, t , where the drug in the device becomes exhausted and Q equals M_o,

$$t_e = \frac{A \cdot a_o^2}{4 \cdot C_s \cdot D_e} \tag{3}$$

rearranging

$$D_e \cdot C_s = \frac{A \cdot a_o^2}{4 \cdot t_e} \tag{4}$$

The derivation of the release-rate equations for rim inserts with the additional coating layer of blank silicone rubber follows a form similar to those derived previously for the uncoated system (based on the Roseman and W. Higuchi model).

Starting with the basic restatement of Fick's First law of diffusion:

$$\frac{dQ}{dt} = -2 \cdot h \cdot \pi \cdot D_e \cdot a \cdot \frac{dC}{da} \tag{5}$$

where $\frac{dQ}{dt}$ = rate of drug release from polymer cylinder

h = height of cylinder (constant)

a = radial distance from center of cylindrical rod

$\frac{dC}{da}$ = concentration gradient along the cylinder radius

and all other variables are as previously defined. Referring to
Figure 2, a diagram of a cross section through the coated rim insert,
the amount of drug depleted per unit time from the core of the
device to the interface between the coating layer and the central
drug-loaded rod was derived by integrating equation (5) and applying
the conditions, $C=C_s$ at $a=a'$ and $C'=C_s'$ at $a=a_o$:

$$\frac{dQ}{dt} = \frac{-2 \cdot \pi \cdot D_e \cdot h \cdot (C_s - C_s')}{\ln (a'/a_o)} \tag{6}$$

The drug release rate across the additional coating layer of the
device was derived by substituting the appropriate conditions into
equation (5), yielding:

$$\frac{dQ}{dt} = \frac{2 \cdot \pi \cdot h \cdot a_o \cdot D_c}{h_c} (C_s' - C_B) \tag{7}$$

where $a = a_o$, radius of central rod

$da = h_c$, thickness of coating layer

C_B = concentration of drug in bulk (eluting) solution

D_c = diffusion coefficient of drug in (blank silicone rubber) coating layer

C_s' = concentration of the drug at the coating-central rod interface

and all other variables are as defined previously.

On the assumption that infinite sink conditions existed, which
was justified in this instance, as gentamicin is highly soluble
in aqueous solutions and there was a relatively rapid turnover of
the sink fluid both in the _in vitro_ test apparatus and the _in vivo_
implantation site, C_B may be set equal to zero, and equation (7)
becomes:

$$\frac{dQ}{dt} = \frac{2 \cdot \pi \cdot a_o \cdot h \cdot D_c \cdot C_s'}{h_c} \tag{8}$$

At steady-state, when the coating layer reaches equilibrium, the
rate of drug release from the core equals the rate of drug transfer
across the coating membrane. Equating equations (6) and (8):

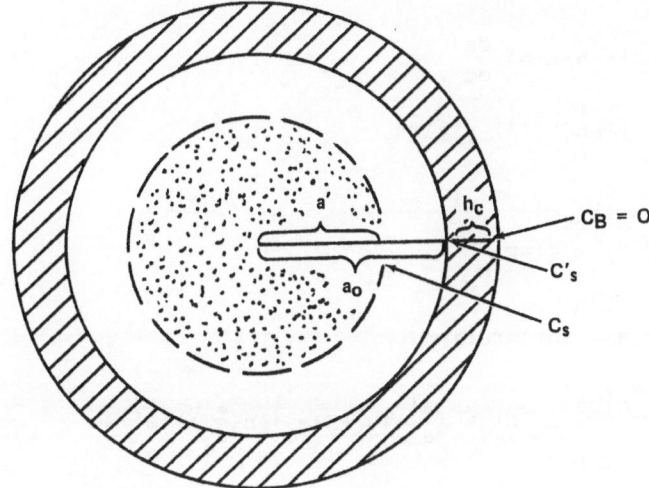

Figure 2.   Diagram of cut edge of coated valve rim insert (see text
            for definition of symbols).

$$\frac{-2\cdot\pi\cdot h\cdot D_e\cdot(C_s-C_s')}{\ln\,(a'/a_o)} = \frac{2\cdot\pi\cdot a_o\cdot h\cdot D_c\cdot C_s'}{h_c} \qquad (9)$$

and solving for C_s'

$$C_s' = \frac{C_s}{(1-\frac{a_o}{h_c}\cdot\frac{D_c}{D_e}\cdot\ln\,(\frac{a'}{a_o}))} \qquad (10)$$

substituting the above equation for C_s' into equation (6)

$$\frac{dQ}{dt} = \frac{-2\cdot\pi\cdot h\cdot D_e\cdot C_s}{\ln\,(\frac{a'}{a_o})} \cdot(1 - \frac{1}{(1-K\cdot\frac{a_o}{h_c}\cdot\ln\,(\frac{a'}{a_o}))}) \qquad (11)$$

where $K = \dfrac{D_c}{D_e}$

By definition,

$$Q = \pi\cdot h\cdot A\cdot(a_o^2 - a'^2) \qquad (12)$$

and differentiating equation (12)

$$\frac{dQ}{dt} = -2 \cdot \pi \cdot h \cdot A \cdot a' \cdot \frac{da'}{dt} \tag{13}$$

Equating (11) and (13) yields,

$$\frac{D_e \cdot C_s}{\ln(\frac{a'}{a_o})} \cdot (1 - \frac{1}{(1 - K \cdot \frac{a_o}{h_c} \cdot \ln(\frac{a'}{a_o}))}) = A \cdot a' \cdot \frac{da'}{dt} \tag{14}$$

Rearranging and integrating,

$$\frac{-K \cdot D_e \cdot a_o \cdot C_s}{A} \int_o^t dt = \int_a^{a'} (h_c - K \cdot a_o \cdot \ln(\frac{a'}{a_o})) \cdot a' \cdot da' \tag{15}$$

Solving the above, substituting in the definition of K and reducing:

$$\frac{D_e \cdot C_s \cdot t}{A} = \frac{-h_c \cdot (a'^2 - a_o^2)}{2 \cdot a_o} \cdot \frac{D_e}{D_c} + \frac{a'^2}{2} \cdot \ln(\frac{a'}{a_o}) + \frac{(a_o^2 - a'^2)}{4} \tag{16}$$

Expressing the above equation in terms of Q and M_o (as defined previously):

$$\frac{4 \cdot D_e \cdot C_s \cdot t}{A \cdot a_o^2} = \frac{Q}{M_o} \cdot (1 + \frac{2 \cdot D_e \cdot h_c}{D_c \cdot a_o}) + (1 - \frac{Q}{M_o}) \cdot (\ln(1 - \frac{Q}{M_o})) \tag{17}$$

Differentiation of equation (17) gives the release rate from the device:

$$\frac{dQ}{dt} = -4 \cdot D_e \cdot C_s \cdot \pi \cdot h / (\ln(1 - \frac{Q}{M_o}) - \frac{2 \cdot D_e \cdot h_c}{D_c \cdot a_o}) \tag{18}$$

These equations were applied to the coated valve-rim insert system by using the measured values of the physical constants h, h_c, a_o, M_o, and A, taking the value of $D_e \cdot C_s$ as solved from the uncoated rim insert and calculating the ratio of D_e/D_c from the transformation of equation (17) when the device becomes exhausted (t = t_e),

$$\frac{D_e}{D_c} = (\frac{4 \cdot D_e \cdot C_s \cdot t_e}{A \cdot a_o^2} - 1) \cdot \frac{a_o}{2 \cdot h_c} \tag{19}$$

Correlation of In Vitro and In Vivo Release Characteristics

To investigate the in vivo efficacy of sustained-release preparations a comprehensive pharmacokinetic model is necessary. The
two basic processes depicted within a given analysis are the primary
diffusive transport of the active agent through the polymer delivery
vehicle into the biological receiving medium and the subsequent
transport, distribution and elimination of the drug. The latter
process has been detailed in numerous pharmacokinetic models relating the observations on absorption, distribution, and elimination
of orally or parenterally administered conventional pharmaceutical
agents. The former process is unique to the topic of sustained
drug release and is related to the physical and chemical characteristics of the drug and its polymer delivery vehicle and the biological response elicited by the implanted system in situ.

Many groups have designed sustained-release devices and
evaluated the systems in vitro. Relatively few investigators have
extended their experiments to include in vivo trials. Only a
handful of reports have attempted to quantitatively correlate the
in vitro release characteristics of sustained release systems with
the performance of these systems in animal testing (Kulkarni et
al.,[9] Saksena et al.,[10] Kent,[11] Chien and Lau,[12] Kalkwarf,[13] Chien
et al.,[14] Winkler et al.,[15] Ho et al.,[16] Chien et al.,[17] Chien et
al.[18]). The article by Chien et al.[17] is the only report in which
sustained drug-release rates were incorporated into a pharmacokinetic
model to yield predictions of drug concentrations in the blood of
the animal test model. Chien et al. described the intravaginal
release of norethindrone from a ring-shaped cylindrical silicone
rubber matrix delivery vehicle. They incorporated the release rate
constants of the T. Higuchi model,[4] calculated from values in their
in vitro experiments, into an open one-compartment pharmacokinetic
model describing absorption of norethindrone from the device through
the vaginal tissues into the bloodstream. The elimination constant
was predetermined by giving the animal an intravenous dose of norethindrone and observing the disappearance of the drug from the
plasma. The accuracy of predictions by Chien's pharmacokinetic
model ranged from 42 to 135% of actual experimentally determined
serum-drug values even when a correction factor for differences
observed between in vitro and in vivo release rates was used.

To couple the in vitro release rate behavior of the gentamicin
releasing prosthetic valve system with observations on serum gentamicin levels after implantation of the valve in dogs, an open one-
compartment pharmacokinetic model was added to the release rate
equations describing in vitro drug delivery. Gentamicin is not
metabolized, and its distribution kinetics can be modeled adequately
(within a 15% error) by a one-compartmental system.[19] Elimination
kinetics and the apparent volume of distribution in the individual

dogs were derived from the gentamicin clearance studies. The general
pharmacokinetic model is as follows:

$$\frac{dC_s}{dt} = \frac{\text{rate of drug release (as predicted by the in vitro kinetic models}}{V_D} - K_e \cdot C_s \qquad (20)$$

where $\dfrac{dC_s}{dt}$ = change in serum gentamicin concentration, C_s, with
                  time, t

V_D = apparent volume of distribution for gentamicin

K_e = first order constant of gentamicin elimination from
         the one compartment volume.

The above analysis assumes:

1.   The drug released from the valve-rim insert is rapidly distri-
     buted at all points equally within the predetermined volume
     of gentamicin distribution.

2.   The gentamicin elimination for this model is described in toto
     by the first-order elimination constant and the elimination
     constant does not vary with time.

3.   There is no significant sequestration of drug in the tissues
     (i.e. outside the central compartment).

4.   Physiological handling of gentamicin is not adversely affected
     by the dog's condition during surgery (including the bypass
     procedure) and the recovery period.

RESULTS

Modeling Results: In Vitro Studies

     Attempts to fit the in vitro release data from the uncoated
rim inserts to the release model of Roseman and W. Higuchi (equation
(2)) are depicted in Figure 3 for a range of diffusion coefficient
values. The physical constants employed in the solution are given
in Table I. No one value for the diffusion coefficient, D_e, fits
all the data points. From the results, D_e appeared to decrease
in magnitude over the release period (assuming C_s, the drug solubility in the rubber matrix, remains constant with time). To better
fit the experimental data, D_e was allowed to decrease with time
by the use of a simple exponential expression incorporating an additional lag-time factor of four days. The revised form of equation
(2) is the following,

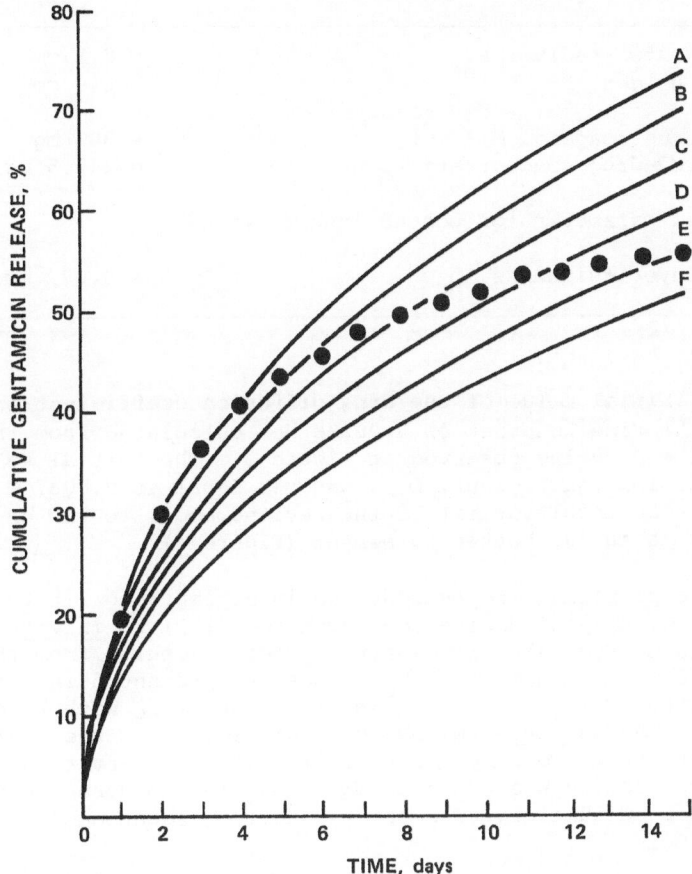

Figure 3. Comparison of the experimental results (●), of in vitro gentamicin release to the Roseman-Higuchi diffusion model predictions (solid lines). Model results for un-coated valve rim insert system over a range of diffusion coefficient values, D_e = ; (A) $0.0037/C_S$; (B) $0.0033/C_S$; (C) $0.0027/C_S$; (D) $0.0023/C_S$; (E) $0.0019/C_S$; (F) $0.0016/C_S$.

$$(1 - \frac{Q}{M_o}) \ln \cdot (1 - \frac{Q}{M_o}) + \frac{Q}{M_o} = \frac{4 \cdot C_s \cdot D_{eo}}{A \cdot a_o^2} \exp(-0.00298 \cdot (t-4)) \cdot t \quad (21)$$

where: t = time (days).

TABLE I.   PHYSICAL CONSTANTS FOR GENTAMICIN DIFFUSION MODEL

Cylinder outer radius, a_o	= 0.2 cm
Cylinder height, h	= 6.9 cm
Initial drug loading, M_O	= 302 mg
Initial rod-drug concentration, A	= 347.5 mg/cm^3
Additional parameter for coated insert system:	
Coating layer thickness, h_c	= 0.072 mm

D_{eo} = initial value of the drug diffusion coefficient in the polymer. The time constant of 0.00298 was calculated from the decrease in the D_e value observed in Figure 3. The initial value of the diffusion coefficient, D_{eo}, was set equal to $0.0037/C_s$ (from Figure 3). The resultant fit of the revised model to the experimental data is in far better agreement (Figure 4).

Similar problems were encountered in attempts to fit the adapted Roseman and W. Higuchi derivation (equation (17)) to in vitro release data for the coated valve rim insert system. Results from the diffusion model for a range of D_e/D_c values are presented in Figure 5 ($D_{eo} = 0.0037/C_s$). A decrease in the value of D_e with time is apparent for the in vitro release of gentamicin from the coated valve-rim inserts. To compensate for the above observation an identical correction was added to equation (17) to describe the decrease in D_e with time. The revised form of equation (17) is the following,

$$(1 - \frac{Q}{M_o}) \cdot \ln (1 - \frac{Q}{M_o}) + \frac{Q}{M_o} \cdot (1 + \frac{2 \cdot h_c \cdot D_{eo} \cdot \exp (-0.00298 \cdot (t-4))}{D_c \cdot a_o})$$

$$= \frac{4 \cdot C_s \cdot D_{eo} \cdot \exp (-0.00298 \cdot (t-4)) \cdot t}{A \cdot a_o^2} \qquad (22)$$

where   t = time (days)

and all other parameters as defined previously.

The use of equation (22) to successfully model the coated valve rim gentamicin release data is depicted in Figure 6. The results of the model are in good agreement with the experimental data except for some slight error in the early and late regions. Best results were obtained using a ratio of D_e/D_c equal to 4.0.

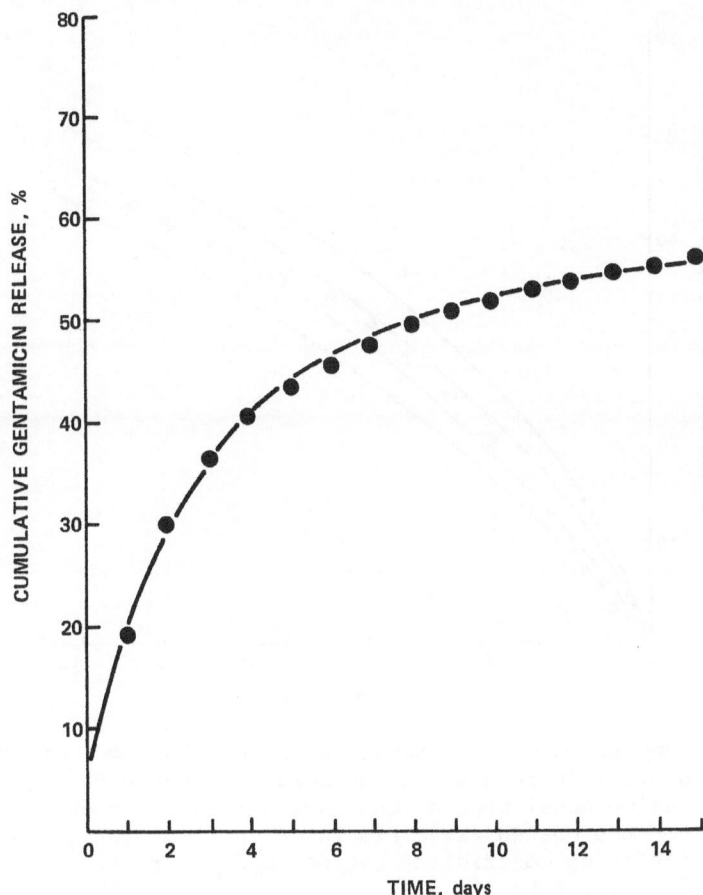

Figure 4. Comparison of the experimental results (●) of in vitro
          gentamicin release to predictions from the revised dif-
          fusion model (solid line). Uncoated valve rim insert
          system.

Comparison of In Vivo Results to Pharmacokinetic Models

     Attempts were made to fit the in vivo serum concentration
results to pharmacokinetic models based on the revised diffusion-
model equations (21 and 22) for the uncoated and coated valve-rim
inserts. To couple the in vitro diffusion equations to an in vivo
simulation, a classical one-compartment model of drug distribution
was employed (equation (20)). The mean apparent volume of distribution, V_D = 5.63 liters, and the first-order elimination constant,

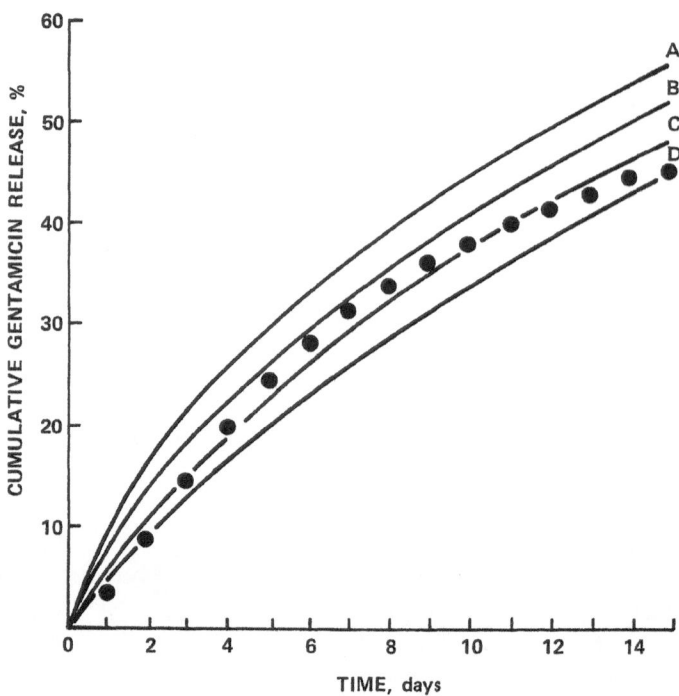

Figure 5.   Comparison of the experimental results (●) of in vitro
             gentamicin release to the adapted Roseman-Higuchi dif-
             fusion model predictions (solid lines). Model results
             for the coated valve rim insert system over a range of
             diffusion coefficient ratios, D_e/D_c = ; (A) 2.0; (B)
             3.0; (C) 4.0; (D) 5.0.

K_e = 0.695/hr, for gentamicin were determined in the intravenous
injection-clearance studies reviewed previously.[3] Diffusion-model
constants were recalculated using the results from in vitro flow-
cell studies with suture punctured, Dacron mesh enclosed, valve-
rim inserts.

    Predictions of serum-gentamicin concentrations by the pharmaco-
kinetic models are presented in Figures 7 and 8 for the revised
Roseman-Higuchi diffusion models of the uncoated and coated valve-
rim insert systems, respectively. The range of model predictions
plotted in Figures 7 and 8 was arrived at by adding or subtracting
the calculated standard deviations to the mean values of V_D and
K_e. In general, all the model results fall short of predicting
the actual serum-gentamicin concentrations determined experimentally
over the observed valve implantation period.

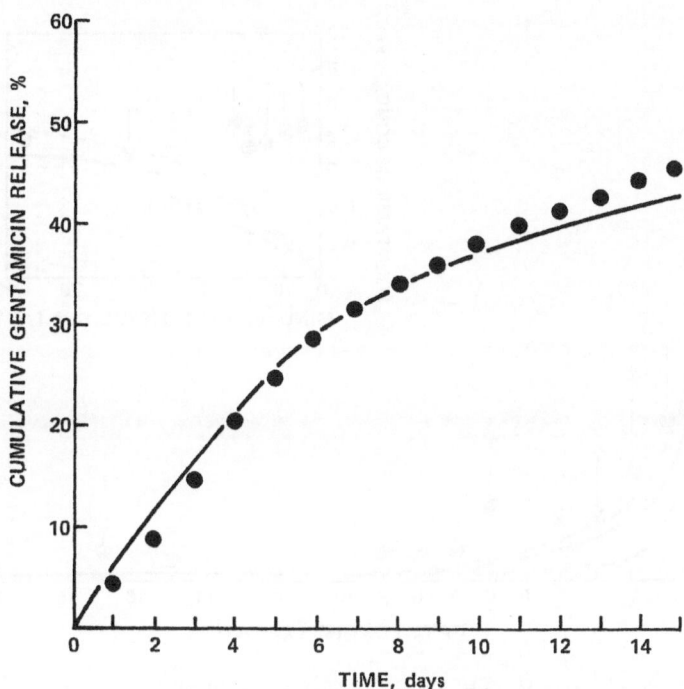

Figure 6.   Comparison of the experimental results (●) of in vitro
gentamicin release to predictions based on the revised
diffusion model (solid line). Coated valve rim insert
system (D_e/D_c = 4.0).

DISCUSSION

     To provide more efficacious application of prophylactic anti-
biotic therapy, an implantable sustained-release system has been
developed for the delivery of gentamicin sulfate from prosthetic
heart valves, which markedly increases survival rates when these
valves are implanted in dogs.[2] There is a significant increase
in both short-term and long-term survival rates for the group of
dogs receiving the uncoated gentamicin-loaded valves compared to
controls. Results from a limited number of coated gentamicin-loaded
valves suggest that the use of a diffusion barrier of drug-free
silicone rubber prolongs the overall release of antibiotic, and
may further increase the long-term survival by facilitating delivery
of low levels of drug over a longer period.

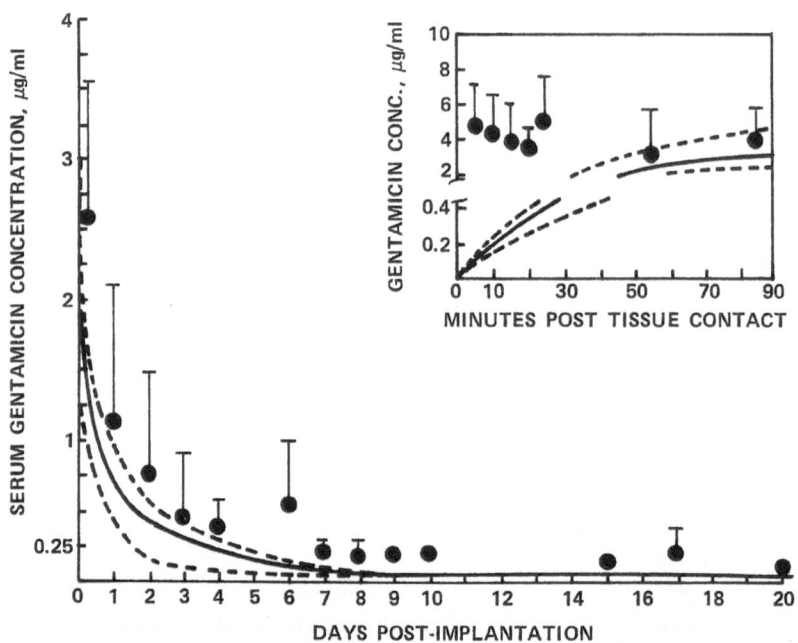

Figure 7.   Comparison of serum gentamicin concentrations ((●)
            mean value ± standard deviation) after implantation of
            a prosthetic valve containing a drug-loaded uncoated
            valve rim insert to predictions from a pharmacokinetic
            model based on the revised Rosman-Higuchi equation of
            drug release for the uncoated valve rim insert system
            ($D_{eo} = 0.0052/C_S$). Key: solid line, V_D = 5.63 liters,
            K_e = 0.695/hr; upper dashed line, V_D = 3.9 liters, K_e =
            0.576/hr; lower dashed line, V_D = 7.4 liters, K_e =
            0.877/hr.

     Although serum gentamicin levels fall below therapeutic concen-
trations within the first two days of valve implantation, a prolonged low level of release is maintained over an additional one
to two months, producing high local concentrations at the desired
tissue site. These long-term, low systemic-drug levels may reduce
the incidence of aminoglycoside related side effects at peripheral
sites (i.e. ototoxicity and nephrotoxicity).

     The ability of a sustained antibiotic releasing prosthetic
valve to selectively deliver optimal amounts of the drug to the
surrounding cardiac tissue offers a promising alternative to conventional prophylactic antibiotic therapy in minimizing postoperative complications of infection following valve replacement.

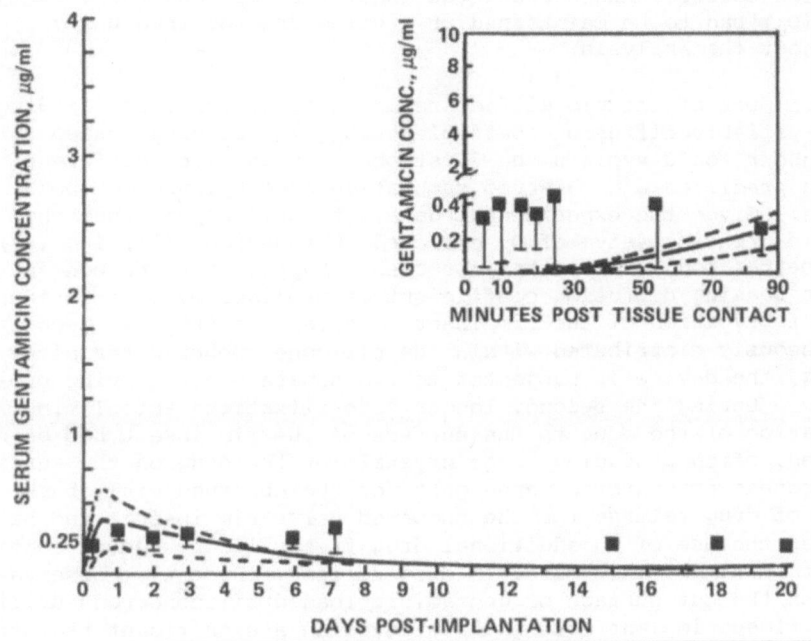

Figure 8. Comparison of serum gentamicin concentrations ((●)
mean value ± standard deviation) after implantation of
a prosthetic valve containing a drug-loaded coated valve
rim insert to predictions from a pharmacokinetic model
based on the revised Rosman-Higuchi equation adapted to
describe drug release from the coated valve rim insert
system (D_{eo} = 0.0052/C_s, D_e/D_c = 4.0). Key: solid line,
V_D = 5.63 liters, K_e = 0.695/hr; upper dashed line,
V_D = 3.9 liters, K_e = 0.576/hr; lower dashed line, V_D =
7.4 liters, K_e = 0.877/hr.

From the results obtained in the attempts to model the in vitro
release of gentamicin from the uncoated and coated valve rim inserts,
it would appear that the actual drug-release process is more complex
than predicted by relatively simplistic numerical analyses.

For the uncoated rim insert system, computer fitting of the
data was good over the early period of release but somewhat less
adequate during the later times when a constant diffusion coefficient throughout the analysis was employed. The same trend was
observed in the analysis of the coated rim insert system under
identical conditions. In addition, to properly describe the gentamicin release from the coated valve rim inserts, the ratio of

diffusion coefficients between the inner rod (D_e) and the coating
layer (D_c) had to be maintained at a value greater than unity
throughout the analysis.

    A number of unexplored factors may account for these findings.
A time-variable diffusion coefficient (D_e) in the drug loaded silicone rubber would explain the first observation, i.e. difference
between predicted and observed cumulative drug release for both
systems. Given the experimental data, it would appear that the
slowly decreasing valve of D_e employed in equations (21) and (22)
would better model the release process. Support for the concept
of a decreasing diffusion coefficient is provided by observations
on the fabrication of the rim insert. After the drug has been
homogeneously distributed within the silicone rubber material by
milling, the device is subjected to two separate autoclaving procedures. During the second, longer "sterilization" autoclaving,
segregation of the drug to the surface of the rim insert has been
observed, often producing large crystals of the drug on the surface.
This process accounts in large part for the observed early burst
effect of drug release for the uncoated valve-rim inserts and has
prompted the use of an additional drug-free silicone rubber coating
layer to minimize this burst in drug release. Recently, observations on the cut surface of gentamicin-loaded silicone rods utilized
in the tissue implant studies have revealed a significant redistri-
bution of drug to the outer layers of the silicone rubber cylinders,
producing a darker colored outer rim of increased drug concentration over 20 to 25% of the rod radius. This layering effect is
probably the result of the second autoclaving procedure, with the
penetration of water vapor into the outer sections of the drug-
loaded silicone rubber devices causing dissolution of the drug in
many small voids and preferentially segregating a portion of the
drug near the surface because of the extremely high affinity of
gentamicin for an aqueous environment. When the water vapor is
withdrawn during the rapid vacuum and drying cycle, macrocrystals
of gentamicin remain in this outer circumferential layer. Early
drug dissolution and release from this area would leave nonchannel-
ing voids which would account for the relatively large early value
of the drug diffusion coefficient. At later times of diffusion,
drug release is largely from the unaffected deeper portions of the
cylinder, and the diffusion coefficient in the absence of the void
spaces would be expected to decrease for the deeper regions. Thus
the observed drug permeability would decrease with time, as is
depicted by the experimental data and the revised theoretical
analysis.

    Similar reasoning can explain the difference observed in the
drug-diffusion coefficients between the inner drug-loaded rod and
the initially drug-free silicone rubber coating layer in the coated
valve-rim insert system. The drug-free coating layer would not

be subject to void formation during fabrication and autoclaving, as it is for the inner rod portion of the device, and the coating layer would thus offer a more intact barrier to the diffusion of the drug molecules, accounting for a reduced value of the diffusion coefficient, D_c with respect to D_e. As in the previous discussion for the uncoated valve-rim insert system, the diffusion front would be expected to advance with time to the deeper layers of the central rod (unaffected by the water vapor induced voids), and the value of the diffusion coefficient, D_e, of the central rod would decrease. This decrease would cause a lowering of the ratio, D_e/D_c with time, which is incorporated into the adapted model of drug release (equation (22)).

Release of gentamicin in vivo is an even more complex process. After implantation of the valve in the dog, the rate of release of the drug from the rim-insert surface would be dependent on such factors as: the relative amounts of surface exposed to the blood and the tissue, blood perfusion of the tissue, intracellular sequestration of the drug (both at the valve site and at peripheral organs), and the biological response of the blood and tissue layers adjacent to the valve surface. The fibrin pseudo-intima which forms early over the blood-contacting surface of the valve sewing ring might offer an additional diffusional resistance to the drug delivery device. At the tissue interface, fibrous capsule formation and the pooling of fluids within the surgically damaged tissue, or either one, may produce similar effects, modifying the release process.

Observation on the serum concentrations of gentamicin in the dogs after valve implantation indicate that these levels are generally greater than predicted by the in vivo pharmacokinetic model. The discrepancy in the early-time serum values are probably the result of reduced drug clearance during and immediately following the cardiopulmonary bypass procedure. The renal clearance of other antibiotics have been reported to decrease during cardiopulmonary bypass surgery, and drug elimination may be prolonged for variable periods postoperatively (Miller et al.,[20] Polk et al.[21]). This effect on drug clearance may be the result of altered renal hemodynamics due to the cardiopulmonary bypass procedure (Porter et al.,[22] Mielke et al.[23]) and changes in drug disposition due to the anesthetic agents employed (Miller et al.[20]), or either one. Porter et al.[22] found that in patients undergoing bypass procedures during prosthetic valve replacement, impaired renal function, observed in the postoperative period, correlated with findings suggesting renal afferent arteriolar vasoconstriction during perfusion. The effects were reversible and normal renal function returned two to four days following surgery. The net result is that the elimination constants employed in the gentamicin model, as measured from the preoperative clearance studies, are not in accord with the true early postoperative physiological handling of the drug.

In the later serum-gentamicin determinations, the elevation of measured serum-drug concentration over levels predicted by the pharmacokinetic model is most likely due to the inability of a one compartment distribution model to properly describe the observed tissue sequestration of gentamicin and the later return of the drug from the tissues to the vascular compartment. This process would delay total drug excretion and cause an elevation of the later-time measurements of serum gentamicin concentration. Over the low serum concentration range observed in the experiments after three to four days of valve implantation, the effects of tissue drug depots on serum gentamicin concentration would become significant.

Future pharmacokinetic models dealing with sustained drug release must take these effects into account through the use of time varying elimination parameters and multi-compartmental simulations. To this end, investigations are being conducted to better measure the tissue handling of gentamicin delivered from intramuscular sustained-release devices with different initial drug loadings and the effect of the cardiopulmonary-bypass procedure on drug-elimination characteristics.

In conclusion, a novel sustained drug release device has been designed which demonstrates an effective method of preventing prosthetic-valve endocarditis in dog implantation studies. This system can serve as a model for antibiotic delivery systems to be utilized in other prosthetic device applications. The pharmacokinetic analysis employed in the investigation of the implanted device offers a means of evaluating the in vivo performance of sustained release devices through the correlation of the processes of in vitro drug diffusion and the physiological distribution and elimination of the drug in a suitable animal model.

ACKNOWLEDGEMENTS

From the Departments of Pathology and Macromolecular Science, Case Western Reserve University, and Division of Surgical Research, St. Luke's Hospital, Cleveland, Ohio. Supported by National Institutes of Health; Grant 1-RO1-HL22888, Medical Scientist Training Program Grant GM-07250, and St. Luke's Hospital Association of Cleveland, Ohio, of the United Methodist Church.

REFERENCES

1. R.D. Jones, L.S. Olanoff, and J.M. Anderson, First European Conference on Evaluation of Biomaterials, Strasbourg, France, September 26-28, 1977, in press.

2. L.S. Olanoff, R.D. Jones, and J.M. Anderson, Trans. Amer. Soc. Artif. Internal Organs 25:334 (1979).
3. L.S. Olanoff, Ph.D. Thesis, Case Western Reserve University (1980).
4. T. Higuchi, J. Pharm. Sci. 50:874 (1961).
5. Y.W. Chien, H.J. Lambert, and D.E. Grant, J. Pharm. Sci. 63:365 (1974).
6. Y.W. Chien, and H.J. Lambert, J. Pharm. Sci. 63:515 (1974).
7. T.J. Roseman, J. Pharm. Sci. 61:46 (1972).
8. T.J. Roseman, and W.I. Higuchi, J. Pharm. Sci. 59:353 (1970).
9. B.D. Kulkarni, T.D. Auila, B.B. Phariss, and A. Scommegna, Contracep. 8:299 (1973).
10. S.K. Saksena, I.F. Lau, and M.C. Chang, Fertil. Steril. 26:126 (1975).
11. J.S. Kent, in: "Controlled Release Polymeric Formulations," D.R. Paul and F.W. Harris, ed, ACS Symposium Series, Vol. 33, American Chemical Society, Washington, D.C. (1976). pp. 157-170.
12. Y.W. Chien, and E.P.K. Lau, J. Pharm. Sci. 65:488 (1976).
13. D.R. Kalkwarf, M.R. Sikov, L. Smith, and R. Gordon, Contracep. 6:423 (1972).
14. Y.W. Chien, H.J. Lambert, and L.F. Rosek, in: "Controlled Release Polymeric Formulations," D.R. Paul and F.W. Harris, eds, ACS Symposium Series, Vol. 33, American Chemical Society, Washington, D.C. (1976). pp. 72-86.
15. V.W. Winkler, S. Borodkin, S.K. Webel, and J.T. Mannebach, J. Pharm. Sci. 66:816 (1977).
16. N.F.H. Ho, L. Suhardja, S. Hwang, E. Owada, A. Molokhia, G.L. Flynn, W.I. Higuchi, and J.Y. Park, J. Pharm. Sci. 65:1578 (1976).
17. Y.W. Chien, S.E. Mares, J. Berg, S. Huber, H.J. Lambert, and K.F. King, J Pharm. Sci 64:1776 (1975).
18. Y.W. Chien, L.F. Rozek, and J.H. Lambert, J. Pharm. Sci. 67:214 (1978).
19. J.C. Pechere, and R. Dugal, Clin. Pharmacokin. 4:170 (1979)
20. K.W. Miller, K.K.H. Chan, H.G. McCoy, R.P. Fischer, W.G. Lindsay, and D.E. Zaske, Clin. Pharmacol. Therap. 26:54 (1979).
21. R.E. Polk, G.L. Archer, and R. Lower, Clin. Pharmacol. Therap. 23:473 (1978)
22. G.A. Porter, F.E. Kloster, R.J. Herr, A. Starr, H.E. Griswold, J. Kimsey, and H. Lenertz, Circ. 34:1005 (1966).
23. J.E. Mielke, F.T. Maher, J.C. Hunt, and J.W. Kirklin, Circ. 32:394 (1965).

CONTROLLED DRUG RELEASE FROM POLYMERIC MATRICES

INVOLVING MOVING BOUNDARIES

P.I. Lee

Central Research
CIBA-GEIGY Corporation
Ardsley, N.Y. 10502

INTRODUCTION

The diffusional release of a dispersed or dissolved drug from a polymeric matrix generally involves the presence of a moving diffusional front separating the undissolved core and the partially extracted region. In the case of an erodible or swellable polymer matrix, the release kinetics is further complicated by the presence of a second moving boundary, namely the eroding or swelling polymer front. The mathematical descriptions of such mass transfer problems involving moving boundaries are known as moving boundary problems, free boundary problems, or simply Stefan problems. Except for some special cases, the presence of a moving boundary introduces a non-linearity so that only a few exact solutions are known.[1-3] In addition to numerical schemes, various approximate analytical techniques have been applied to moving boundary problems developed in other areas such as freezing and melting with varying degree of success.[2,3] However, only very simple pseudosteady state approximations have been used to analyze the release of a dispersed drug from a polymeric matrix.[4,5]

A familiar example is Higuchi's treatment[5] for a rigid matrix under perfect sink condition. Higuchi's results have been frequently applied to controlled drug release whenever the initial drug loading per unit volume, A, is greater than the drug solubility in the matrix, C_s. Recently Paul and McSpadden[6] pointed out that Higuchi's result for planar geometry does not match the exact result by an amount of 11.3% in the limit of $A \to C_s$. This discrepancy was removed by Paul and McSpadden utilizing the exact solution for a semi-infinite system. However, the exact solution involves a transcendental

expression which is cumbersome for routine usage. For the release
of a dispersed drug from an erodible polymeric matrix, Hopfenberg[7]
treated the case of no diffusional contribution, whereas Baker and
Lonsdale[8] presented a brief pseudosteacy state analysis of the more
general system including diffusional contribution. For drug release
from a swellable polymeric matrix, Peppas et al.[9] recently presented
theoretical and experimental results taking into account the counter-
current diffusion of solvent. However, a steady state assumption
was also made in the treatment.

The pseudosteady state approach employed in these systems
assumes a linear drug concentration profile which is valid only
when the drug loading is in great excess of the drug solubility
$(A \gg C_s)$. In reality, however, one often encounters situations where
the polymer hydrophilicity, drug solubility, dosage level, and rate
requirements limit the loading to be not in great excess of the
solubility. The direct application of pseudosteady state results
to such systems is certainly undesirable. It is therefore the
purpose of this study to develop more practical and accurate analytical solutions applicable to all A/C_s values for the kinetics
of drug release from these systems. For the sake of simplicity,
only planar geometry will be considered here.

ANALYSIS

For a planar polymeric matrix with uniform initial drug loading per unit volume A and equilibrium drug solubility C_s, the general diffusion equation describing the kinetics of drug release under
perfect sink condition is

$$\frac{\partial C}{\partial t} = \frac{\partial}{\partial x} \left(D \frac{\partial C}{\partial x} \right) \tag{1}$$

where x = o at the center and x = a at the surface, the initial
and boundary conditions involved are

$$C[S(t),t] = 0 \tag{2}$$

$$C[R(t),t] = C_s \tag{3}$$

$$D\frac{\partial C}{\partial x} = (A-C_s)\frac{dR}{dt} \text{ at } x = R(t) \tag{4}$$

$$S(0) = a \tag{5}$$

and

$$R(0) = a \tag{6}$$

where D is the drug diffusion coefficient in the matrix, R(t) the
time dependent position of the moving diffusion front, and S(t)
the time dependent position of the eroding or swelling front. To
illustrate the system under consideration, the physical situation
of drug release from an erodible membrane is shown in Figure 1.
The same illustration is also applicable to rigid and swellable
matrices with different time dependence of S(t). Equations (1)
to (6) are not amenable to exact analysis except in the special
case of a rigid matrix.

In the present study, based on a refined version of Goodman's
heat balance integral method[10] due to Volkov and Li-Orlov,[11] approximate analytical solutions for the kinetics of drug release from
(a) rigid, (b) surface erodible, and (c) swellable polymeric matrices
in planar geometry are obtained. The heat balance integral method
and its refinement have been demonstrated to be particularly effective in obtaining approximate solutions to transient heat and mass
transfer problems, especially those involving phase changes.[10 13]

The concentration dependence of the drug diffusion coefficient,
D, and the external mass transfer resistance are neglected in the
current treatment. But they can readily be incorporated through
the use of a concentration dependent diffusion coefficient and
an external mass transfer coefficient.[6] A more detailed description
of the mathematics involved for both the rigid and surface erodible

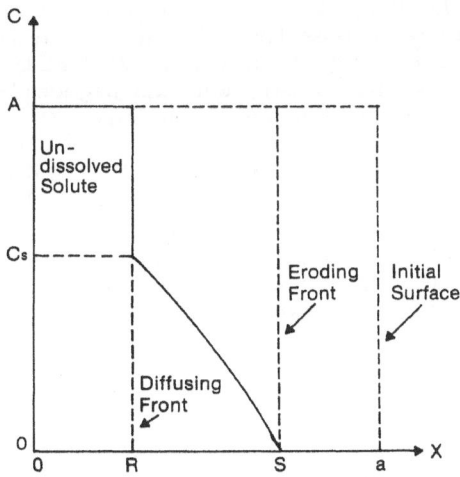

Figure 1.   General schematic profile for the release of a dispersed
            drug from an erodible polymer matrix.

systems has been given elsewhere.[14] The analysis is now extended
to the case of a swellable polymer matrix. Only the resulting
equations and their utilities are presented here.

Rigid Matrix

This matrix is identical to the problem modeled by Higuchi[5]
and later refined by Paul and McSpadden.[6] The only moving boundary
involved is the diffusion front R(t) whereas the polymer surface
is stationary, i.e. S(t) = a. The solution to this problem is:

$$M = \frac{1+H}{\sqrt{3H}}[C_s \sqrt{Dt}] \tag{7}$$

where

$$H = 5(\frac{A}{C_s}) - 4 + \sqrt{(\frac{A}{C_s})^2 - 1}$$

This equation also predicts the amount of solute released per unit
area, M, to be linear in square root time similar to the Higuchi
equation and the exact solution. However, the dependencies on A/C_s
are not the same. These are compared in Table I for various values
of A/C_s. For the present work, the percentage deviations from the
exact solutions are consistently one order of magnitude smaller
than those of Higuchi's results. In the limit of $A \rightarrow C_s$, equation
(7) is only 2.33% over the exact solution as compared with Higuchi's
equation which is 11.38% too small. In fact, as $A/C_s > 1.04$ equation (7) accurately describes the release within 1% of the exact
solution and as $A/C_s > 4.5$ equation (7) is virtually identical to
the exact solution (within 0.1%), whereas Higuchi's equation requires $A/C_s > 10$ to have an accuracy within 1%.

Therefore the new approximate analytical solution, equation
(7) can be considered as uniformly valid over all the A/C_s values.
In addition to the accuracy and simplicity, it is particularly
useful in controlled-release systems where the polymer hydrophilicity, drug solubility, dosage level, and rate requirements limit
A to a loading not in great excess of C_s.

Surface Erodible Matrix

The mechanisms of polymer erosion have been discussed in detail
recently by Heller and Baker.[15] The situation where polymers erode
by surface erosion is of special interest because the drug release
from such devices having constant geometry will be zero order.
In this case the eroding front moves at a constant velocity in the

TABLE I.   COMPARISON OF ANALYSES FOR THE DRUG RELEASE
FROM A PLANAR MATRIX

$\dfrac{A}{C_s}$	$M/[C_s\sqrt{Dt}]$				
	Exact (6)	Higuchi (5)	% Error	This Work	% Error
50.668	10.0333	10.0186	− 0.15	10.0333	0
13.170	5.0667	5.0337	− 0.65	5.0661	− 0.013
6.230	3.4336	3.3853	− 1.41	3.4317	− 0.055
3.806	2.6340	2.5713	− 2.38	2.6302	− 0.14
2.086	1.8686	1.7812	− 4.68	1.8605	− 0.44
1.501	1.5205	1.4150	− 6.94	1.5101	− 0.68
1.246	1.3390	1.2217	− 8.76	1.3306	− 0.63
1.060	1.1849	1.0579	− 10.72	1.1909	+ 0.51
1.000	1.1284	1.0000	− 11.38	1.1547	+ 2.33

same direction of the diffusion front. With some manipulations
the resulting solutions for $A>C_s$ can be simplified to:

$$\frac{M}{M_\infty} = [1 - \frac{1}{2}(\frac{C_s}{A})]\delta + (\frac{Ba}{D})\tau \tag{8}$$

and

$$\tau = \frac{1}{6h}[3(\frac{A}{C_s}) - 2][\delta - \frac{1}{2h}\ln(1 + 2\,\delta h)] \tag{9}$$

where

$$h = \frac{1}{2}(1 - \frac{A}{C_s})(\frac{Ba}{D}) \text{ and } \tau = \frac{Dt}{a^2}$$

With M_∞ defined as the total amount released per unit area, M/M_∞
represents the fractional release.

The surface-erosion rate constant, B, has the dimension of a velocity. And δ is the relative separation between the diffusion
and eroding fronts defined as $[S(t)-R(t)]/a$. It can easily be shown
that the rate of movement of diffusion front is

$$-\frac{1}{a}\frac{dR}{d\tau} = \frac{1}{\delta(\frac{A}{C_s} - 1)} \tag{10}$$

In the limit of $A \rightarrow C_s$, or a dissolved drug system the current method gives

$$\frac{M}{M\infty} = \sqrt{\frac{4\tau}{3}} + (\frac{Ba}{D})\tau \qquad (11)$$

and the rate of movement of the diffusion front is

$$-\frac{1}{a}\frac{dR}{d\tau} = \frac{6}{\sqrt{\tau}} + (\frac{Ba}{D}) \qquad (12)$$

The parameter Ba/D is essentially the erosion rate to matrix permeability ratio which measures the relative contribution of erosion and diffusion processes. For a fixed Ba/D = 1, the fractional release as a function of time and A/C_s calculated from equations (8) and (9) is shown in Figure 2 together with the analytical results of Peterlin,[16] where Peterlin's results were reported for the sorption of solvent in a glassy polymer membrane undergoing Case II swelling. The mathematical problem posed is identical to the special case of A/C_s = 1, or the dissolved drug, considered here. It can be seen from Figure 2 that in the limiting case of A/C_s = 1, the results predicted here agree quite well with those of Peterlin's. The deviation starts to appear only after the diffusion fronts have met. As A/C_s increases, the zero-order release region extends substantially, and the moment when the diffusion fronts meet shifts toward the tail end of the release.

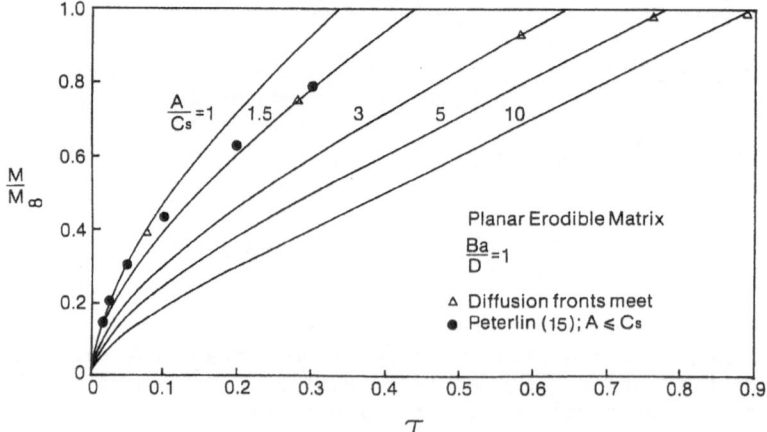

Figure 2.   Fractional release vs. time for a dispersed drug in a planar erodible polymer matrix (Ba/D = 1) with various drug loading levels.

The fractional release as a function of time and Ba/D predicted from equations (8) and (9) for the case of A/C_s = 5 is presented in Figure 3. It shows that, as the erosion process dominates the diffusion process, e.g. Ba/D = 10, almost total zero-order release results. The release generally starts with a typical first-order kinetics, then shifts toward a zero-order one with a limiting slope approaching Ba/D. Similar to the results of Baker and Lonsdale[8] the zero-order release is primarily contributed by the identical rate of movement of the diffusing and eroding fronts at large time. This synchronization of front velocities is illustrated in Figure 4 for the same example considered in Figure 3. It is seen that the larger the value of Ba/D the sooner the synchronization can be reached. This synchronizing behavior perhaps can best be realized by examining equations (11) and (12) for the special instance of $A \rightarrow C_s$ where the fractional release is expressed as a combination of $\sqrt{\tau}$ and τ dependencies and the diffusion front velocity as a combination of a constant, Ba/D, and a $1/\sqrt{\tau}$ dependent term. At large τ the linear time dependence will dominate the fractional release and a constant diffusion front velocity will prevail.

Swellable Matrix

The method of solution for the surface-erodible matrix can easily be extended to the case of a swellable matrix. The swelling polymer surface now moves in an opposite direction to that of the

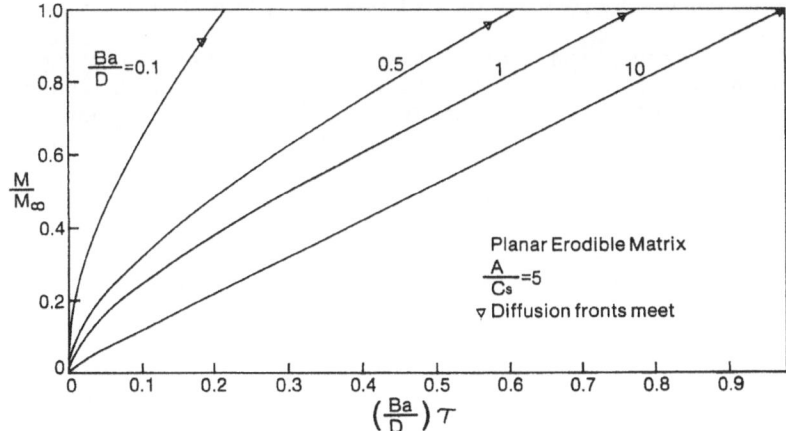

Figure 3.   Fractional release vs. time for a dispersed drug in a planar erodible polymer matrix (A/C_s = 5) with various erosion rate to matrix permeability ratios.

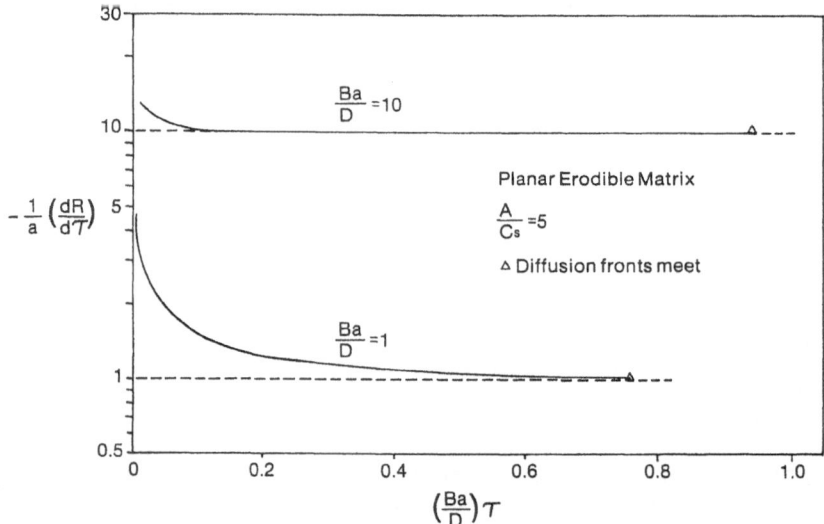

Figure 4. Time dependency of diffusion front velocity in a planar
erodible polymer matrix (A/C_s = 5) with various erosion
rate to matrix permeability ratios.

diffusion front. This situation is generally encountered in the
drug release from a hydrogel or hydrophilic polymer matrix.

With the assumption that Fickian diffusion is obeyed and the
increase in linear dimension of the planar membrane is proportional
to the solvent uptake, i.e. proportional to the square root of
time $S(t) - a = L\sqrt{t}$ with a proportionality constant L having the
same dimension as the square root of diffusion coefficient, the
following solutions are obtained

$$\frac{M}{M_\infty} = [\beta(1 - \frac{1}{2}\frac{C_s}{A} - (\frac{L}{2\sqrt{D}})]\sqrt{\tau} \qquad (13)$$

where

$$\beta = [-(1 - \frac{A}{C_s})(\frac{L}{2\sqrt{D}}) + \sqrt{(1 - \frac{A}{C_s})^2(\frac{L}{2\sqrt{D}})^2 + 2(\frac{A}{C_s}) - \frac{4}{3}}]/(\frac{A}{C_s} - \frac{2}{3})$$

$$(14)$$

Equation (4) predicts square root time dependence of the fractional release from a swellable matrix undergoing Fickian diffusion.
This agrees qualitatively with the experimental results reported
by Peppas et al.[9] for the release of KCl from a highly swellable
hydroxypropyl methyl cellulose matrix.

For systems involving non-Fickian diffusion mechanism, the
method of analysis can still be applied as long as an exact time
dependence of boundary position of the swellable matrix can be formulated.

DISCUSSION

The general moving boundary problems encountered in the controlled drug release from a planar polymeric matrix have been successfully treated using a refined heat balance integral method.
The resulting analytical solutions presented here are much more
accurate than the pseudosteady state results and more convenient
to use than the exact solutions. The results can also be the basis
for solutions of more complicated systems such as those involving
concentration dependent diffusion coefficient and external mass
transfer resistance.

For a dispersed drug, the results presented here are particularly applicable to cases where the drug loading is not in great
excess of the drug solubility in the matrix. This situation occurs
quite often in controlled release systems involving hydrophilic
polymers and drugs of high water solubility.

REFERENCES

1. J. Crank, in: "Mathematics of Diffusion," 2nd ed., Clarendon
    Press, Oxford (1975).
2. J.R. Ockendon and W.R. Hodgkins, in: "Moving Boundary Problems
    in Heat Flow and Diffusion," Clarendon Press, Oxford (1975).
3. D.G. Wilson, A.D. Solomon, and P.T. Boggs, in: "Moving Boundary
    Problems," Academic Press, New York (1978).
4. R.W. Baker and H.K. Lonsdale, in: "Controlled Release of Bio-
    logically Active Agents," Vol. 47 of Advances in Experimental
    Medicine and Biology, A.C. Tanquary and R.E. Lacey, eds.,
    Plenum Press, New York (1974). pp. 15-72.
5. T. Higuchi, J. Pharm. Sci. 50:874 (1961).
6. D.R. Paul and S.K. McSpadden, J. Membrane Sci. 1:33 (1976).
7. H.B. Hopfenberg, in: "Controlled Release Polymeric Formula-
    tions," Vol. 33 of ACS Symposium Series, ACS, Washington (1976).
    pp. 26-32.

8. R.W. Baker and H.K. Lonsdale, Div of Organic Coatings and Plastics Preprints, ACS 3(1):229 (1976).

9. N.A. Peppas, R. Gurny, E. Doelker, and P. Buri, J. Membrane Sci. 7:241 (1980).

10. T.R. Goodman, Trans ASME 80:335 (1958).

11. V.N. Volkov and V.K. Li-Orlov, Heat Transfer Sov. Res. 2:41 (1970).

12. T.R. Goodman, Adv. Heat Transfer 1:51 (1964).

13. P.I. Lee, in: "Controlled Release of Bioactive Materials," R.W. Baker, ed., Academic Press, New York (1980). pp. 135-153.

14. P.I. Lee, J. Membrane Sci. 7:255 (1980).

15. J. Heller and R.W. Baker, in: "Controlled Release of Bioactive Materials," R.W. Baker, ed., Academic Press, New York (1980). pp. 1-17.

16. A. Peterlin, J. Polym. Sci., Polym. Phys. Ed. 17:1741 (1979).

ANTHRACYCLINE-DNA COMPLEXES AS SLOW-RELEASE PREPARATIONS

IN THE TREATMENT OF ACUTE LEUKEMIA

Curt Peterson

Department of Pharmacology
Karolinska Institute
S-104 01 Stockholm, Sweden

Christer Paul and Gösta Gahrton

Section of Oncology and Hematology
Department of Medicine
Huddinge Hospital
S-141 86 Huddinge, Sweden

INTRODUCTION

The anthracycline antibiotics daunorubicin (DNR) and doxoru-
bicin (DOX, adriamycin) play a prominent role in the treatment of
acute leukemia.[1,2] The most successful programs for treatment of
acute non-lymphoblastic leukemia (ANLL) in adults now cause remission in about 70-80% of previously untreated patients. But most
patients relapse despite maintenance therapy given at certain intervals. The response rate is then much lower and most of these
patients are resistant to the drugs which initially caused remission.

Chemically, the anthracyclines are built up of a tetracyclic
aglycone linked to an aminosugar. DOX is the 14-hydroxy derivative
of DNR (Figure 1). The drugs probably enter the cells by diffusion[3]
and exert their cytotoxic effects by intercalation in the DNA double
helix, thereby inhibiting replication and transcription.[4] The association constant for the binding of DNR to double-stranded DNA in
vitro is about $0.1 - 0.3 \times 10^6 M^{-1}$ and somewhat higher for the interaction between DOX and DNA.[5] Clinically, DNR is used against acute
leukemia only, whereas DOX has a very broad activity spectrum.[2]

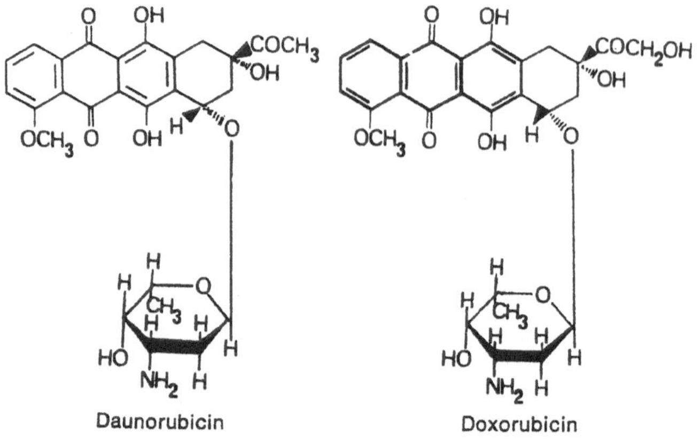

Figure 1. Formulae of DNR and DOX.

The reason for this difference is not known. Distinct differences have been observed, however, in cellular uptake and subcellular localization between DNR and DOX.[6,3]

The dose-limiting factor of the anthracyclines in inducing remission in ANLL is the toxic effects on normal hematopoetic stem cells. Maintenance therapy is restricted by a serious cardiotoxicity, which clinically and morphologically resembles a congestive cardiomyopathy.[7] The mechanism behind this effect is unknown. The cardiotoxic effect is dose dependent, and the risk of developing a manifest cardiomyopathy becomes substantial at an accumulated dose level of 750 mg DNR[8] or 550 mg DOX per sq.m. body surface.[9] Therefore, treatment is generally discontinued at these total dose levels.

In an attempt to increase the selectivity of the anthracyclines in cancer chemotherapy, Trouet and coworkers suggested that the drugs be administered linked to DNA as a carrier.[10] According to the concept of lysosomotropic cancer chemotherapy, the cellular uptake of the anthracycline-DNA complexes occurs by endocytosis, and the carrier is then digested by acid deoxyribonucleases in the lysosomes.[10] Thereafter the liberated drug diffuses to the nucleus and exerts its cytotoxic effects. According to this concept, the effect of DNA-linked DNR or DOX on a certain normal or malignant cell type is dependent on the endocytic activity of that cell type. In certain experimental systems the DNA complexes have been shown to exert higher antitumoral and reduced toxic effects as compared to the free anthracyclines.[11,12] Experimentally, the DNA-complexes have also been found less cardiotoxic than the free anthracyclines.[13]

In late 1976 the Leukemia Group of Central Sweden (LCS) started a randomized clinical study to compare the therapeutic and toxic effects of free and DNA-linked DNR in combination with cytosine arabinoside (ARA-C) in the treatment of ANLL in adults.[14] Sixty patients with newly diagnosed, previously untreated ANLL were randomized for treatment with one of three different regimens (Figure 2).

Parallel with the clinical trial of the LCS, we have compared the pharmacokinetics of free and DNA-linked DNR in plasma, leukemic cells, and urine. Some patients, who for certain reasons (e.g. previous chemotherapy) were excluded from the randomized study, have been treated with free or DNA-linked DOX, and therefore the pharmacokinetics of these drugs have also been studied.

METHODS AND MATERIALS

Patients

Ten patients with ANLL and 8,000-200,000 blast cells/mm^3 in the peripheral blood were studied during 14 treatment courses with i.v. infusions of free or DNA-linked DNR or DOX, 1.5 mg/kg body weight. The DNA-complexes were prepared as described by Gahrton et al.[15]

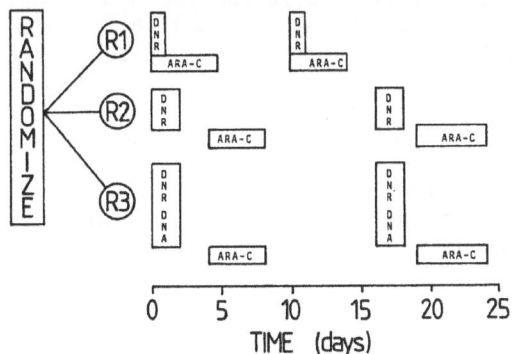

Figure 2. Treatment program (760920) of the Leukemia Group of
           Central Sweden for induction of remission in patients
           with ANLL.

Collection of Blood and Urine

Before, during, and at certain time intervals after the drug infusions, venous blood samples (five ml) were collected and immediately cooled on ice. The leukemic cells were isolated (>85% pure) by centrifugation on sodium metrizoate/Ficoll (Lymphoprep, Nyegaard & Co, AS, Oslo, Norway), washed, and suspended in phosphate buffered (pH 7.4) saline (PBS) as earlier described.[16] Leukemic cells, plasma, and urine samples were stored at -20°C until the day of analysis.

High-Performance Liquid Chromatography

After thawing, the cell samples were sonicated for 20 s at 50 W with a Branson B-12 sonicator (Branson Sonic Power Company, Danbury, CT). A 0.2-ml aliquot of cell sample, plasma, or urine was added to 0.2 ml of 0.1 M borate buffer (pH 9.8) containing 0.2 μM of DOX as internal standard if the patient had received DNR or DNR if the patient had received DOX. The drugs were extracted with 1.8 ml of chloroform/methanol (4:1 by volume). 25-200 μl of the organic phase was injected in the Model U6-K injector (Waters Associates, Inc, Milford, MA). The Lichrosorb Si-60 column (Hibar, 25 cm x 4 mm, from E. Merck, Darmstadt, FRG) was eluted by a mixture of chloroform, methanol, glacial acetic acid, and 0.3 mM $MgCl_2$ (720:210:40:30 by volume) at a flow rate of 1.5 ml/min obtained with a Waters Associates Chromatography Pump. The column outlet was connected to a Gilson model FL-1B fluorometer (Gilson Medical Electronics, Inc, Middleton, WI) and the fluorescense (λ_{ex}480 nm, λ_{em}560 nm) signal integrated by a Chromatopac data processor (Shimadzu Seisakusho Ltd, Kyoto, Japan). Figure 3 shows a chromatogram of an equimolar (1 μM) standard mixture of DNR, DOX and their reduced metabolites daunorubicinol (DOL) and doxorubicinol (DOXOL). The detection limit in our system is about 0.2 pmol, corresponding to a sample concentration of 8 nM.

Subcellular Fractionation

Our subcellular fractionation technique involves the preparation of a cell homogenate and the centrifugation of the various components of this homogenate to their equilibrium densities in a sucrose gradient.

Isolated leukemic cells were suspended in RPMI 1640-medium with 20 mM HEPES buffer (pH 7.4) (Gibco Bio-Cult, Glasgow, U.K.). Two hundred ml of the suspension (3×10^6 cells/ml) was incubated in a shaking water-bath (+37°C) for two hours with free or DNA-linked DNR (1.75 μM). At the end of the incubation, the cells were harvested by centrifugation (1000 x g, +5°C, five min) and then washed once

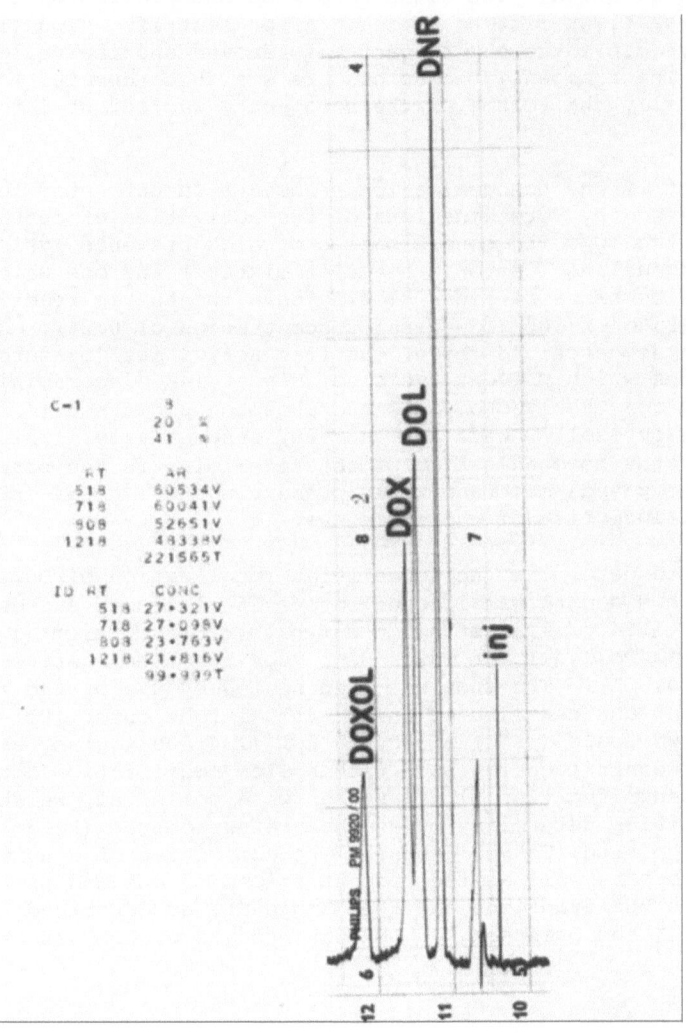

Figure 3.   Separation of an equimolar (1 μM) standard mixture of
            DNR, DOX, and their reduced metabolities, DOL and DOXOL,
            by HPLC as described in Methods and Materials.   The
            retention times were: 5.18 min (DNR), 7.18 min (DOL),
            8.08 min (DOX), and 12.18 min (DOXOL).   The relative
            peak areas were 27.3%, 27.1%, 23.8%, and 21.8%,
            respectively.

in ice-cold PBS. After resuspension in 0.25 M sucrose (pH 7.4)
containing 1 mM EDTA, the cells were transferred to a Dounce glass
homogenizer (volume 7 ml), washed once, and resuspended in 1.5 ml
of the sucrose solution. The cells were then homogenized by ten
strokes with the tight-fitting pestle. After centrifugation (1000
x g, +5°C, five min), the supernatant was removed and the pellet
resuspended. The homogenization procedure was then repeated four
times, and finally the volume of the homogenate was adjusted to
10 ml.

The effect of the homogenization procedure on untreated leukemic
cells was assessed by determinations of the activities of certain
enzymes under two opposite conditions: one which prevents lysis
of the cell organelles (isotonic reaction mixture) and one which
suppresses the membrane barriers slowing down the enzyme reactions
(addition of Triton X-100 to a final concentration of 0.2%). After
homogenization as described above, the free activities (measured
under conditions which prevent lysis) of N-acetyl-β-glucosaminidase
(marker enzyme for the lysosomes)[17] and phosphoglucomutase (marker
enzyme for the cytosol)[17] were 28% and 90%, respectively. This
indicates that the homogenization procedure eliminates the barrier
function of the plasma membrane while preserving to a great extent
the structural integrity of the lysosomes.

In order to determine the subcellular localization of DNR,
7.5 ml of the homogenate was layered onto a 26-ml linear sucrose
gradient (1.10-1.24 g/ml) resting on a 6-ml sucrose cushion (1.34
g/ml) in a 38-ml Pollyallomer Quick-Seal tube (Beckman Instruments
Inc., Palo Alto, CA). The tube was then sealed by use of the Tube
Sealer (Beckman) and centrifuged in a vertical tube rotor (VTi-50,
Beckman) for two hours (+5°C) at 40,000 rpm (134,000 x g) by a Beckman L5-65 ultracentrifuge equipped with a Slow Acceleration Accessory. After centrifugation, 15 fractions were collected, weighed,
and their densities determined by an Abbe refractometer (Atago
Optical Works Co. Ltd, Tokyo, Japan). The activities of a number
of marker enzymes as well as the concentrations of DNA and protein
were assayed in the fractions and the homogenate as described by
Tulkens et al.[18] and Quintart.[17] DNR was assayed by HPLC as described above.

RESULTS

Typical concentration curves of DNR, DOX, and their main metabolites in plasma and leukemic cells from patients treated with free
or DNA-linked drug are shown in Figures 4-8.

Figure 4 shows the plasma concentrations of DNA and DOL in
a patient with acute myeloblastic leukemia (S.-A. H., female, 63
years old) after intravenous infusion of DNR (1.5 mg/kg body weight

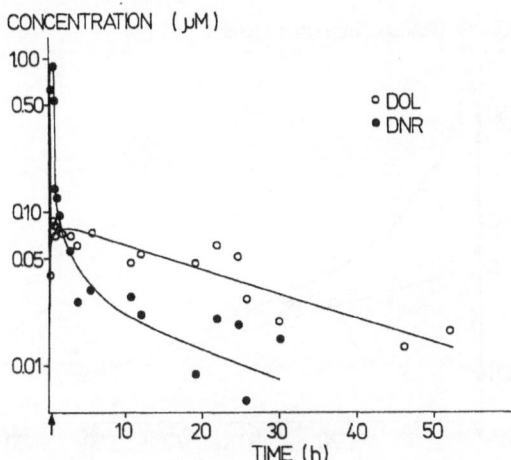

Figure 4.   Plasma concentrations of DNR and DOL in patient S.-A.H.
            after an i.v. infusion of DNR, 1.5 mg/kg during 40 min.

during 40 min). The plasma disappearance of DNR was at least biphasic with an initial rapid decay (t½ about two min) followed by
a slow phase with a t½ of more than ten hours. Within a few minutes
after the infusion, the plasma concentration of DOL exceeded that
of the parent compound. The concentration then declined slowly
(t½ about 20 hours), and the metabolite could be detected after
more than 50 hours.

     The corresponding drug concentrations in the leukemic cells
from peripheral blood, expressed as nanomoles per mg cell protein,
are shown in Figure 5. Assuming that one mg of cell protein corresponds to a cell volume of five µl,[19] it can be calculated that
the concentration of DNR in the leukemic cells at the end of the
infusion was about 175 times higher than in plasma. Thirty hours
later the ratio increased to about 500. In contrast to what was
found in plasma, DOL did not reach the same concentration in the
leukemic cells as that of the parent compound until about 50 hours
after the infusion. Immediately after the infusion, it can be calculated that the concentration of DOL in the leukemic cells exceeded
that in plasma by a factor of 120, and 30 hours later the ratio
was 150.

     During the first hours after the infusion, high concentration
of DNR appeared in the urine. The excretion of DOL was initially
low but continued for at least 100 hours, whereas significant
amounts of DNR only were found in urine during the first 24 hours.
Taken together, the amount of DNR and DOL recovered in urine within
one week only accounted for about 15% of the administered dose.

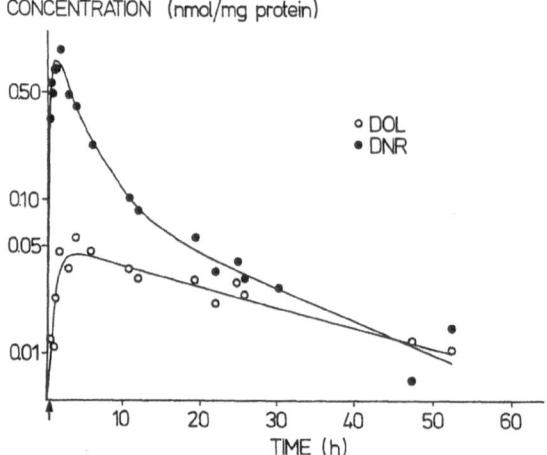

Figure 5.   Concentrations of DNR and DOL in the leukemic cells in
peripheral blood from patient S.-A.H.

Figures 6 and 7 show the concentrations of DNR and DOL in
plasma and leukemic cells from another patient with acute myeloblastic leukemia (G.A., male, 69 years old) after infusion of the
DNR-DNA complex (1.5 mg/kg during four hours). Although the DNR-
DNA solution, because of high viscosity, was infused much slower
than the free drug, the plasma concentrations of DNR and DOL reached
higher values than those observed during treatment with the free
drug. After the infusion, the plasma decay of DNR was slower (t½
of the initial phase: five to 10 min) than after infusion of free
DNR. The peak level of DNR in the leukemic cells was lower during
treatment with the DNR-DNA complex; but the drug was somewhat better
retained intracellularly, and the appearance of DOL was more pronounced.

Two patients, who had been excluded from the randomized clinical trial, were treated with free DOX in one course and DOX-DNA
in the following course (in both cases 1.5 mg/kg, free drug infused
during 40 min and the DNA-complex during four hours). The interval
between the courses was about three weeks, and no remaining DOX
could be detected in blood samples obtained immediately before the
second infusion. Figure 8 shows the plasma concentrations of DOX
after infusion of free and DNA-linked DOX to one of the patients
(T.G., male, 60 years old). In both infusions,, the plasma decay
seemed biphasic. DOX reached a higher peak concentration and could
be detected longer after treatment with the DNA-linked drug, DOXOL
could only be detected after infusion of the DNA-complex. As compared to treatment with free and DNA-linked DNR, DOX gave higher

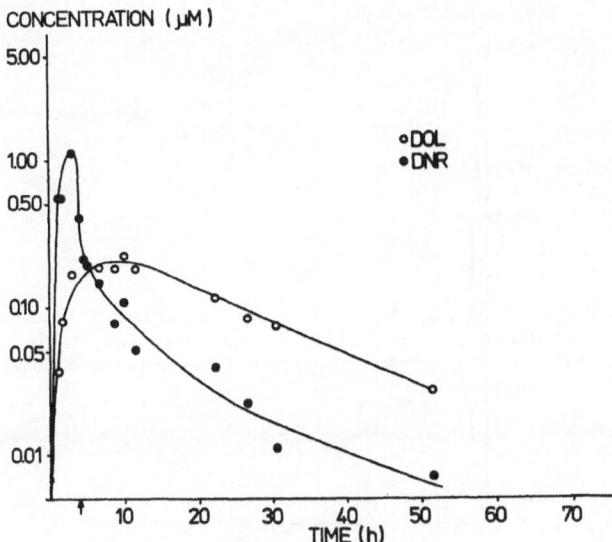

Figure 6.   Plasma concentrations of DNR and DOL in patient G.A. after an i.v. infusion of DNA-linked DNR, 1.5 mg/kg during 4 hours.

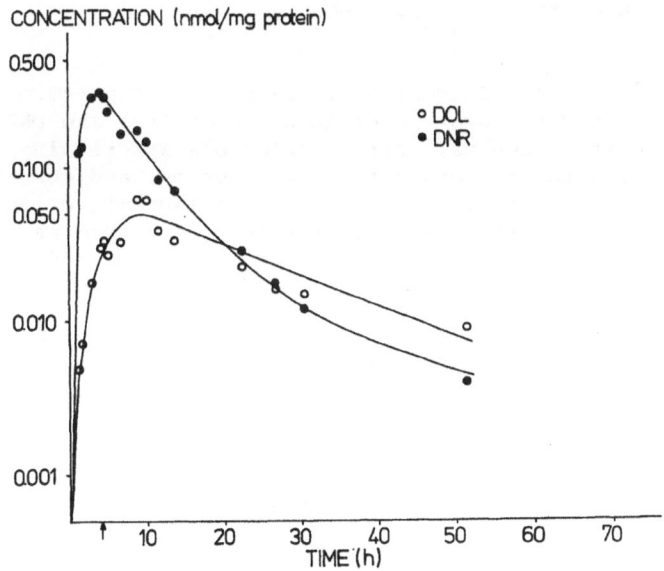

Figure 7.   Concentrations of DNR and DOL in the leukemic cells in peripheral blood from patient G.A.

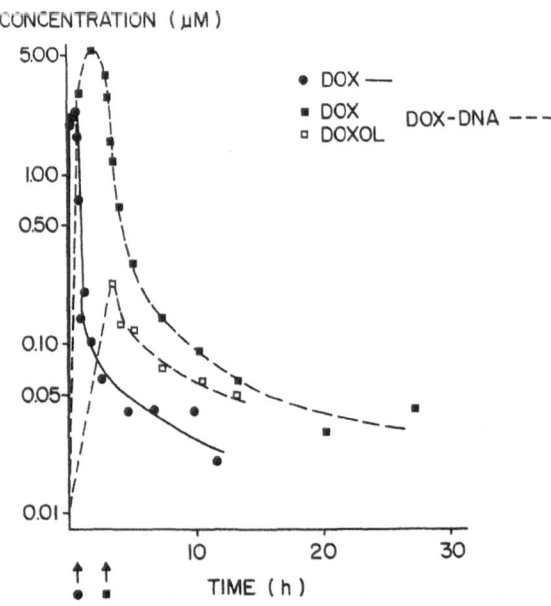

Figure 8.   Plasma concentrations of DOX and DOXOL in patient T.G.
            after i.v. infusions of free and DNA-linked DOX, 1.5
            mg/kg. The free drug was given during 45 min and the
            DNA-linked during 4 hours.

plasma peak levels. In contrast, the peak concentrations in the
leukemic cells were lower after infusion of free and DNA-linked
DOX (Figure 9). However, intracellular DOX was retained much longer
than DNR. Ten to 15 hours after the infusion, and for at least
30 hours, the concentration of DOX in the leukemic cells was about
three times higher after administration of the drug as a DNA-complex
than with free drug. No metabolite could be detected in the cells.
After treatment with free DOX, only 10% of the drug could be recovered in urine within one week. The urinary excretion was marginally higher after treatment with the DNA-linked drug. In both
treatments, 85% of the excreted DOX was identified as unchanged
drug, the rest being DOXOL. Treatment with DNA-linked DOX caused
a greater reduction of the number of leukemic cells in peripheral
blood than treatment with free DOX (Figure 10). Very similar results
were found when samples from the other patient (K.S., male, 56 years
old) treated with free and DNA-linked DOX were analyzed.

     Figure 11 shows the density distribution of DNR and a number
of subcellular markers after isopyknic centrifugation of a homogenate of leukemic cells previously incubated with DNR in vitro.
Phosphoglucomutase (marker enzyme for the cytosol) equilibrated

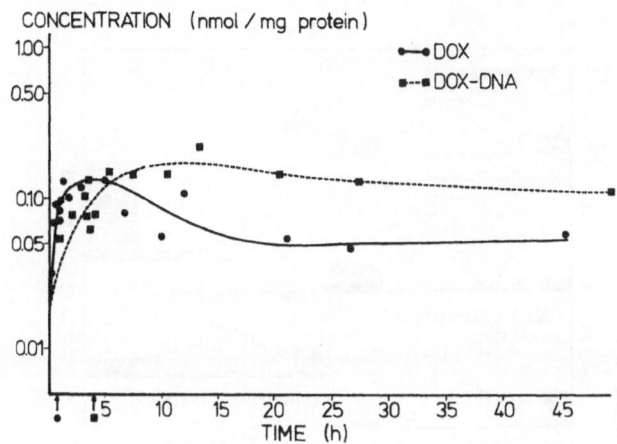

Figure 9.   Concentration of DOX in the leukemic cells in peripheral
            blood from patient T.G. after treatment with free and
            DNA-linked DOX, respectively.

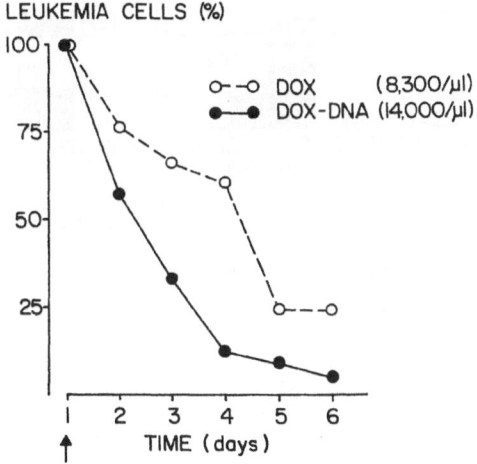

Figure 10. Effect of free and DNA-linked DOX on the number of
            leukemic cells in peripheral blood from patient T.G.
            The cell counts before treatment given within brackets.

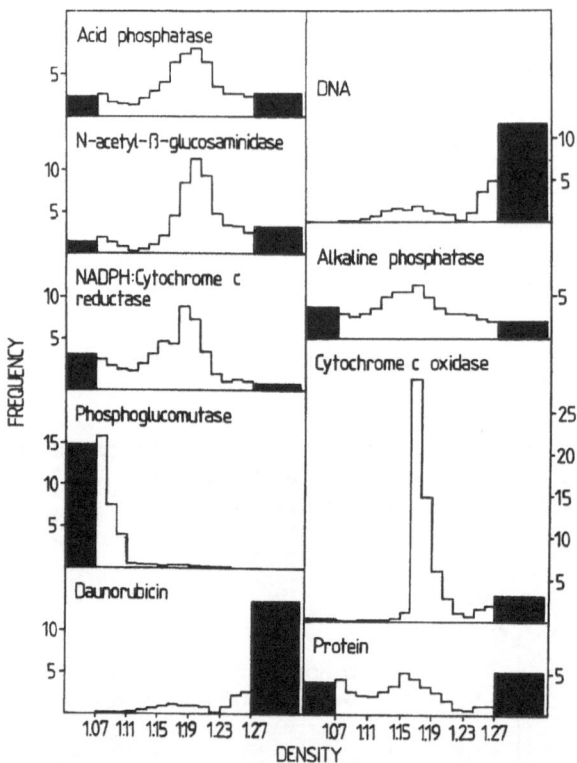

Figure 11. Distribution of DNR, marker enzymes, cell protein and
            DNA after isopyknic centrifugation of a homogenate of
            leukemia cells. The isolated cells had previously
            been incubated with DNR (1.75 μM for two hours at
            +37°C). The results are plotted in the form of
            normalized histograms (25). The frequency (ordinate)
            is $Q/(\Sigma Q \times \Delta\delta)$ where Q is the amount of constituent in
            the section and ΣQ the total amount in all sections.
            $\Delta\delta$ represents the density increment (0.013) between
            the sections. Solid areas on each side of the distri-
            bution profile represent materials recovered at den-
            sities below 1.07 g/ml and above 1.27 g/ml, respectively.

in the lightest fractions below a density of 1.07 g/ml; most DNA
was localized in fractions with densities above 1.27 g/ml. Cyto-
chrome c oxidase (mitochondria) showed a distinct peak around 1.17
g/ml; the distribution of NADPH:cytochrome c reductase (endoplasmic
reticulum) was broader with the highest concentration around 1.18
g/ml. The highest concentrations of acid phosphatase and N-acetyl-
β-glucosaminidase (lysosomes) were found in fractions around 1.19
g/ml. The distribution of alkaline phosphatase (plasma membrane)
was very broad with no distinct peak. The distribution of DNR was
almost identical to that of cellular DNA and Figure 12 shows that
the drug distribution was very similar when the cells had been
incubated with DNA-linked DNR. In both instances very little drug
was found in fractions containing high concentrations of the lysosomal enzymes N-acetyl-β-glucosaminidase and acid phosphatase.
The total cellular accumulation of free DNR was about three times
higher than of the DNA-linked drug. No metabolites could be detected after the in vitro incubations.

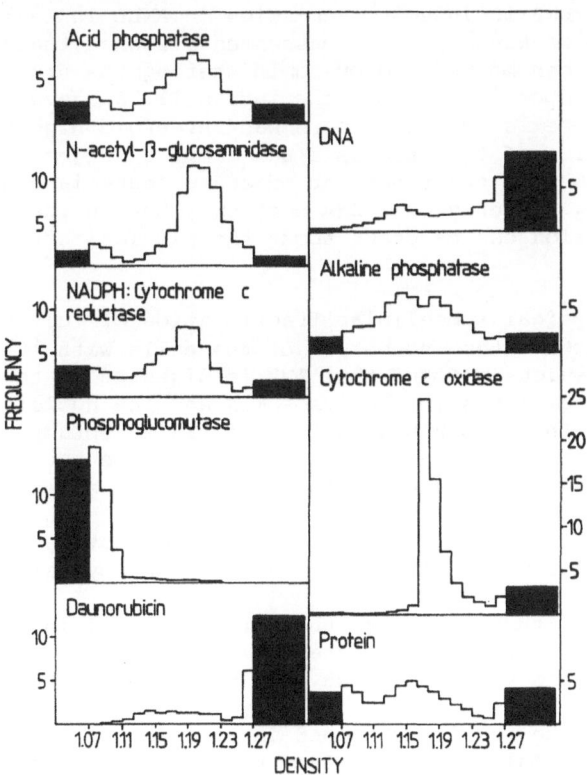

Figure 12.   Same as Figure 11 except that the isolated leukemia
             cells had been incubated with DNA-linked DNR.

DISCUSSION

Reports have previously been presented on the plasma pharmacokinetics of the anthracyclines.[20,21] However, the drugs exert their
effects intracellularly and are used under non-steady-state conditions. We have, therefore, determined the pharmacokinetics of free
and DNA-linked DNR and DOX not only in plasma but also in a compartment, which is a target for the drugs, namely the circulating leukemic cells. The results show that the drugs are highly concentrated intracellularly, and that there is no simple relationship
between the levels of DNR, DOX, and their reduced metabolites in
plasma and leukemic cells.

The pharmacokinetics of DNR and DOX can be modified by administering the drugs as DNA-complexes. This modification was more
pronounced for DOX than for DNR. The consequences of the pharmacokinetic differences between free and DNA-linked anthracyclines for
the therapeutic and toxic effects of the drugs are not yet clear.
The clinical trial of the LCS indicates that DNR-DNA has the same
potency as free DNR in inducing remission in ANLL in adults (Table
I).[14] However, we have recently presented evidence that the cardiotoxicity of DNR can be reduced by administering the drug as a DNA
complex.[22] The observation that the intracellular level of DOX
in the leukemic cells for many hours was threefold higher after
the administration of the drug as a DNA-complex suggests that the
selectivity of DOX in the treatment of acute leukemia can be enhanced by giving the drug as a DNA complex. But in the present
study no conclusion can be drawn about the clinical effects of DOX-
DNA.

Using analytical subcellular fractionation of cultured rat
embryo fibroblasts after incubation of the cells with ^{125}I-DNA-linked
DNR, we have previously found that DNA is digested by these cells
and that DNR accumulates in the lysosomes and the nuclei.[23] These
results support the hypothesis that the cellular uptake of DNA-linked
anthracyclines occurs by endocytosis. However, we have found that
both DNR and DOX also accumulate in the lysosomes and the nuclei
during incubation of the fibroblasts with the drugs in free form.[6]
Therefore, the lysosomal accumulation of DNR cannot be used as proof
that the DNR-DNA complex enters the cells by endocytosis.

The present study indicates that virtually all intracellular
DNR is localized in the nuclei after in vitro incubations of leukemia
cells with free and DNA-linked DNR. In both, very little drug was
localized in the lysosomes. It is not yet quite clear if this difference between the results obtained in rat fibroblasts and human
leukemia cells is only due to different properties of the cells or,
at least to some extent, can be explained by the lower incubation
concentration used in the present study. It has previously been

TABLE I.   INDUCTION OF REMISSION IN ANLL WITH DNA
AND DNR-DNA

Treatment		Number of Patients	Number in CR	% in CR
DNR x 1 + ARA-C	(R1)	20	14	70
DNR x 2 + ARA-C	(R2)	18	13	72
DNR-DNA x 2 + ARA-C	(R3)	22	15	68
Total		60	42	70

found that the lysosomal accumulation of anthracyclines in fibroblasts is much more prominent at higher incubation concentrations.[3]

If cellular uptake of DNA-linked anthracyclines occurs by endocytosis, it is difficult to understand why the accumulation of DNA-
linked DNR and DOX in leukemic cells in vitro is lower than of the
free drugs,[16] and, as shown in the present study, it is higher (at
least of DOX) in vivo. In vitro, the ratio between the cellular
uptake of free and DNA-linked DOX is very similar to that between
free and DNA-linked DNR,[16] whereas the intracellular accumulation
of DOX in vivo was much more influenced when the drug was given as
a DNA-complex than was the uptake of DNR. Furthermore, after the
injection of ^{125}I-DNA-linked drugs to mice, the discrepancy between
the plasma decays of radioactivity and DNR was much greater than
between radioactivity and DOX.[24]

In our opinion, there is strong evidence that the anthracycline-
DNA complexes mainly serve as slow-release preparations of the anthracyclines. Since DOX has higher affinity for DNA, the pharmacokinetics of DOX will be more influenced than that of DNR by the administration of the drug linked to DNA. This pharmacokinetical modification might enhance the drug selectively in the treatment of leukemia. Therefore, the LCS now will study the clinical effects of
DOX-DNA in ANLL in adults.

ACKNOWLEDGEMENTS

This study was supported by grants from the Swedish Cancer
Society (No. 1015-B80-03X), the Karolinska Institute and Åke Wibergs
Foundation. We are indebted to Miss Britt Sundman, Miss Irène
Granath, and Mrs. Sif Hultgren for excellent technical assistance.

REFERENCES

1. M. Weil, O.J. Glidewell, C. Jacquillat, R. Levy, A.A. Serpick, P.N. Wiernik, J. Cuttner, B. Hoogstraten, L. Wasserman, R.R. Ellison, S. Gailani, K. Brunner, R.T. Silver, V.B. Rege, M.R. Cooper, L. Lowenstein, N.I. Nissen, F. Hauarni, J. Blom, M. Boiron, J. Bernard, and J.F. Holland, Cancer Res. 33:921 (1973).
2. S.K. Carter, Cancer Chemother. Rep. 6:389 (1975).
3. C. Peterson and A. Trouet, Cancer Res. 38:4645 (1978).
4. W.J. Pigram, W. Fuller, and L.D. Hamilton, Nature New Biol. 235:17 (1972).
5. Y.-J. Schneider, R. Baurain, A. Zenebergh, and A. Trouet, Cancer Chemother. Pharmacol. 2:7 (1979).
6. G. Nöel, C. Peterson, A. Trouet, and P. Tulkens, Eur. J. Cancer 17:363 (1978).
7. L. Lenaz and J.A. Page, Cancer Treat. Rev. 3:111 (1976).
8. D.D. von Hoff, M. Rozencweig, M. Layard, M. Slavik, and F.M. Muggia, Am. J. Med. 63:200 (1977).
9. C. Praga, G. Beretta, P.L. Vigo, G.R. Lenaz, C. Pollini, G. Bonadonna, R. Canetta, R. Cavtellani, E. Villa, C.G. Gallagher, H. von Melchner, M. Hayat, P. Ribaud, G. De Wasch, W. Mattsson, R. Heinz, R. Waldner, K. Kolaric, R. Beuhner, W. Ten Bokkel-Huywinck, N.I. Perevodchikova, L.A. Manziuk, H.J. Senn, and A.C. Mayr, Cancer Treat. Rep. 63:827 (1979).
10. A. Trouet, D. Deprez-De Campeneere, and C. De Duve, Nature New Biol. 238:110 (1972).
11. A. Trouet, D. Deprez-De Campeneere, M. De Smedt-Malengreaux, and G. Atassi, Eur. J. Cancer 10:405 (1974).
12. C. Deckers, F. Mace, L. Deckers-Pauuau, and A. Trouet, in: "Molecular Base of Malignancy," George Thieme Publishers, Stuttgart 254 (1976).
13. A. Langslet, I. Øye, and S.O. Lie, Acta Pharmacol. Toxicol. 35:379 (1974).
14. C. Paul et al, Proc. from the 5th Meeting of the Int. Soc. of Haematology, European and African Division, 36 (1979).
15. G. Gahrton, M. Björkholm, G. Brenning, I. Christenson, L. Engstedt, S. Franzén, B. Gullbring, G. Holm, C. Högman, P. Hörnsten, S. Jameson, A. Killander, C. Simonsson-Lindemalm, D. Lockner, B. Lönnquist, H. Mellstedt, J. Palmblad, C. Paul, C. Pauli, C. Peterson, P. Reizenstein, B. Simonsson, K.-O. Skårberg, A.-M. Udén, and B. Wadman, Cancer Chemother. Pharmacol. 2:73 (1979).
16. C. Paul, C. Peterson, G. Gahrton, and D. Lockner, Cancer Chemother. Pharmacol. 2:49 (1979).
17. J. Quintart, Ph.D. Thesis, Universite Catholique de Louvain, Belgium (1977).
18. P. Tulkens, H. Beaufay, and A. Trouet, J. Cell Biol. 63:383 (1974).
19. P. Tulkens and A. Trouet, Arch. int. Physiol. Biochem. 80:623 (1972).

20. S. Eksborg, H. Ehrsson, B. Andersson, and M. Beran, J. Chromat. 153:211 (1978).
21. R. Hulhoven, G. Sokal, and C. Harvengt, Cancer Chemother. Pharmacol. 3:243 (1979).
22. C. Paul, B. Lönnquist, G. Gahrton, and C. Peterson, Cancer, in press.
23. C. Peterson, G. Noël, A. Zerebergh, and A. Trouet, Cancer Chemother. Pharmacol. 2:3 (1979).
24. D. Deprez-De Campeneere, R. Baurain, M. Huybrechts, and A. Trouet, Cancer Chemother. Pharmacol. 2:25 (1979).
25. F. Leighton, B. Poole, H. Beaufay, P. Bandhuin, J.W. Coffey, S. Fowler, and C. de Duve, J. Cell Biol. 37:482 (1968).

BIOLOGICAL ACTIVITIES AND TARGETING OF

SOLUBLE MACROMOLECULES

Josef Pitha and John W. Kusiak

Section on Macromolecules, National Institutes of
Health, National Institute on Aging
GRC-Baltimore City Hospitals
Baltimore, Maryland 21224

Macromolecules differ from small molecular-weight compounds
in many aspects, and that has been the main reason for delays in
their study and practical applications. Macromolecules may form
an important class of drugs, but their potential in that respect,
with the exception of polypeptidic hormones, still has not been
realized. This review deals with the similarities in pharmacodynamic phases (drug-receptor interactions) of small and large
molecular-weight compounds and the considerable differences these
two classes show in pharmacokinetic phases (drug distribution) of
their action. The results obtained both on synthetic and natural
macromolecules are used as examples because of the interests of
authors in synthetic macromolecules and their interactions with
the cell or their components in vitro and in the field of enzyme
replacement therapy, where effects of the introduction of enzymes
into animals are studied. There is only a limited formal overlap
between these fields; nevertheless, examination of respective
results leads to similar conclusions, a situation which perhaps
may be compared to a description of the same phenomena in different
languages.

BIOLOGICAL MEMBRANES

Drugs, in order to be effective, must get to their proper
targets, i.e. drug receptors; macromolecules differ profoundly from
conventional drugs in that ability, i.e. pharmacokinetic aspects.
From an anatomical point of view an organism or body is compartmenta-
lized physically into separate areas. Some of the barriers separating organs seem formidable but can be penetrated by macromolecules,

e.g. peritoneal membrane, while some others, e.g. the lining of
capillaries in the brain, represent a completely insulating element.
The penetrability of membranes to macromolecules is due to water-
filled channels crossing the membrane through which macromolecules
may diffuse. These channels represent only a small fraction of
the total surface; for example, in the lining of capillaries in
muscle this area was estimated to be 0.2% of the total surface.[1]
Channels in different membranes vary in size. To study the size
of channels the permeation rates of a series of compounds are
compared with their rate of diffusion in aqueous media; above some
molecular size an unproportionate and sizable decrease in permeation
rate is observed. This molecular size approximates the size of
aqueous channels. The following sequence gives an example of the
sizes of channels as measured by the described method:[1]

> glomerular capillaries in kidney > sinusoidal capillaries in
> liver > capillaries in muscle (about 30 Å) > capillaries in
> brain (about 8 Å)

From these values it is apparent that some macromolecules may penetrate the capillary wall in muscle but none have the potential to
penetrate into the brain. Macromolecules, compared to conventional
drugs, are thus rather limited to certain compartments in the
organism. There is an additional limitation to permeation rates
which is not obvious from the above data. The sizes given above
were measured using electroneutral compounds; the charged molecules
have a much lower ability across a membrane. For example, the
electroneutral sucrose penetrates to a limited extent into brain
while anions of sulfosalicylic acid are completely excluded.[1]

Distribution of macromolecules in the organism is limited not
only on the organ level but also on the cellular and subcellular
levels. The cytoplasmic membrane, which separates the interior
of a cell from its surroundings, does not have suitable aqueous
channels and thus prevents entry of many foreign compounds into
cells. The lipid bilayer, which is one component of the cytoplasmic membrane, is the main barrier to this entry. Many compounds
and conventional drugs dissolve to some extent both in water and
in lipids and may penetrate the cytoplasmic membrane by phase-phase
transfer. In this process a drug is transferred by a concentration
gradient from the external aqueous phase into the lipid phase of
the membrane and again into the aqueous phase of intracellular
space. Penetration through this lipid bilayer is proportionate
to the partition coefficient of the compound between non-polar
solvent and water. Compounds smaller than 15 Å penetrate somewhat
faster than larger compounds, suggesting that some very limited
transport through aqueous channels also exists.[1]

A large majority of water soluble macromolecules, both synthetic and natural, have negligible solubility in lipids, which
excludes them from penetrating effectively through lipid bilayers.
However, macromolecules can enter cells via various endocytic processes. In these processes the macromolecules which enter the cell
are contained in vesicles and thus still isolated by the membrane
of the vesicle from cytoplasm.

Membranes which are located intracellularly also represent
a barrier to homogenous distribution of compounds. The nuclear
membrane has aqueous channels about 40 Å in size[2] and thus enables
limited access of macromolecules to nuclear material. Membranes
of mitochondria were found to be permeable to polynucleotides,[2]
but a specific transport mechanism may be involved in this process.

Membranes very effectively limit distribution and interactions
of macromolecules in the body. A large portion of injected macromolecules is barred from organs possessing blood-organ barriers,
like those present in brain or sex organs; foreign macromolecules
are also excluded from the majority of the cytoplasmic space of
the entire body. Nevertheless, there are two important sites in
an organism which macromolecules may affect. Injected macromolecules may interact with components of body fluids, e.g. with
blood proteins, and accessible cell surfaces. Both these interactions are of critical importance for the further fate and effects
of macromolecules.

A number of interactions between macromolecules and components
of body fluids or membrane surfaces are of low specificity. An
example of such non-specific binding are interactions based on electric charges. The surface of membranes is dominated by polyanionic
regions with only a few polycationic sites. The major blood proteins are also polyanions, antibodies being the main exception.
Thus injected polycationic macromolecules will adhere very strongly
to the surface of membranes and will associate with and aggregate
blood proteins. Limited benefits may be derived from these interactions, since they are nearly universal; yet these interactions,
owing to their considerable strength, are very important. The interactions which are based on electric charge are, in contrast to
specific interactions, insensitive to steric strains, usually complicating attempts to diminish their considerable strength.

Specific interactions, on the other hand, may transform a compound into a magic bullet of Paul Ehrlich; these interactions are
as elusive and sensitive to steric factors as the comparison implies.
Strong and specific binding of macromolecules to membranes invari-
ably produces remarkable biological responses; some of these responses have therapeutic potential, but the high toxicity of some
compounds is also a result of such binding ability. In this context

it may be noted that specific binding of insulin to its cell surface
receptor is about the same strength as specific binding of a toxic
macromolecular organomercurial to cell surface cysteine residues.

SYNTHETIC MACROMOLECULES

In the field of synthetic macromolecules we prepared and
studied compounds in which a small molecular-weight drug or toxic
agent was attached to an inert macromolecular carrier. Such attachment in some cases sustained and in other cases abolished the corresponding biological effects. The mechanism by which these changes
occur was investigated using derivatives which were either prone or
resistant to hydrolysis; these compounds were evaluated using relatively simple systems, i.e. cell-membrane preparations and cells in
culture. All the results are consistent with the view that the
cytoplasmic membrane is the main cause of the observed differences
between effects of drugs and their conjugates. Hydrophilic macromolecules cannot cross the cytoplasmic membrane, and consequently
they may affect only the external surface of cells.

The polysaccharide dextran was used as an inert, hydrophilic
carrier for the active species. The studies done previously with
tritiated dextran show clearly that this polysaccharide is well
excluded and only negligibly bound to cells in culture.[3] When drugs
which have cell-surface receptors were attached by non-hydrolyzable
bonds to dextran, their binding abilities and biological effects
were principally sustained, while drugs which have their receptors
located intracellularly, after attachment to dextran, regularly
lost their effects.

Alprenolol, a drug which is used in the treatment of hyper-
tension and binds strongly to beta-adrenergic receptors located
on the cell surface, was used in our studies as the representative
of the first group of compounds.[4] Interestingly enough, the properties of alprenolol-dextran conjugates depend strongly on the
length of the chain connecting the drug to the polysaccharide.
When a chain having 13 atoms was used, the conjugate was bound very
strongly both to the drug receptor and to the drug-specific antibody. Shortening of the arm resulted in qualitative changes in
the binding pattern. The alprenolol-dextran conjugate, in which
the connecting arm contained only four atoms, was also well bound
to the antibody but not at all to the receptor.[4] Similar changes
in binding properties were also found for other alprenolol derivatives—those in which the drug is directly incorporated into a
polyacrylamide chain via its allyl group.[5]

Toxic agents were studied as other representatives of membrane
active compounds. Main attention was given to organomercurials
and reactive diazonium salts. Preference of the organomercurial

for coordination to sulfur is so great that under suitable conditions nearly a quantitative specific binding to sulfhydryl residues can be achieved. The surface of living cells grown in culture contains cysteine residues, and thus there are cell surface receptors for ogranomercurials.[6,7] Both ionic mercury and macromolecular organomercurial were found to bind to cells, and these mercury derivatives were highly toxic when added directly to the cell-growth medium.[6] When cells and mercury compounds were separated by a semipermeable membrane, the macromolecular organomercurial lost its toxicity; the toxicity of small molecular-weight organomercurials was not changed.[6,7] Thus the observed toxicity of macromolecular organomercurial cannot be due to the release of mercury salt.

Macromolecular diazonium salts were studied as another example of agents acting on the cell surface. In slightly basic solutions diazonium ions react in an irreversible manner with tyrosine and histidine residues of proteins and possibly also with amino groups present on proteins and phospholipids. Anilin residues were attached by non-hydrolyzable bonds to dextran, and the resulting anilin-dextran was converted by nitrous acid to the corresponding diazonium derivative. The macromolecular diazonium salt, in contrast to anilin-dextran, was considerably cytotoxic.[6] When the reactive diazonium-dextran derivative was at first deactivated by treatment with tyrosine and cells were treated with that compound, only low cytotoxic effects were detected. The results are thus consistent with the view that the toxic effects of diazonium-dextran are entirely due to the reaction of that compound with the components of the cell surface which are critical for cell metabolism.

In context with studies on membrane-macromolecule interactions it was of some interest to prepare and study macromolecular detergents. Non-ionic detergents do not have specific binding sites; they dissolve in the lipid bilayer of the cytoplasmic membrane, penetrate it, and then dissolve and damage the intracellularly located membranes. The non-ionic detergent, Triton X-100, was attached to a polysaccharide, insulin.[8] The resulting compound was found to have zero-critical micelle concentration, i.e., even a single macromolecule possessed a micellar space and was able to solubilize natural phospholipids. Similarly to Triton X-100 the macromolecular detergent was cytotoxic to cells, but the cytotoxic effect occurred at a noticeably slower rate; apparently the diffusional processes necessary for the ultimate cell damage occurred at a much slower rate.[8] Obviously even compounds which have only non-specific receptors fully conform to the above rules on bioactivity.

In contrast to agents acting on the cell surface, drugs which have intracellular receptors, after irreversible attachment to macromolecules, almost completely lose their potency. This phenomenon was observed while we were studying two groups of compounds.

The first group studied consisted of aromatic bases which
strongly interact with deoxyribonucleic acids. Many such compounds
have been used as antiparasitic and antineoplastic drugs and presumably act on target cells by penetrating into nuclear regions
of cells and interfering with replication processes occurring there.
The following compounds were tested: proflavine, acridine orange,
primaquine, fluorescent dye Hoechst 33258, and daunorubicin.[6,9]
Toxicities of all these compounds to cells in culture decreased
by two to three orders after they were affixed with non-hydrolyzable
bonds to dextran.

The second group of compounds studied were steroids with gluco-
corticoid activity. These hormones are known to easily cross the
cytoplasmic membrane, and subsequent binding to intracellular receptors then mediates transfer of the hormone to the nuclear region
of cells. These hormones stimulate cell division in fibroblastic
cells in culture. Two potent glucocorticoids, hydrocortisone and
dexamethasone, after irreversible attachment to dextran, completely
lost their ability to stimulate division in fibroblasts.[10]

It is important to note that the situation is rather different
when some of these same compounds are attached to dextran by a hydrolyzable bond. This type of attachment did not abolish, but retained
or even slightly potentiated the respective bio-effects, e.q., the
cytotoxic effects of daunorubicin[9] or the stimulation of cell division by hydrocortisone.[10] Similar observations were also made for
a compound with vitamin A activity, retinal.[11]

ENZYMES AND THEIR DERIVATIVES

Enzyme therapy may be a useful approach in the treatment of
various disease states including inherited disorders of carbohydrate, nucleic acid, amino acid, and glycolipid metabolism, various
asparagine dependent tumors, and certain inflammatory states. Un-
fortunately, the purified enzymes required for these therapies
sometimes lack the physical and pharmacological qualities necessary
to be of therapeutic benefit. Purified enzymes, when injected
intravenously into experimental animals or patients, are in general,
rapidly cleared from the circulation and sequestered by the liver
into lysosomes, small vesicles located in the cytoplasm of cells
but separated from it by enveloping membranes. In these lysosomes
entrapped enzymes rapidly lose their activity due to hydrolysis
by proteases present there. While in certain disease states hepatic
uptake of exogenously supplied enzymes is desirable, rapid cataho-
lism is not, and some means to prolong enzymic activity must be
found for therapy to be effective. For other applications of enzyme
therapy, however, increased circulation time of administered enzyme
is desirable, and enzymes must be altered to reduce uptake by liver

and other organs containing reticulo-endothelial cells. For most
applications of enzyme therapy the enzymes will probably have to
be considerably modified to achieve the desired effectiveness.

A number of techniques are available to enhance the stability
of biologically active molecules, including covalent coupling of
enzymes to water-soluble carrier molecules such as albumin or polysaccharides and intermolecular and intramolecular crosslinking of
enzymes. Effective targeting of enzymes to diseased tissues can
be achieved by taking advantage of receptors on cell surfaces
specific for certain proteins or glycoproteins that enhance delivery
to these cells. Enzymes can be modified by the addition or removal
of specific targeting moieties (monosaccharides, charged groups
of amino acid side chains) that would lead to altered tissue distribution. Some recent evidence suggests that alternative targeting
of enzymes may be accomplished by covalently attaching specific
recognition markers of other molecules (i.e. the B subunits of
cholera toxin or glycopeptides of plasma glycoproteins) to enzymes,
thereby directing these chimeras to different cell types.

A number of methods have been utilized to stabilize purified
enzymes to inactivation and enzymatic hydrolysis. Poznanski prepared soluble enzyme polymers of uricase[12] and α-1,4-glucosidase[13]
by covalently crosslinking these enzymes with an excess of serum
albumin using glutaraldehyde. With this treatment, about 50% of
the enzyme activity was retained, and the conjugates exhibited
enhanced stability in vitro. Furthermore, the circulation half-
time of the uricase-albumin polymer in dogs was increased approximately six-fold above that of the native enzyme. Also, the albumin
seemed to have masked antigenic sites on the unicase, since no
hypersensitivity reactions were noted upon repeated injections of
the uricase-albumin polymer, while after the third injection of
native uricase an anaphylactic reaction was observed. These results
suggested that condensation of uricase with albumin may enhance the
therapeutic usefulness of this enzyme since its activity is prolonged
in vitro, its antigenicity is reduced, and most importantly the
circulation time in vivo is increased. Wang and Tu [14]modified
glycogen phosphorylase b by treating purified enzyme with glutaraldehyde. While their final product had only about 4% of the original
activity, that which remained was considerably more stable to heat
and urea denaturation. As others have pointed out,[15,16] care must
be taken in assigning the enhanced stability of polymeric enzymes
to intermolecular crosslinking, since the manipulations and reagents
used in the crosslinking process may also result in intramolecular
crosslinking which could also stabilize enzymatic activities.

Marshall and co-workers stabilized the activities of a number
of enzymes by coupling them to soluble dextrans that had been acti-
vated by low concentrations of cyanogen bromide.[17] In all these

reactions there was an enhanced stability to heat denaturation;
with trypsin, attachment to dextran prevented rapid denaturation
by urea and 2-mercaptoethanol. The effects of this coupling procedure probably resulted from the multipoint attachment of enzymes
to the dextran, thereby stabilizing the tertiary and in the case
of β-amylase, the quaternary structure of the enzymes. In a more
recent publication,[18] this group showed, in addition to enhanced
heat stability of α-amylase- and catalase-dextran complexes, an
increased circulation lifetime upon intravenous injection into rats
and acatalesmic mice respectively.

Essentially the same results were obtained by Davis and co-
workers,[19] who prepared adducts of phenylalanine ammonia-lyase and
polyethylene glycol. These conjugates were more resistant to proteolytic digestion and had an increased circulation; although they
induced antibody formation in mice, the antibodies had apparent
low specificity for the antigen (i.e. the polyethylene glycol
adduct) when tested in vitro. In another study, von Specht and
Brendel[20] prepared poly(vinylpyrrolidone) adducts of trypsin and
chymotrypsin. Both were more stable to autolysis, but there was
some decrease in the activity of these derivatives towards large
molecular-weight substrates.

The specific recognition of foreign or modified foreign enzymes
by receptors located on cell membranes may lead to their selective
accumulation by these cells. Recently, a number of these receptors
have been delineated having specificity for the carbohydrate portion
of glycoproteins. The presence of these receptors creates the
potential to selectively target glycoproteins to different cell
types by either modifying the terminal non-reducing sugar moiety
of the oligosaccharide or covalently coupling an oligosaccharide
containing the proper monosaccharide terminus to the protein.
Examples of each of these approaches will be given to demonstrate
their feasibility.

Plasma glycoproteins generally contain sialic acid as a terminus
of their oligosaccharide chains and have a very long half-life in
the circulation. Ashwell and his co-workers showed that if the
sialic acid was removed, exposing the penultimate galactose, the
modified glycoproteins were rapidly cleared from the circulation
and sequestered in hepatocytes, where they were rapidly catabo-
lized.[21] This rapid removal from the circulation was due to the
specific, high affinity binding of these galactose terminated glycoproteins by a receptor associated exclusively with hepatocytes.
This specific recognition mediated the rapid internalization and
ultimate deposition of these glycoproteins in the lysosomes where
they were degraded. If galactose was removed from the oligosaccharide exposing N-acetylglucosamine, the glycoproteins were still
cleared rapidly from the circulation by a receptor mediated

process,[22] but in this case they accumulated in cells of the
reticulo-endothelial system, primarily in liver. Numerous groups
showed that lung,[23] peritoneal macrophages,[24] and isolated rat liver
Kupffer cells,[25] all components of the recticuloendothelial system,
contained receptors that specifically bound glycoproteins whose
oligosaccharides terminated in either N-acetylglucosamine or
mannose. Other investigators discovered receptors on hepatocytes
that recognized fucose containing glycoproteins.[26] The mutiplicity
of receptors on different cell types theoretically would allow for
precise targeting of exogenously supplied enzymes not only to
specific organs but to different cell types within organs.

The same mechanisms apply to the recognition of lysosomal
enzymes. Sly and others[27,28] have shown that most injected human
lysosomal enzymes are cleared rapidly from the circulation of rats
by a receptor mediated process. This clearance is carbohydrate
dependent; it is specific in that glycoproteins terminated only
in mannose or N-acetylglucosamine or the respective monosaccharides
will block the rapid clearance. Subsequently, Steer et al.[25] showed
that ^{125}I-β-hexosaminidase A was specifically taken up by isolated
rat liver non-parenchymal cells but not by isolated hepatocytes
and that this uptake was also blocked by mannose or N-acetylglu-
cosaminyl terminated glycoproteins. In another study of a lysosomal
enzyme, glucocerebrosidase, it was shown that the purified native
enzyme was slowly cleared from the circulation ($t_{1/2}$ = 21 minutes)
and was taken up by both hepatocytes and non-parenchymal cells.
After neuraminidase treatment of the enzyme to remove the sialic
acid, the half-life in the circulation was reduced to less than
two minutes, while the uptake by hepatocytes was greatly increased
and the uptake by non-parenchymal cells was decreased.[29] If glucocerebrosidase was then treated with β-galactosidase to expose N-
acetylglucosamine, its clearance was still very rapid, but appreci-
ably more enzyme was found in the non-parenchymal cell fraction.[30]
Further covalent modifications of the oligosaccharide by removal
of the N-acetylglucosamine and fucose with specific glycosidases
may increase the selectivity of the targeting for this enzyme.

The identification of saccharide residues as signals for
specific uptake of glycoproteins by cells led to attempts to attach
these residues to proteins synthetically. Lee,[31-33] Youle,[34]
Wilson,[35] and Marsh[36] have developed methodology for attachment
of various sugars and oligosaccharides to non-glycosylated proteins.
The glycoconjugates they synthesized had the clearance characteristics and binding specificity expected of glycoproteins having
the respective monosaccharide termini. The same end result was
also achieved by coupling glycoproteins with non-glycosylated
proteins; the former then targeted the latter to specific cell
types.[37,38]

A number of recent studies indicate that cellular uptake of proteins may also be considerably changed by modification of their amino acid side chains. Low-density lipoprotein has been shown to bind specifically to cultured fibroblasts, lymphocytes, and adrenal cells, where it is then internalized and degraded releasing cholesterol for cellular metabolism.[39] Modification of the lysine and arginine residues on low density lipoprotein with acetic anhydride abolished its uptake by fibroblasts and lymphocytes but stimulated its uptake by peritoneal macrophages which do not recognize native low-density lipoprotein.[40] In vivo, low-density lipoprotein, whose basic amino acids had been altered by acetoacetylation, was cleared from the circulation much more rapidly than native low-density lipoprotein, and approximately 80% of the injected dose was found in the liver within 1/2 hour after injection.[41]

CONCLUSION

Utilization of the numerous synthetic techniques reviewed here will lead to the development of many new macromolecular conjugates of both small molecular-weight drugs (steroids, vitamins, neurotransmitters) and large molecular-weight enzymes. These new adducts are being designed to have therapeutic properties that are more beneficial in terms of enhanced activity and/or reduced toxicity. The macromolecular derivatives of small molecular-weight drugs should have a limited cellular distribution due to their impermeability to cell membranes. Also, these types of drugs could be derivatized to obtain a slow release of active drug to tissue sites. On the other hand, enzyme derivatives can be designed for stability to degradation, enhanced targeting to specific cell types, and the abolishment or at least a reduction of the immunological response of an organism to challenge by these foreign macromolecules. Any one or a combination of these altered characteristics can lead to more effective therapeutic potential of exogenously administered enzymes.

REFERENCES

1. A. Goldstein, L. Aaronow, and S.M. Kalman, in: "Principles of Drug Action," John Wiley & Sons, Inc., New York, (1974). pp. 166-192.
2. J. Pitha, in: "Targeted Drugs,", E.L. Goldberg, L.G. Donaruma, and O. Vogl, eds., John Wiley & Sons, Inc., New York, in press.
3. G.D. Press and J. Pitha, Mech. Ageing Dev. 3:323 (1974).
4. J. Pitha, J. Zjawiony, R.J. Lefkowitz, and M.G. Caron, Proc. Natl. Acad. Sci. USA 77:2219 (1980).
5. J. Pitha, J. Zjawiony, R.J. Lefkowitz, and M.G. Caron, Makromol. Chem., in press.

6. J. Pitha, Eur. J. Biochem. 82:285 (1978).

7. J. Pitha, B. Hughes, and N.A. Berger, manuscript in preparation.

8. J. Pitha, K. Kociolek, and M.G. Caron, Eur. J. Biochem. 94:11 (1979).

9. E. Hurwitz, M. Wilchek, and J. Pitha, J. Appl. Bichem. 2:25 (1980).

10. J. Pitha, J. Zjawiony, B. Rosner, and V. Cristofalo, manuscript in preparation.

11. J. Pitha, S. Zawadzki, F. Chytil, D. Lotan, and R. Lotan, J. Natl. Cancer Inst. 65:1011 (1980).

12. M.J. Poznansky, Life Sci. 24:153 (1979).

13. M.J. Poznansky and D. Bhardwaj, Can. J. Physiol. Pharmacol. 58:322 (1980).

14. J.H.-C. Wang and J.-I. Tu, Biochemistry 8:4403 (1969).

15. K. Martinek, A.M. Klibanov, V.S. Goldmacher, and I.V. Berezin, Biochim. Biophys. Acta 485:1 (1977).

16. A.M. Klibanov, Anal. Biochem. 93:1 (1979).

17. J.J. Marshall and M.L. Rabinowitz, Arch. Biochem. Biophys. 167:777 (1975).

18. J.J. Marshall, J.D. Humphreys, and S.L. Abramson, FEBS Letters 83:249 (1977).

19. K.J. Wieder, N.C. Palczuk, T. van Es, and F.F. Davis, J. Biol. Chem. 254:12579 (1979).

20. B.-U. Von Specht and W. Brendel, Biochim. Biophys. Acta 484:109 (1977).

21. G. Gregoriadis, A.G. Morell, I. Sternlieb, and I.H. Scheinberg, J. Biol. Chem. 245:5833 (1970).

22. D.T. Achord, F.E. Brot, and W.S. Sly, Biochem. Biophys. Res. Commun. 77:409 (1977).

23. P.D. Stahl, J.S. Rodman, M.J. Miller, and P.H. Schlesinger, Proc. Natl. Acad. Sci. USA 75:1399 (1978).

24. J.W. Kusiak, J.M. Quirk, and R.O. Brady, Biochem. Biophys. Res. Commun. 94:199 (1980).

25. C.J. Steer, J.W. Kusiak, R.O. Brady, and E.A. Jones, Proc. Natl. Acad Sci. USA 76:2774 (1979).

26. J.-P. Prieels, S.V. Pizzo, L.R. Glasgow, J.C. Paulson, and R.L. Hill, Proc. Natl. Acad. Sci. USA 75:2215 (1978).

27. D. Achord, F. Brot, A. Gonzalez-Noriega, W. Sly, and P. Stahl, Pediat. Res. 11:816 (1977).

28. D.T. Achord, F.E. Brot, C.E. Bell, and W.S. Sly, Cell 15:269 (1978).

29. F.S. Furbish, C.J. Steer, J.A. Barranger, E.A. Jones, and R.O. Brady, Biochem. Biophys. Res. Commun. 81:1047 (1978).

30. C.J. Steer, F.S. Furbish, J.A. Barranger, R.O. Brady, and E.A. Jones, FEBS Letters 91:202 (1978).

31. Y.C. Lee, C.P. Stowell, and M.J. Krantz, Biochemistry 15:3956 (1976).

32. M.J. Krantz, N.A. Holtzman, C.P. Stowell, and Y.C. Lee, Biochemistry 15:3963 (1976).

33.   C.P. Stowell and Y.C. Lee, J. Biol. Chem. 253:6107 (1978).
34.   R.J. Youle, G.J. Murray, and D.M. Neville, Jr., Proc. Natl. Acad. Sci. USA 76:5559 (1979).
35.   G. Wilson, J. Biol. Chem. 253:2070 (1978).
36.   J.W. Marsh, J. Denis, and J.C. Wriston, Jr., J. Biol. Chem. 252:7678 (1977).
37.   J.C. Rogers and S. Kornfeld, Biochem. Biophys. Res. Commun. 45:622 (1971).
38.   G. Schmer, J.S. Holcenberg, and J. Roberts, Biochim. Biophys. Acta 538:397 (1978).
39.   J.L. Goldstein and M.S. Brown, Ann. Rev. Biochem. 46:897 (1977).
40.   J.L. Goldstein, Y.K. Ho, S.K. Basu, and M.S. Brown, Proc. Natl. Acad. Sci. USA 76:333 (1979).
41.   R.W. Mahley, K.H. Weisgraber, T.L. Innerarity, and H.G. Windmueller, Proc. Natl. Acad. Sci. USA 76:1746 (1979).

HYDROPHILIC/HYDROPHOBIC CONTROL OF STEROID RELEASE FROM A CORTISOL - POLYGLUTAMIC ACID SUSTAINED RELEASE SYSTEM

N. Tani, M. Van Dress, and J. M. Anderson

Department of Macromolecular Science
Case Western Reserve University
Cleveland, Ohio 44106

INTRODUCTION

Biodegradable polymer formulations which allow delivery of biologically active agents to a target organ or organism at controlled rates over a prolonged period of time have been developed and studied.[1,2] These biodegradable controlled-release systems offer the distinct advantage that no residual polymer remains following release of the drug and degradation of the polymer.

Earlier studies have focused on erosion-type devices in which active agents are dispersed within the biodegradable polymer matrix. However, some of those devices showed very high release rates. To overcome this problem, we have developed a biodegradable polymer system for the controlled release of steroids using the pro-drug concept.[3]

In this type of system, the drug is covalently bound to the side chain of a biodegradable polymer via a labile, easily degradable bond. The polymer backbone was chosen so that it degrades at a much slower rate than the rate of cleavage of the labile bond. A spacer unit separates the steroid from the polymer backbone, and its properties (length, hydrophilicity, etc.) assist in controlling the release rate, while the labile bond plays the major role in determining the release rate of the drug.

In spite of their advantages, the development and application of biodegradable pro-drug systems have been limited. Release kinetics of these systems are more complicated than those of diffusional systems, and little work has been done on the kinetics of the pro-drug systems.[4,5] This complexity in pro-drug devices arises

79

because not only diffusion but also the hydrolysis of the labile
bonds control the release behavior, and this hydrolysis can be
affected by many factors in the local molecular environment. For
example, "neighboring effects" such as catalysis by adjacent groups
may be produced as the hydrolysis proceeds. This catalysis may
be due to the direct involvement of such groups in the hydrolysis
or indirectly due to the hydrophilicity of such groups.[6-9]

The system presented in this paper was designed for possible
use in the control of the symptoms of chronic inflammation. Polyglutamic acid (PGA) was chosen as the polymer backbone for the
system. The biodegradability of homopolymers and copolymers of
L-glutamic acid has been widely studied in our laboratories.[10]
These earlier studies have shown that the side-chain carboxyl group
of the L-glutamic acid can provide sufficient hydrophilicity required for biodegradation. The side-chain carboxyl groups also
serve as points of attachment for the labile bonds. Cortisol was
chosen as the drug because of its anti-inflammatory activity and
the presence of functional groups on the molecule to which the
labile bond could be attached. Since cortisol has two types of
functional groups, i.e. keto and hydroxyl, the drug molecule can
be bound to PGA side chains via various labile bonds.

Our initial attempts were directed toward preparing ester bonds
between the hydroxyl groups of cortisol and the side-chain carboxyl
groups of PGA, using dicyclohexylcarbodiimide (DCC). Although
cortisol has three hydroxyl groups, only the 21-hydroxyl group,
a primary hydroxyl, was found to be capable of coupling. While
small amounts of cortisol could be coupled to PGA, the coupled
polymer showed a very slow cortisol release rate upon hydrolysis.

Previous work in our laboratories has shown that the oximino
bond is suitable as a labile bond for steroid-PGA systems.[3] To
form this system, a keto group of cortisol must be transformed to
an oxime with hydroxylamine; then the cortisol oxime can be coupled
to the PGA side-chain carboxyls by DCC. Since cortisol has two
keto groups, the selective preparation of a mono-oxime derivative
was necessary. The 3-mono-oxime derivative of cortisol was successfully prepared by an enamine method[11] (see Figure 1). Loading
levels (percentage of esterified PGA side chains) were controlled
by changing the steroid/PGA ratios in the coupling reaction. Thus
four polymers with various loading levels were obtained.

The release behavior of these coupled polymers was studied
using buffer/ethanol mixtures at 37°C. Ethanol was added in order
to improve upon the poor solubility of cortisol in water. Since
the coupled polymers exist in a solid or semi-solid state during
most of the hydrolysis, both film and powder samples of the polymers
were hydrolyzed in order to evaluate possible surface area effects

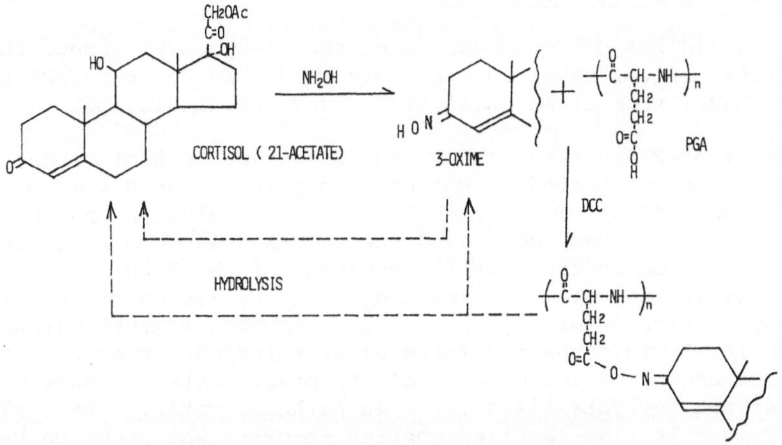

Figure 1. Synthesis and hydrolysis of the PGA-cortisol oxime
controlled-release system.

on the cortisol release rate. Radioactive tracer techniques were
also employed to evaluate the importance of diffusion to the overall release rate in the various hydrolysis media.

METHODS AND MATERIALS

Polyglutamic Acid (PGA)

PGA[12] was prepared by debenzylation of poly-γ-benzyl-L-glutamate, which was prepared by polymerization of γ-benzyl-L-glutamate-
N-carboxyanhydride in benzene-methylene chloride (1:1) solution
using n-hexylamine as the initiator. Poly-γ-benzyl-L-glutamate,
4.3 g, was dissolved in 500 ml of dry benzene. Hydrogen bromide
was bubbled into this solution under vigorous stirring for two hrs.
This reaction mixture was tightly sealed and allowed to stand at
room temperature for two days. The volume of the reaction mixture
was reduced to 150 ml, and the reaction mixture was poured into
dry ether. The resulting PGA was washed with ether in a Soxhlet
extractor for four days. The PGA was obtained as a white powder,
yield 2.0 g, and its molecular weight was ca. 12,000 as determined
by light scattering in pH 7.3 buffer solution containing 2M NaCl.[12]
The ultraviolet spectrum of the PGA showed no residual benzyl
groups in the polymer.

Cortisol 21 Acetate-3-Oxime

To avoid the direct coupling of the 21-hydroxyl group, the
21-acetate derivative of cortisol was used. The cortisol-21-acetate
was purchased from Sigma Chemical Company, St. Louis, MO.

Cortisol-21-acetate, 1.0 g, was dissolved in 5 ml of methanol.
This solution was heated to the boiling point; then 0.4 ml of pyrrolidine was added. To the resultant yellow solution, another 0.4
ml of pyrrolidine was added, and the solution was cooled to room
temperature. On cooling, yellow crystals of the 3-enamine derivative precipitated. To this reaction mixture, 190 mg of hydroxyl-
amine-hydrochloride was added, and the reaction mixture was heated
to 50°C for 5 min. The resulting clear solution was poured into
an excess amount of ice water, and the precipitated product was
filtered and recrystallized twice in methanol-water. The yield
was 780 mg. Tritium-labelled cortisol-3-oxime was prepared by the
same method.

PGA Coupled Cortisol-21-Acetate-3-Oxime

PGA (170 mg) and 500 mg of cortisol-21-acetate-3-oxime was
dissolved in 6 ml of dry dimethylformamide (DMF). To this solution,
0.5 ml of acetonitrile was added and the solution was cooled to
-5°C. Dicyclohexylcarbodiimide (272 mg) was dissolved in 1 ml of
dry DMF and added to the PGA, cortisol-21-acetate-3-oxime solution.
This solution was kept at -5°C for two hours then 0°C to 5°C for
two days. After the reaction, the precipitated dicyclohexyl urea
was filtered out, and the filtrate was reduced to a small volume.
Ethylacetate was added to this solution to precipitate the coupled
polymer. The polymer was reprecipitated twice more using DMF and
ethylacetate and once using dioxane and water. The yield was 430
mg.

Loading Level Determination

The coupled polymer was dissolved in dioxane, and the absorbance of this solution at 245 nm was measured. Loading levels were
calculated by comparing this absorbance to those obtained for
standard solutions of cortisol-21-acetate-3-oxime in dioxane.

Hydrolysis of Coupled Polymers

Films were cast from dioxane solution. A film was placed on
the bottom of a 5-ml vial and 1 ml of hydrolysis solvent (buffer/
ethanol mixture) was added. The vial was tightly sealed and placed

in a 37°C water bath. The hydrolysis solvent was replaced by fresh solvent every one to three days. The steroid concentration in the sample solution was measured by UV spectroscopy.

Coupled polymer powder samples were used as obtained by the reprecipitation process. The powder (5 to 10 mg) was placed in a small test tube and 1 ml of hydrolysis solvent was added. The test tube was tightly sealed and placed in a 37°C water bath. In order to avoid loss of any powder on sampling, the mixture was centrifuged, and only an aliquot from the upper half of the solvent was taken as a sample and replaced by fresh solvent every one to three days. The amount of released steroid was calculated by comparing the steroid concentration of one sample to that of the previous sample.

Both pH 2 and pH 7.4 buffer/ethanol mixtures were used in this experiment; the former was used to accelerate the hydrolysis. These buffers were used in both 95/5 and 50/50 v/v mixtures with ethanol. To insure that the high water content 95/5 mixtures were not becoming saturated with steroid during hydrolysis, the solubilities of both the cortisol-21-acetate and the 3-oxime derivative were checked in these 95/5 mixtures. The limiting solubilities at room temperature were found to be ca. 500 µg/ml and ca. 800 µg/ml respectively. These levels are well above the maximum steroid concentration of 80 µg/ml observed during hydrolysis.

Tritium-labelled cortisol for use in the diffusion studies was purchased from New England Nuclear (1,2,6,7-^{3}H-labelled cortisol, specific activity 93.1 Ci/mmol). Films of the coupled polymers, in which tritium-labelled cortisol was dispersed, were prepared by casting from a solution containing non-labelled coupled polymer and tritium-labelled free cortisol in dioxane. Released radio-labelled cortisol was measured by liquid scintillation counting, with Scintisol (Isolab Inc.) as a fluorescent agent.

Precoated alumina GF (Analtech Inc.) and precoated silicagel 60F-254 plates (Merck) were used for the thin-layer chromatography (TLC). A mixture of chloroform/dioxane/acetic acid (87/10/3) was used as the developing solvent.

RESULTS AND DISCUSSION

Coupling Reaction

The formation of a chemical bond between PGA and cortisol-21-acetate-3-oxime was evident from the infrared spectra of the carefully purified coupled polymer (Figure 2). Strong absorptions were

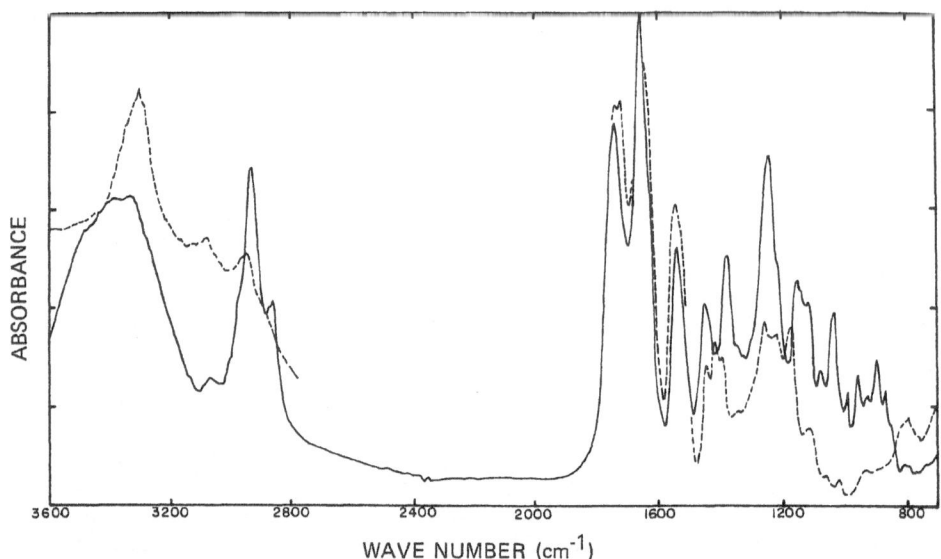

ABSORBANCE

WAVE NUMBER (cm^{-1})

Figure 2. IR spectra of PGA-cortisol oxime (———) and PGA (---).

present from 2850 to 2950 cm^{-1} because of the steroid C-H bonds, and a shift of the PGA carboxyl absorption because of the formation of ester bonds between PGA side chains and cortisol-21-acetate-3-oxime can be seen.

The reaction between cortisol-21-acetate and PGA gave virtually no coupling. Therefore, the 11- and 17-hydroxyl groups of cortisol were found to be incapable of forming an ester bond with the PGA side-chain carboxyl groups under our conditions.

The solubility properties of the coupled polymers were also markedly different from that of PGA. The coupled polymers were soluble in dioxane and insoluble in water, whereas PGA was soluble in water but not in dioxane. Thin-layer chromatography of the purified coupled polymer showed no free steroid remaining in the polymer.

The results of the coupling reactions are listed in Table I. The loading level can be varied from 15 to 90% by changing the initial steroid/PGA mole ratio from 0.5 to 2, respectively.

Hydrolysis Studies

The preliminary hydrolysis of the coupled polymer showed that not only cortisol-21-acetate but also cortisol-21-acetate-3-oxime

TABLE I. VARIABLE LOADING LEVELS FROM THE COUPLING REACTION

No.	PGA	Used Steroid	Mole Ratio Steroid/PGA	Loading (%)
1	LMw	Cortisol-21-Acetate-3-Oxime	0.5/1	15 ± 2
2	LMw	Cortisol-21-Acetate-3-Oxime	1/1	60 ± 5
3	LMw	Cortisol-21-Acetate-3-Oxime	2/1	90 ± 7
4	LMw	Cortisol-3-oxime	1/1	30 ± 3
5	HMw	Cortisol-21-Acetate-3-oxime	1/1	---

was produced by hydrolysis (See Figure 1). Both result from the hydrolysis of the oxime-coupled polymer. The first is released by the cleavage at the ester bond and the second by the cleavage at the imino bond. It has been reported that cortisol-21-acetate-3-oxime also has anti-inflammatory activity.[13] Although two forms of the steroid are released, both have the same extinction coefficient and λ max, and differ only slightly in molecular weight; therefore, UV spectroscopy was used to measure the total steroid released, i.e. the sum of both forms.

Hydrolysis in the 95/5 (v/v) buffer/ethanol mixture. The results for the hydrolysis studies of the films and powder samples are given in Table II. As shown in Figure 3, the release rates for 90% and 60% loaded films in the pH 2 buffer mixture gradually increase for the first 20 to 30 days, finally reaching a constant rate of release. After 70 days, the release rate of the 60% loaded film starts to decrease, while the 90% loaded film continues to hydrolyze at a constant release rate until 120 days. The constant release rates are 0.8% of the total loaded steroid per day for the 60% loaded film and 0.4% of the total loaded steroid per day for the 90% loaded film.

Powder samples of the 60% and 90% loaded polymers showed essentially the same type of release behavior as the films of these polymers (Figure 4). However, the constant release rates of the powder samples were higher, and the duration times over the constant release periods were shorter than those of the film samples. The higher release rates of the powder samples are considered to be due to the larger surface areas of the powder samples as compared to the films. On the other hand, the 15% loaded polymer did not exhibit a constant release rate. A film sample of this material was not tested because of difficulty in fabricating the film. But a powder sample showed a rapidly increasing release rate for the first 17 days followed by a rapidly decreasing release rate.

TABLE II. HYDROLYSIS OF PGA – CORTISOL OXIME SUSTAINED RELEASE SYSTEM IN 95/5 (v/v) BUFFER/ETHANOL MIXTURE

No.	Loading (%)	Surface Area[a] (cm^2)	Weight (mg)	Buffer pH	Constant Release Period (days)	Constant Release rate	Duration[b] Period (days)
1 film	90	0.24x2	7.24	2.0	95	85 $\mu g/cm^2 \cdot day$	120
2 film	90	0.29x2	8.43	7.4	60	120 $\mu g/cm^2 \cdot day$	105
3 film	60	0.18x2	4.14	2.0	48	100 $\mu g/cm^2 \cdot day$	70
4 film	60	0.29x2	6.10	7.4	--	---	30
5 powder	90	--	5.03	2.0	45	5.5 $\mu g/day \cdot mg$ polymer	65
6 powder	90	--	4.90	7.4	75	4.7 $\mu g/day \cdot mg$ polymer	105
7 powder	60	--	6.08	2.0	30	7.0 $\mu g/day \cdot mg$ polymer	50
8 powder	60	--	4.88	7.4	--	---	30
9 powder	15	--	6.26	2.0	--	---	21
10 powder	15	--	6.31	7.4	--	---	immediately dissolved

a   x2 stands for both sides of the film used in the hydrolysis studies.

b   period between the start and the time point when polymer dissolves or the release rate rapidly decreases.

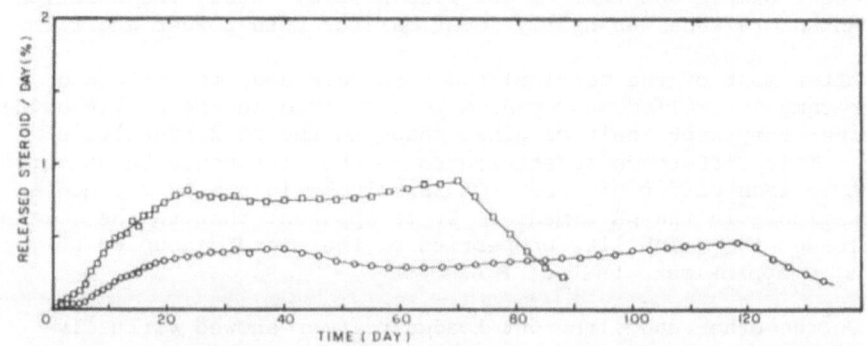

Figure 3.   Hydrolysis of PGA-cortisol oxime films in 95/5 (v/v)
             pH 2 buffer/ethanol mixture: o 90% loading;   □ 60%
             loading.

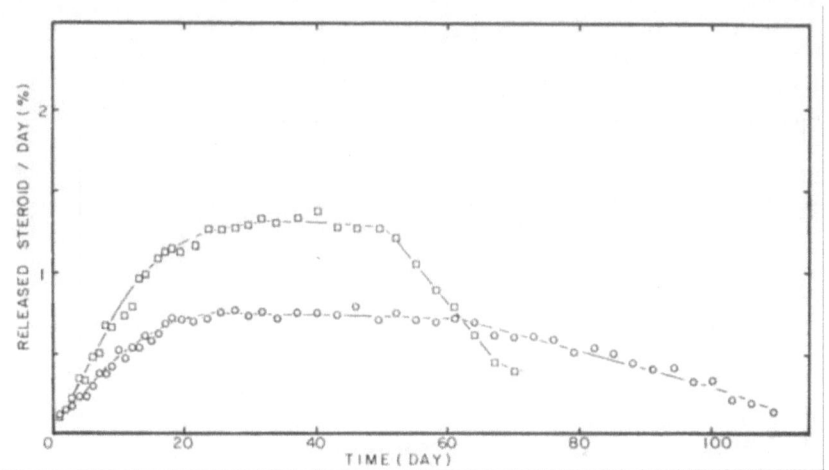

Figure 4.   Hydrolysis of PGA-cortisol oxime powder in 95/5 (v/v)
             pH 2 buffer/ethanol mixture: o 90% loading;   □ 60%
             loading.

    In the pH 7.4 buffer mixture, the 90% loaded film and powder
samples showed release curves somewhat similar to those in the pH
2 buffer mixture (Figures 5 and 6). However, unlike the pH 2 buffer
mixture, there was little difference between the release rate of
the powder sample and that of the film sample. Also, the duration
at constant release was nearly identical for both powder and film.

    After most of the cortisol had been released, the film and
powder samples swelled and eventually dissolved in the pH 7.4 buffer
mixtures; they kept their original shape in the pH 2 hydrolysis
media. This difference is attributed to the difference in solubility
of PGA in each buffer mixture; PGA is soluble in the pH 7.4 media
and insoluble in the pH 2 media. It is apparent that as the cortisol
is released the solubility properties of the steroid coupled polymer
begins to approximate that of PGA.

    On the other hand, the 60% loaded polymer showed virtually
no constant release in the pH 7.4 buffer mixture. Its release rate
rapidly increased and the polymer dissolved within 30 days. According to the TLC analysis, no polymer or decomposed compounds other
than cortisol-21-acetate and cortisol-21-acetate-3-oxime were found
in the sample solution until the polymer swelled.

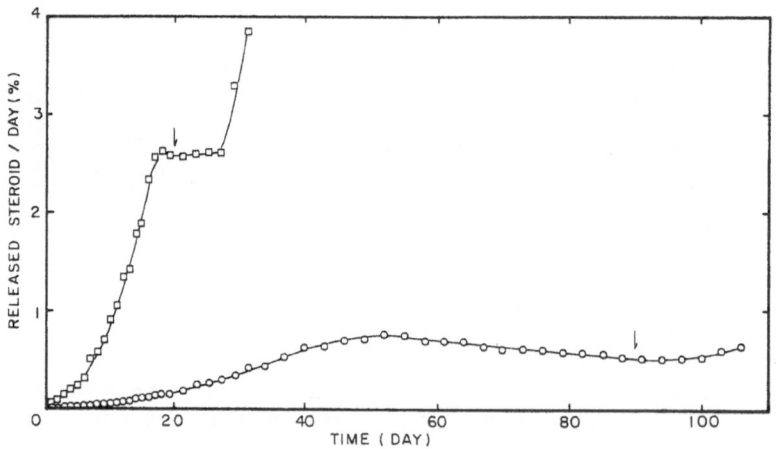

Figure 5.   Hydrolysis of PGA-cortisol oxime films in 95/5 (v/v)
            pH 7.4 buffer/ethanol mixture: o 90% loading;   □ 60%
            loading, the arrow indicates the swelling point.

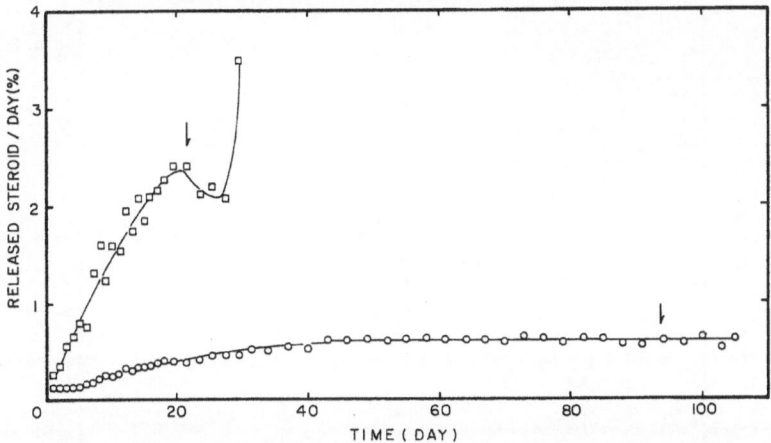

Figure 6.   Hydrolysis of PGA-cortisol oxime powder in 95/5 (v/v)
            pH 7.4 buffer/ethanol mixture: o 90% loading;   □ 60%
            loading; the arrow indicates the swelling point.

Hydrolysis in 50/50 (v/v) buffer/ethanol mixture. The release
behavior of the coupled polymers was totally different in this
solvent mixture.   Typical release curves are shown in Figure 7.
The release patterns of all the polymers showed initial bursts which
rapidly decreased with time. Unexpectedly, powder and films of
all samples showed similar release rates. This similarity suggests
that the surface area is not an important factor in determining
the release rate in this solvent mixture. In other words, the
hydrolysis reaction in this solvent mixture is not surface controlled as in ordinary solid-liquid reactions, but appears to be closer
to a homogeneous reaction. This phenomenon is also suggested by
the fact that the release kinetics are first-order (Figure 8).
No sample exhibited an autocatalytic effect.[8] As shown in Figure
8, however, coupled polymers with lower loading levels have larger
rate constants. This result was attributed to the difference of
steroid-carboxyl sequences in the polymers.[14] The absence of autocatalytic effects in the hydrolysis was further confirmed by the
following analysis. Figure 9 compares the percentage of loaded
residues remaining for three differently loaded polymers versus
time, where the initial point for each loading is time zero for
that loading. As shown in Figure 9, the polymer having an initial
loading of 90% releases cortisol and, at a certain time, has decreased its loading to 60%. At this point, if one compares the
release rate of this polymer to that of the polymer with a 60%
initial loading, the latter has a faster initial release rate.
This difference is considered to be due to the difference of steroid-

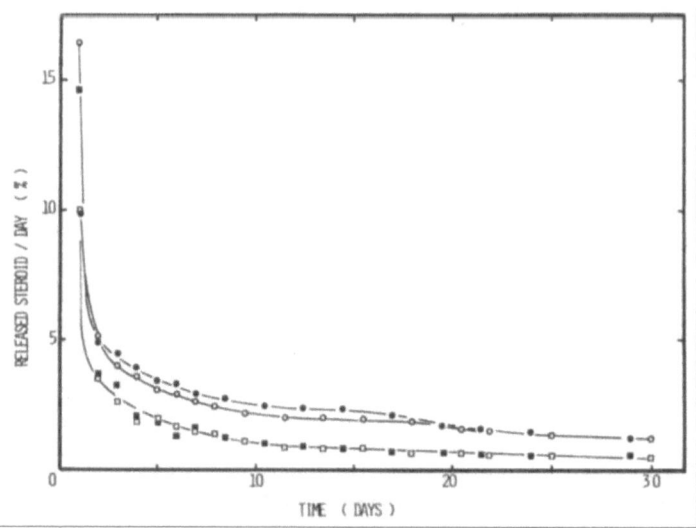

Figure 7. Hydrolysis of 30% loaded PGA-cortisol oxime in 50/50
           (v/v) buffer/ethanol mixture: o film, pH 2;   • powder,
           pH 2;   □ film, pH 7.4;   ■ powder, pH 7.4.

carboxyl sequences in the polymers. A similar result is obtained
by comparing the 60% and 15% loaded polymers.

Release Mechanism

     As described above, the release behavior changes with loading,
pH, and hydrolysis media. In attempting to understand these results,
we must consider a three-component release mechanism as shown in
Figure 10. The three components of the release mechanism are:
  I) Permeation of Buffer into the Polymer Matrix
 II) Hydrolysis of Bound Drug to Produce Free Drug
III) Diffusion of Free Drug out of the Polymer Matrix.
The overall release rate can be determined by any one of these steps
or any combination of these steps.

     To evaluate the diffusion step (step III), two films of 90%
loaded polymer were cast in which a very small amount (0.05 wt %)
of free tritium-labelled cortisol was dispersed. These films are
similar to monolithic devices, in which free drug is dispersed in
a polymer matrix. The films were hydrolyzed in 95/5 and 50/50 (v/v)
pH 2 buffer/ethanol mixtures. In this experiment, the hydrolysis
and the release of bound drug (nonradioactive) and the diffusion

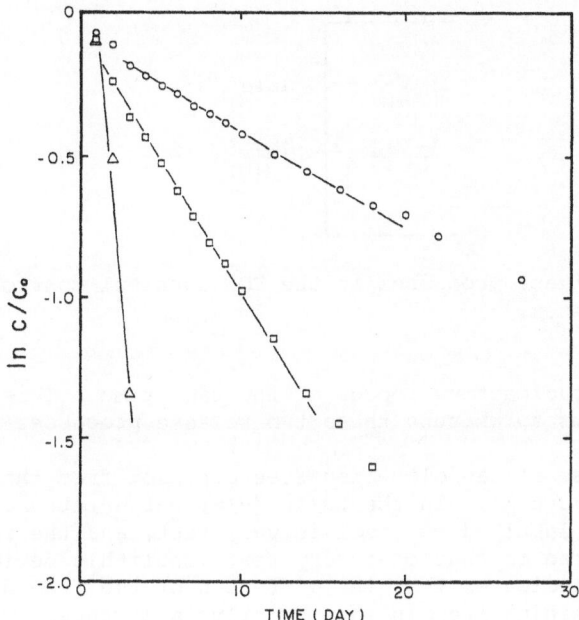

Figure 8. First-order plot for the hydrolysis of PGA-cortisol oxime powder in 50/50 (v/v) pH 7.4 buffer/ethanol mixture: o 90% loading; □ 60% loading; △ 15% loading.

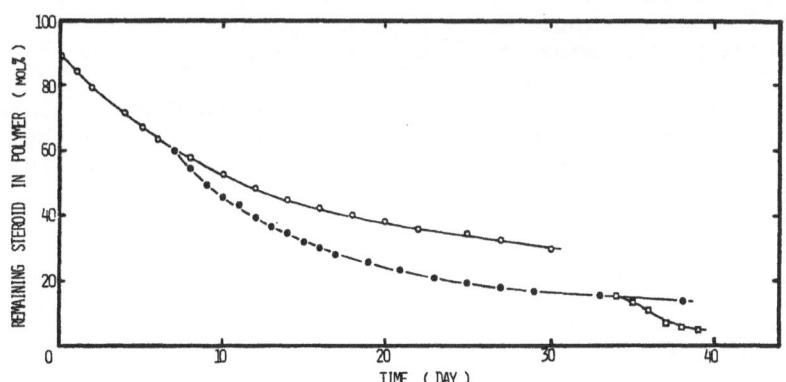

Figure 9. Hydrolysis of PGA-cortisol oxime powder in 50/50 (v/v) pH 2 buffer/ethanol mixture: o 90% loading; ● 60% loading; □ 15% loading.

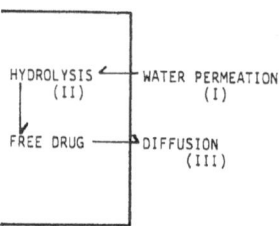

Figure 10.   Release processes in the PGA-cortisol controlled-release
             system.

of free drug (radioactive) occur at the same time. This tracer
study enabled us to measure these two release processes separately.

     The release of radiolabelled free cortisol from the polymer
is shown in Figure 11. In the 50/50 (v/v) buffer/ethanol mixture,
the release of labelled cortisol is very fast, and the release curve
might be compared to that of a very fast monolithic device.[15] This
rapid release indicates that the diffusion of the free drug is not
the rate-determining step in this hydrolysis mixture. Water permeation (step I) should be at least as fast as step III, because it
is also a diffusion process and the water molecule is much smaller
than the cortisol and thus diffuses faster. If diffusion (step
I and/or III) is the rate-determining step, the release rate should
be dependent on surface area; however, no surface area dependency
was found in this solvent mixture. Therefore, the hydrolysis reaction is considered to be the rate-determining step. Since the
release of bound cortisol can be approximated by first-order kinetics,
the hydrolysis is considered to be a first-order reaction.

     On the other hand, in 95/5 (v/v) buffer/ethanol mixture, the
release of radiolabelled cortisol was much slower than for the 50/50
mixture, and the release rate was almost constant. Thus diffusion
is important in determining the release behavior in the 95/5 (v/v)
buffer/ethanol mixture. However, this release behavior is far from
that of a monolithic device which is controlled by simple diffusion.
Instead, it is relatively close to Higuchi's model.[16] But the free
drug concentration is too small to apply Higuchi's model, and this
release behavior should be explained by a model which takes not
only diffusion but also the hydrolysis of bound drug into consideration.

Model Studies

     To explain the release behavior of the free radiolabelled
cortisol in the diffusion studies in the 95/5 (v/v) pH 2 buffer/

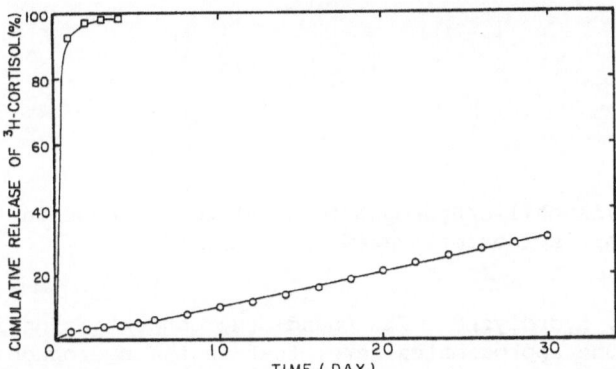

Figure 11.   Release of free radioactive cortisol from 90% loaded
             PGA-cortisol oxime films: o 95/5 (v/v) pH 2 buffer/
             ethanol mixture;   □ 50/50 (v/v) pH 2 buffer/ethanol
             mixture.

ethanol mixture, a hydrophilic/hydrophobic model is proposed and
is shown in Figure 12. Since the hydrolysis of bound cortisol is
suggested to start from the surface of the film, the film is considered to exist in two zones during hydrolysis. One zone, in which
hydrolysis of the bound drug has already begun, is hydrophilic.
The other zone, in which water has not yet penetrated and hydrolysis
has not yet occurred, is hydrophobic. The hydrophilic zone might
be considered to be similar to a hydrogel; thus it may be reasonable
to assume that the diffusion of the free radioactive cortisol in
the hydrophilic zone is much faster than in the hydrophobic zone.
Only free cortisol in the hydrophilic zone will diffuse out of the
film. If the diffusion is rapid, the cumulative release of free
radioactive cortisol is proportional to the volume of the hydrophilic zone (V_w). If V_w increases at a constant rate (dV_w/dt =
constant), the release rate for the free steroid will be constant,
which could explain the zero-order release of the free steroid in
95/5 (v/v) pH 2 buffer/ethanol mixture.

     If we now define R_w as the rate of water permeation into the
hydrophobic zone, i.e. $R_w = dV_w/dt$, the release of the bound cortisol
in the 95/5 (v/v) pH 2 buffer/ethanol mixture (Figure 3) can also
be explained. In order to do this, one must consider the hydrolysis
rate R_h in relation to R_w. There are three major hypothetical cases:
1) $R_h \gg R_w$; 2) $R_h \simeq R_w$; and 3) $R_h \ll R_w$.

     In the first case, where $R_h \gg R_w$, the hydrolysis reaction
(R_h, step II) is much faster than the water permeation (R_w, step
I), so the bound cortisol at the hydrophilic/hydrophobic interface

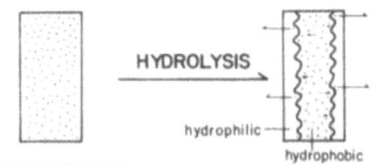

Figure 12. Hydrophilic/Hydrophobic Model for release in the PGA-
            cortisol oxime system.

is immediately hydrolyzed. The bound-drug concentration in the
hydrophilic zone approximates zero; that in the hydrophobic zone
remains at the initial concentration C_O (Figure 13). Therefore,
the release rate of the bound drug (R_r) is determined by R_w, rate
of water permeation, and expressed in equation (1), which gives
zero-order release until the hydrophobic zone finally disappears.

$$R_r = R_w C_O \qquad\qquad\qquad (1)$$

Similar equations have been derived by Hophenberg for erosion
devices.[17] Obviously, the release rate curve defined by this equation does not fit that of Figure 3. In particular, this model cannot explain the induction period and the tailing.

    In the second case, where R_h approximates R_w, the overall
release rate is controlled by the combination of these two rates.
In this case, the bound cortisol is not immediately hydrolyzed at
the hydrophilic/hydrophobic interface, but bound cortisol remains
in the hydrophilic zone and continues to hydrolyze. Therefore,
the drug concentration in the hydrophilic zone is not zero, and
that in the hydrophobic zone remains at C_O (Figure 13). Since the
combination of R_w and R_h determines the release rate, the shape
of the release curve and the drug concentration diagram is dependent
on the kinetics which define R_h (R_w is assumed to be constant).
We consider two sub-cases.

    If R_h is constant and independent of drug concentration, the
drug concentration diagram looks like Figure 13-2a at a given
time, t. The hydrophilic/hydrophobic interface proceeds to the
depth of $R_w t/S$, where S is the surface area. The bound drug concentration at the interface, where hydrolysis has just begun, is
C_O. At the surface, where hydrolysis has occurred for a time, t,
the bound drug concentration is $C_O - R_h t$. The drug concentration
at any point between the surface and the interface is proportional
to the distance from the surface. Therefore, the cumulative
release, M, is expressed as equation (2).

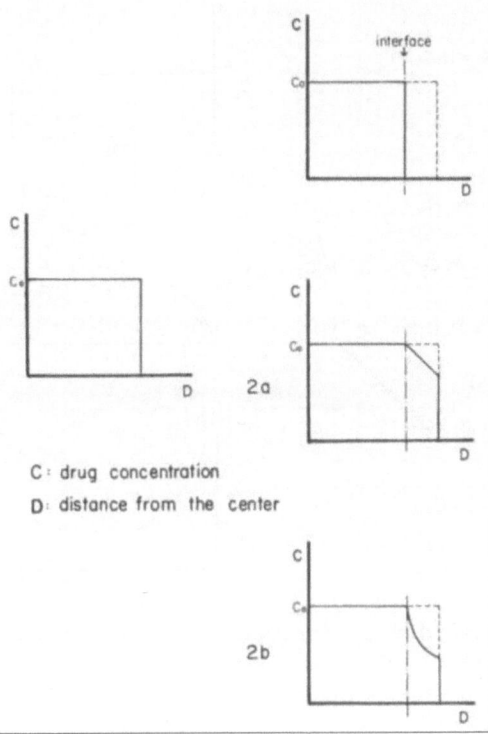

Figure 13. Drug concentration diagrams for the hydrolysis of PGA-cortisol oxime.

$$M = 1/2 \ R_w t \cdot R_h t = 1/2 \ R_h R_w t^2 \qquad (2)$$

where:

$$M = \int_0^t R_r dt \qquad (3)$$

$$dM/dt = R_r = R_h R_w t \qquad (4)$$

R_r constantly increases with time until the drug concentration at the surface becomes zero (dotted line in Figure 14-2). After that point, R_r becomes constant which is the same as the case in which $R_h \gg R_w$ (Equation (1)). This constant release continues until the hydrophobic zone disappears. After that point, R_r decreases with time.

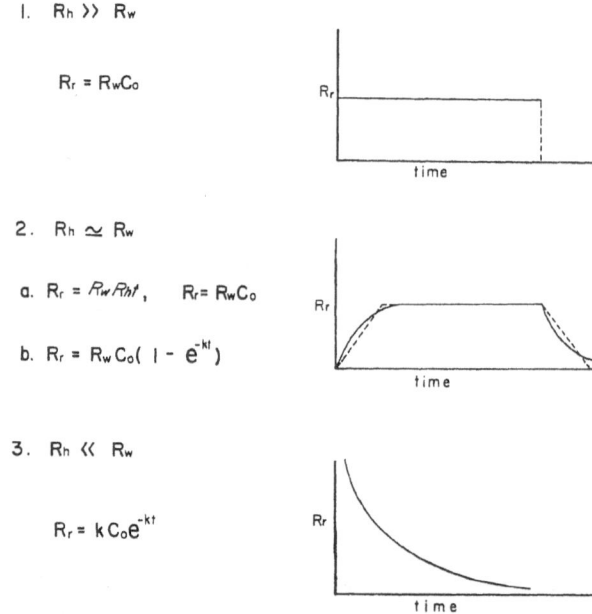

Figure 14.   Release curves derived from the hydrophilic/hydrophobic
             models.

This model can explain the induction period and the tailing
which are observed in Figure 3.   However, the shape of the release
curve is still far from that of Figure 3.

The second sub-case is where R_h = kC.   It has been suggested
that the hydrolysis reaction follows first-order kinetics in 50/50
buffer/ethanol mixtures.   Therefore, it is reasonable to assume
a first-order hydrolysis reaction in the 95/5 buffer/ethanol mixtures.

In this case, the drug concentration diagram is expressed in
Figure 13-2b.   The drug concentration, C, at the interface is C_O,
and it is $C_o e^{-kt}$ at the surface.   The drug concentration at any
point a distance, ℓ, from the surface is expressed in equation (5).

$$C_\ell = C_o e^{-k(t-\ell/R_w)} \tag{5}$$

therefore:

$$M = \int_o^{R_w t} (C_o - C_\ell) \, d\ell = \int_o^{R_w t} C_o \, [1 - e^{-k(t-\ell)/R_w}] d\ell$$

and

$$M = C_o R_w (t + 1/k \ e^{-kt})$$ (6)

R_r is expressed in equation (7).

$$dM/dt = R_r = C_o R_w (1-e^{-kt})$$ (7)

The release rate is expressed as given in equation (7) until the hydrophobic zone disappears. After that point, R_r exponentially decreases. The theoretical release curve is shown as the solid line in Figure 14-2, but a true constant release does not exist; however, it should be noted that if the time is large enough, R_r may be expressed as equation (1), which is the same as the first case. Obviously, the release curve derived from this model is not far from that seen in Figure 3. In fact, this model can explain all aspects of the observed release behavior of highly loaded films in the 95/5 pH 2 buffer/ethanol mixture, including the induction period, constant release, and tailing phenomena.

The water permeation rate in 50/50 buffer/ethanol mixtures is fast, $R_w \gg R_h$, and therefore, R determines the release rate. Since R_h follows first-order kinetics, R_r is expressed as equation (8).

$$R_r = kC_o e^{-kt}$$ (8)

This difference in release behavior between hydrolysis in 50/50 mixtures and hydrolysis in 95/5 mixtures is considered to be due to the difference in the affinity of the solvent mixture for the polymer. That is, the 50/50 mixture is more compatible with the polymer because of the increased EtOH concentration.

In conclusion, 1) highly loaded polymer showed a constant release for considerably long periods, 2) total release kinetics can be explained on the basis that hydrolysis of the bound cortisol occurs only in the hydrophilic portion with the release rate being determined by a combination of hydrolysis (R_h) and water permeation (R_w).

REFERENCES

1. K.R. Sidman, W.D. Steber, and A.W. Burg, in: "Proceedings Drug Delivery Systems," H.L. Gabelnick, ed., Bethesda (1976).
2. C. Pitt, D. Christensen, R. Jeffcoat, G.L. Kimmel, A. Schindler, M.E. Wall, and R.A. Zweidinger, ibid., pp. 141-192.

3. S. Mitra, M. Van Dress, J.M. Anderson, unpublished results.

4. A.N. Neogi and G.G. Allan, in: "Controlled Release of Biologi-
    cally Active Agents," A.C. Tranquary and R.E. Lacey, eds.,
    Plenum Press, New York (1974). pp. 195-224.

5. G.G. Allan, C.S. Chopra, A.N. Neogi, and R.M. Wilkins, Nature
    234:349 (1971).

6. H. Morawetz, Israel J. Chem. 17:287 (1978).

7. G. Smets, Angew. Chem. 74:337 (1962).

8. F.W. Harris, J.W. Thompson, and S. Amdur, in: "Proceedings of
    6th International Symposium on Controlled Release of Bioactive
    Materials," R.W. Baker, ed, New Orleans (1979). pp. III22.

9. I.H. Shaw, C.G. Knight, and J.T. Dingle, Biochem. J. 158:473
    (1976).

10. J.M. Anderson, D.F. Gibbons, R.L. Martin, A. Hiltner, and R.
    Woods, J. Biomed. Mater. Res. Symposium 5:197 (1974).

11. A.H. Janoski, F.C. Shulman, and G.E. Wright, Steroids 23:49
    (1974).

12. M. Idelson and E.R. Blout, J. Amer. Chem. Soc. 80:4631 (1958).

13. G.I. Poos and L.H. Sarret, U.S. Patent, 3,074,979 (1963).

14. G. Smets and W. Van Humbeck, J. Polymer Sci., A, 1:1227 (1963).

15. R.W. Baker and H.K. Lonsdale, in: "Controlled Release of Bio-
    logically Active Agents," A.C. Tranquary and R.E. Lacey, eds.,
    Plenum Press, New York (1974). pp. 195-224.

16. T. Higuchi, J. Pharm. Sci., 50:874 (1961).

17. H.B. Hopfenberg, in: "Controlled Release Polymeric Formula-
    tions," D.R. Paul and F.W. Harris, eds., ACS Symposium Series
    33:26 (1976).

POTENTIAL DELIVERY OF CONTRACEPTIVE AGENTS TO THE
FEMALE REPRODUCTIVE TRACT

David L. Gardner, David J. Fink, and Craig R. Hassler

Battelle Columbus Laboratories
505 King Avenue
Columbus, Ohio 43201

INTRODUCTION

Vaginal contraceptives have played a positive role in fertility planning for years. Prior to the introduction of intrauterine devices (IUDs) and oral contraceptives (OCs), jellies, creams, and suppositories were used, sometimes in conjunction with the diaphragm or condom, but usually they served as the sole barrier.[1] The higher failure rates of the vaginal contraceptives in relation to other contraceptive devices (IUDs and OCs) were believed to be due primarily to the inconsistent use of the method rather than to failure of the method during use.

Disadvantages cited with IUDs include: (a) increased menstrual bleeding and spotting; (b) expulsion soon after insertion; (c) unwanted pregnancies that are more likely to be ectopic; and (d) increased frequency of pelvic infection.[2] Problems noted with OCs have included: (a) the requirement for daily administration; (b) the subsequent daily variation in blood steroid concentrations; and (c) association with circulatory system diseases.[3]

OCs possess two distinct advantages over other fertility control methods. They are the most effective method of preventing pregnancy currently available, and they facilitate more satisfactory sexual relations.[3] However, vaginal contraceptives have been of continuing interest because of some of the disadvantages associated with OCs and IUDs and because recent clinical data have shown that the newer preparations (e.g., foams in aerosol and pressurized containers) can provide substantial protection if used correctly and regularly.[1]

Increased effort is being placed on improving the present status of vaginal antifertility agents with regard to their contraceptive efficacy, mode of administration, and general aesthetic acceptability. An approach which we believe has some promise in this regard is a self-administered microcapsule drug-delivery system for the female reproductive tract.

The primary factors affecting the rate of sperm transport through the reproductive tract include (a) muscular activity, (b) composition and physical characteristics of the fluids, (c) female orgasm, and (d) directional swimming activity of the spermatozoa.[4] The last factor may be of importance in assisting gamete movement past the cervical canal and in fertilization of the egg. However, passive sperm transport is indicated by (a) the rapid transport of sperm to upper segments of the reproductive tract in various animals, including humans, (b) by the passage of seminal plasma constituents, dead sperm, and inert material following vaginal insertion in animals, and (c) the inability of sperm to cover that distance in so short a time period, if left to their normal swimming progression rates.[5]

The concept of a particulate drug-delivery system is further supported by studies in humans, which demonstrate the movement of inert particles through the reproductive tract. Following placement in either the vagina, cervix, or uterus, particles such as carmine or carbon black have been observed to migrate into the fallopian tubes or peritoneal cavity.[6,9]

The advantages of a microcapsular dosage form as a drug-delivery system might include the following: (1) flexibility in controlling the rate of drug delivery from the microcapsules by alteration of microcapsule size, membrane polymer, and wall thickness; (2) the potential for encapsulating antifertility drugs or therapeutic agents separately, but administering them simultaneously, and (3) the possibility of modifying the membrane surface properties or microcapsule size to permit pretargeting of the microcapsules to specific areas of the reproductive tract.

METHODS AND MATERIALS

To determine the feasibility of using a microcapsule drug-delivery system for the female reproductive tract, studies were undertaken to determine the fate of microcapsules following insertion in the vagina of stumptail monkeys (21 experiments) or baboons (10 experiments) at different phases of the menstrual cycle. To follow migration of the dosage form in the primate reproductive tract, tracer microcapsules (containing either soluble ^{125}I-human serum albumin or ^{85}Sr-microspheres) were monitored using a well-collimated detector system (Figures 1, 2, and 3). The collimator

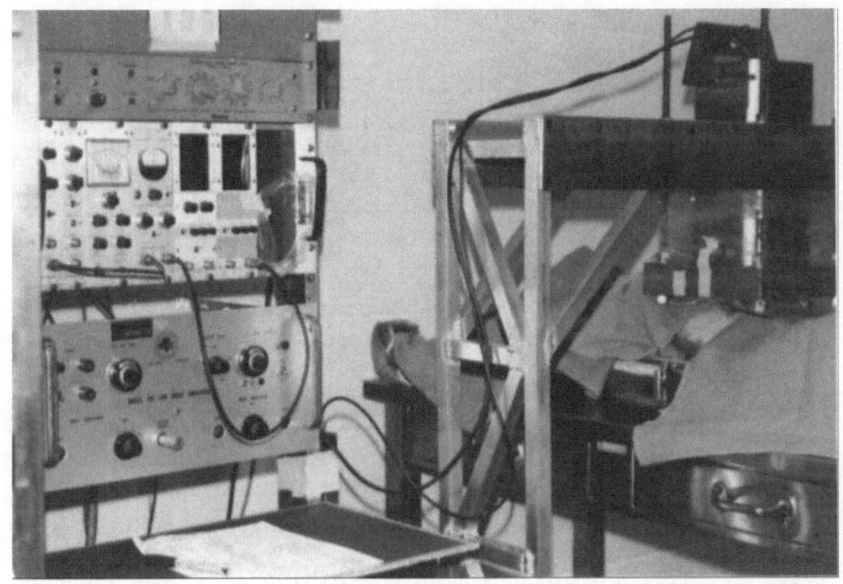

Figure 1.   Physical set-up for monitoring distribution of micro-
            capsules.

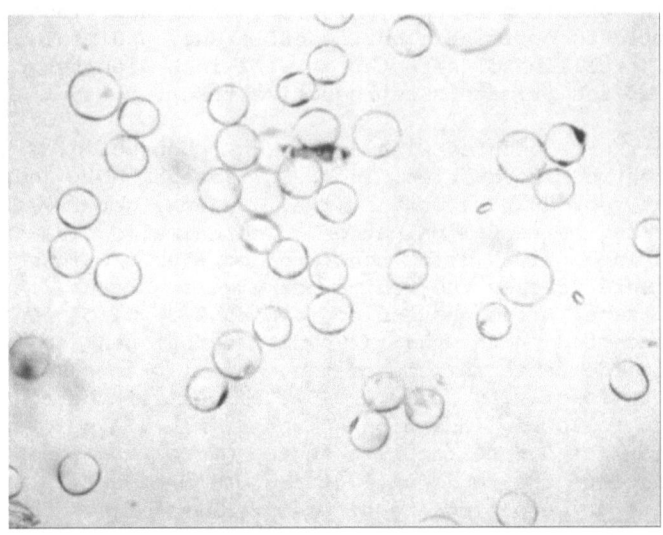

Figure 2.   Tracer microcapsules containing ^{125}I-human albumin.
            Capsules are 50±10 μm diameter. Magnification = 81X.

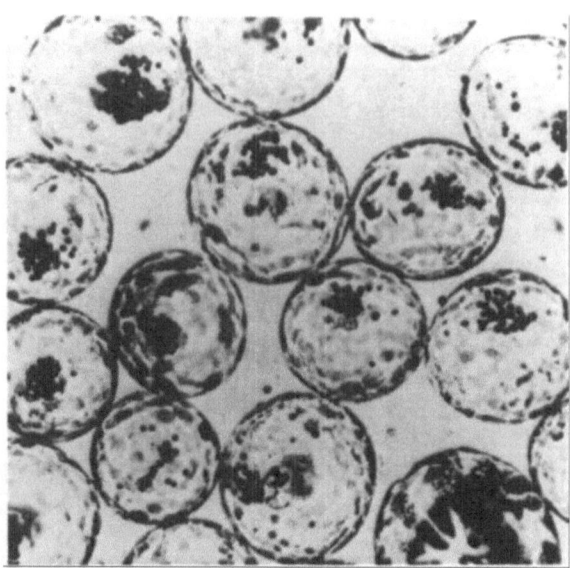

Figure 3.   Tracer microcapsules containing [85]Sr-microspheres
(15±5 μm). Magnification = 51X.

consisted of a 1/2-inch diameter aperture through five inches of
lead. A 2-inch NaI crystal and photomultiplier tube were connected
to a Hamner detection system. Discrimination and window settings
were selected to optimize counting efficiency and minimize background. The collimator detected a 1-1/2-inch diameter circle at
the plane of the primate's reproductive tract.

Animals were sedated with Sernylan® (phencyclidine hydrochloride, Bioceutic Laboratories, Inc., St. Joseph, MO), and the location of the reproductive organs (i.e., vagina, cervix, and uterus)
was determined by rectal palpation. The animal's abdomen was then
demarcated into grids (grids consisted of five 1/2-inch diameter
circles) centered over the vagina, cervix, or uterus. Approximately
1 gram of tracer microcapsules containing 2-3 μCi of radioactivity
was then inserted in the vaginal canal so that peak counts were
obtained in the center circle of the vaginal grid. Even with this
amount of radioactivity, only 0.2-0.4 percent of the counts could
be detected following insertion at zero-time. This low percentage
of detection was due to the high degree of collimation necessary
to differentiate the reproductive-tract segments. All grids were
then counted at zero-time and at predetermined times thereafter.
Total counting time for each grid was five minutes. The tracer
microcapsules were placed in the primate's vagina by either placing
the tracer microcapsules in a frozen or unfrozen plug (approximately

one inch). The plug (capsules were packed in hollow glass tubing
(1/4-inch O.D. x 7 inches)) was delivered by a solid-glass plunger.

A secondary study involved extirpating the reproductive tract
in a single baboon to obtain a more accurate assessment of tracer
microcapsule distribution following insertion in the vagina.

A mixture (0.3 g each) of two tracer capsule types (^{125}I and
^{85}Sr) was used to determine if a particular capsule diameter would
migrate preferentially. The ^{125}I capsules were 20-37 µm in diameter
and the ^{85}Sr capsules were 297-420 µm in diameter. An unfrozen
plug (containing both capsule types homogeneously dispersed) was
placed in the baboon's vagina near the external os of the cervix.
The animal was in the early pre-ovulatory phase of its menstural
cycle (12 days postmenses) and was kept sedated in a horizontal
plane during the course of the experiment.

The animal was sacrificed at the end of six hours, and the
reproductive tract was removed in toto. Each area of the reproductive tract (i.e., vagina, cervix, uterus, and fallopian tubes) was
sectioned transversely into approximately 1/4-inch serial strips
and counted simultaneously on a dual-channel counter for ^{125}I and
^{85}Sr by standard gamma counting techniques.

RESULTS

Stumptail Monkey Studies

The results obtained in stumptail monkeys are presented in
Figures 4 and 5. Figure 4 illustrates studies with pre-ovulatory
phase animals (Days 1-9, with the initiation of menses constituting
the first day), while Figure 5 summarizes the results obtained from
animals during the mid-cycle phase.

Capsule retention in the vaginal grid area of pre-ovulatory
animals (Figure 4) averaged approximately 70 percent for capsule
diameters larger than 200 µm in five experiments. However, for
capsules between 63-200 µm in diameter, an average retention of
25 percent was obtained in the vaginal grid area in six experiments.

Transcervical migration from the vagina to the uterus (24 hours
post-insertion) was observed to some degree in six out of eleven
animals. In these studies it appeared that capsule diameters less
than 300 µm in diameter showed preferential migration. However,
one animal out of three at the largest capsule diameter did show
migration of greater than three percent of the inserted microcapsules.

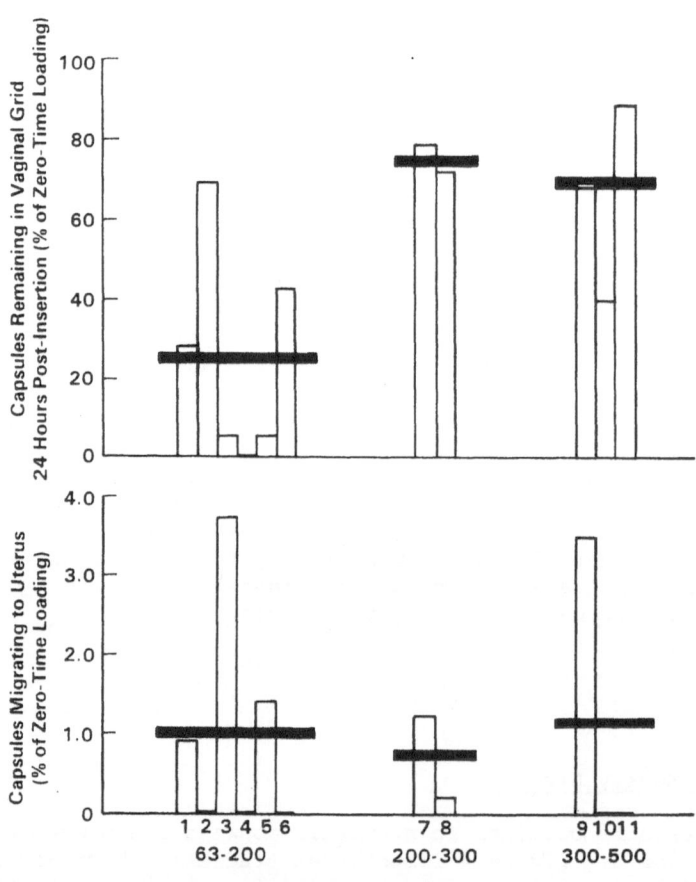

Figure 4. Distribution of microcapsules in stumptail monkeys
           (preovulatory phase).

In the studies with mid-cycle animals (Figure 5), both the
percentage of capsules remaining in the vaginal grid (24 hours post-
insertion) and the amount migrating into the uterus decreased with
increasing capsule diameter.

In the limited number of studies conducted, the average percent
of capsules remaining in the vaginal grid after 24 hours was much
lower for the mid-cycle studies (22.1 percent) than for the pre-
ovulatory studies (44.7 percent). The difference between the two
menstrual phases was also reflected in a similar difference in
transcervical migration. In the pre-ovulatory phase studies, the

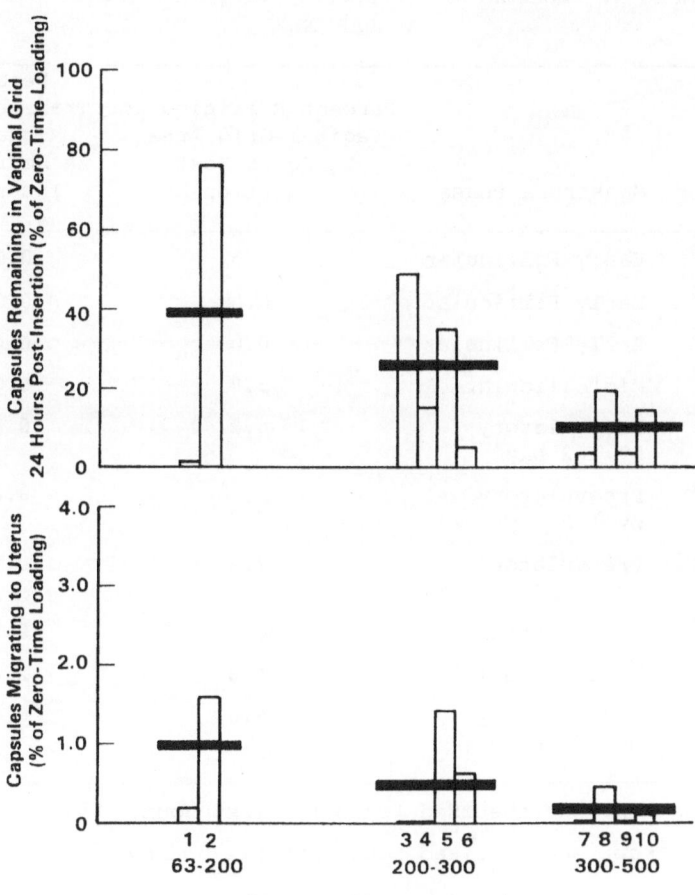

Figure 5.   Distribution of microcapsules in stemptail monkeys
            (mid-cycle phase).

overall transcervical migration percentage was 0.98; for the mid-
cycle phase studies, 0.42 percent was observed in the uterus after
24 hours.

Baboon Studies

     Microcapsule distribution in the baboon reproductive tract
is presented in Table I. In these studies, the percentage of capsules detected in the vaginal grid after 24 hours was much lower

TABLE I.   SUMMARY OF TRANSCERVICAL MIGRATION STUDIES
IN BABOONS

Capsule Diam., μm	Menstrual Phase	Percent Remaining in Vaginal Grid Area 24 Hours Post Insertion	Percent Transcervical Migration 24 Hours Post Insertion
63–105[a]	Early Follicular	1.5	0.0
63–105[a]	Early Follicular	0.0	0.0
63–105[a]	Early Follicular	0.0	0.0
63–105[b]	Midfollicular	3.8	0.0
105–210[b]	Preovulatory by 1–2 Days	4.2	0.0
105–210[b]	Preovulatory by 1–2 Days	3.1	0.0
105–210[b]	Preovulatory by 1–2 Days	2.9	0.57
105–210[b]	Early Luteal	30.8	0.75
105–210[b]	Early Luteal	4.8	2.42
297–420[b]	Preovulatory by 304 Days	6.0	0.0

[a] Baboons kept anesthetized for only first hour.

[b] Baboons kept anesthetized for first six hours.

than in comparable stumptail monkey experiments. However, when the animals were kept anesthetized and in a horizontal plane for six hours, the percentage remaining in the vaginal grid generally increased.

Only three out of ten animals exhibited any transcervical migration, with two of the three migration occurrences during the early luteal phase of the menstrual cycle.

The single experiment in which the baboon was sacrificed six hours after insertion of two different tracer microcapsules is summarized in Table II. These results indicate that (a) there is essentially no difference in transcervical migration between the two sizes, (b) migration occurs relatively rapidly (within six hours) into the cervix, uterus, and fallopian tubes, (c) almost 60 percent

TABLE II.   PLACEMENT OF TWO DIFFERENT MICROCAPSULE SIZES
IN A SINGLE BABOON

	Net CPM	
	^{125}I	^{85}Sr
Vagina	3,235,161	3,472,193
Cervix	22,648	27,078
Uterus	3,460	3,411
Fallopian Tubes	1,713	1,796

Total ^{125}I Net CPM Placed in Vagina = 5,929,837
Total ^{85}Sr Net CPM Placed in Vagina = 5,793,150

	Percentage of Migration After 6 Hours	
	^{125}I	^{85}Sr
Cervix	0.38	0.47
Uterus	0.05	0.06
Fallopian Tubes	0.03	0.03
Total	0.46	0.56

of the microcapsules were still present in the vagina at sacrifice.
Capsules not accounted for in Table II may have been lost in the
exudate observed around the vaginal exterior during removal of the
reproductive tract.

This experiment also points out a problem with the use of the
highly collimated, external-detector system used in the studies
described above. When the baboon was sacrificed six hours after
insertion of the capsules, 0.4 percent of the inserted capsules
were detected in the extirpated cervix. However, external measurements taken six hours post-insertion but prior to sacrifice detected
no capsules in the cervical grid. This observation demonstrates
the generally low sensitivity of the external counting system, which
was employed to gain adequate resolution between the three reproductive segments monitored.

DISCUSSION

These preliminary results in the primate confirm that microcapsules placed in the vagina do migrate across the cervix. Although the percentage of vaginal retention and transcervical migration was low and variable in these studies, the data suggest the
possibility of developing a controlled-release contraceptive system
for the female reproductive tract. Such a system could be based
upon microcapsules for delivery of fertility-control or therapeutic

agents, especially if the required effective local dose is low
(e.g., micrograms per day delivered locally to the uterus or cervix).

It is clear that contraceptive or therapeutic systems based
upon the transcervical migration of drug-containing particles will
require the controlled manipulation of several complex processes.
The primary factors controlling the local rate of drug delivery
at each reproductive site (i.e., vagina, cervix, uterus, or fallopian tubes) can be related as shown in equation (1).

$$LDR = M \times F \times R \tag{1}$$

where LDR is the desired local delivery rate (μg drug/day), M is
the mass of drug-containing particles initially administered (g),
F is the fraction of the administered capsules that migrate to the
selected site, and R is the actual in vivo release rate of drug
from the carrier particles (μg drug/g capsules/day).

Each of the independent factors (M, F, and R) is subject to
unique sets of constraints and relationships which affect the actual
local delivery rate. For example, M will probably be subject to
an upper limit, based on constraints imposed by the vaginal vault
and hygienic factors such as minimal leakage following insertion.
In the studies described above, M was approximately one gram of
wet or frozen capsules/treatment.

The fraction, F, of particles migrating to the target organ,
which was studied in this program, appears to be controlled by many
factors. These probably include the phase of the menstrual cycle
in which the particles are administered, the fluid properties of
the reproductive-tract contents, and the physical characteristics
of the particles. It seems possible, also, that F could depend
on the amount of carrier particles administered, M, and the method
used for particle insertion.

The in vivo release rate of the contraceptive agent, R, is
dependent upon the physical properties of the particles, including
diameter, wall thickness, concentration of drug in the particles,
solubility of the drug in the wall polymer, and the capsule interior
fluid. Transcervical migration contraception efficacy is further
complicated by the contribution of secondary drug release by particles that do not migrate to the target organ. Thus, determination
of the therapeutic dosage must include the contribution of carrier
particles at all sites of the reproductive tract.

Many aspects of a particulate delivery system still need to
be addressed, including (1) determination of the final destiny of
the carrier particles following insertion, (2) the local concentration of drug required at each site for effectiveness, (2) the effect

of menstruation, and (4) the duration of contraceptive effectiveness (e.g., Is a single administration adequate for only a few days
surrounding ovulation or for a full menstrual cycle, or could it
suffice as a post-coital contraceptive?). Nonetheless, in spite
of the obvious complexity associated with the proposed microcapsule
drug-delivery system, we believe that development of the proposed
drug-delivery system could lead to a convenient, safe, and reliable
contraceptive system.

ACKNOWLEDGEMENT

     The investigations described in this report were supported
by Contract No. N01-HD-1-2230 from the National Institute of Child
Health and Human Development.

REFERENCES

1.   G.S. Berstein, Contraception 9:333 (1974).
2.   P.T. Piotrow, W. Rinehart, and J.C. Schmidt, Population Reports,
     Series B, No. 3, May (1979).
3.   W. Rinehart and P.T. Piotrow, Population Reports, Series A,
     No. 5, January (1979).
4.   R.J. Blandau, in: "The Mammalian Oviduct," E.S.E. Hafez and
     R.J. Blandau, eds., The University of Chicago Press, (1969).
     p. 129.
5.   D.W. Bishop, in: "Pathways to Conception," A.I. Sherman and
     Charles C. Thomas, eds., (1971). p. 99.
6.   R. Amersbach, Munchen. Med. Wchnschr 77:225 (1930).
7.   J. Trapl, Zentralbl. Gynak 67:547 (1943).
8.   G.E. Egli and M. Newton, Fert. and Steril., 12(2):151 (1961).
9.   C.H. Deboer, J. Reprod. Fert. 28:295 (1972).

RELEASE OF DRUGS FROM IUDS USING AN ETHYLENE VINYL

ACETATE MATRIX

R.G. Wheeler and P.G. Friel

International Fertility Research Program
Research Triangle Park, North Carolina

INTRODUCTION

The work of the International Fertility Research Program (IFRP) in the clinical evaluation and development of contraceptive methods is aimed primarily at meeting the needs of the developing world. In many places where the contraceptive need is greatest, the IUD is the only reliable method acceptable to many of the women desiring protection. A reduction of the explosive population growth in these countries could result from an improvement in the acceptance of IUDs or from the introduction of effective alternatives to the IUD. Contraceptives whose design is based on the sustained release of drugs may provide the needed improvement. Specifically, the purpose of this paper is to encourage more research and use of the sustained release of drugs from inert polymers in which the connectivity of the drug particles within the matrix is the principal avenue for drug release.

The development of an IUD with sustained release of an anti-fibrinolytic drug is described in detail in this report. The most common reason for removal of IUDs is a dysfunctional increase in menstrual blood loss and accompanying pain. It is thought that the sustained release of antifibrinolytic drugs from the IUD may reduce these side effects, particularly during the first several months of use when excess bleeding is normally the greatest. Other types of contraceptive systems that could benefit from the sustained release of drugs are also suggested in this report.

BACKGROUND

Systems Based on Particle Connectivity

Two of the antibleeding drugs we investigated are trans-4-aminomethyl cyclohexanecarboxylic acid (AMCA) and the polypeptide aprotinin, molecular weight = 6,512. A system based on diffusion of AMCA through a polyurethane membrane (Estane 5716)[1] and one based on the diffusion of aprotinin from a hydrogel matrix[2] were developed via subcontracts with the Southern Research Institute and Bend Research Laboratories, respectively. A system based on the connectivity of particles in an inert matrix, as described here, was developed at the IFRP because only relatively simple laboratory facilities were required. And, of further interest to the IFRP, the simplicity of manufacture would make the technology easy to transfer to developing countries. We first became aware of the possibilities of this mode of release by means of a report by Folkman and Langer.[3]

A review of the literature on sustained-release systems reveals a lack of research in the area of connectivity and a failure to recognize the potential importance of this mode of release. Connectivity of particles in a matrix becomes significant in the release process any time the loading of the matrix exceeds a few volume percent. Two-phase or multiple-phase systems are usually viewed microscopically on a plane section through the material. Under such viewing, it is possible to observe only one phase as being continuous when, in fact, any number of the other phases could be continuous. For example, a plane vertical section through a tree would show a continuous phase of air with widely dispersed spots of the wood phase whose connectivity would not be apparent from the section alone.

Systems based on connectivity of particles offer a great deal of design latitude in matrix material, drug, and release rate because they do not depend upon diffusion of the drug through a matrix or a membrane. How a system based on connectivity of particles can provide complete release of the drug and a variety of release rates is neatly illustrated by a model in which the particles in the matrix are assumed to be soft spheres.[4] In Figure 1, the curve marked 0 represents the percent of spheres contacting no other sphere. Curve 1 represents the percent of spheres contacting one other sphere, and so on. As the volume fraction of spheres (drug) approaches 40%, the number of spheres with zero contact approaches zero, and the highest frequency of contact with neighboring spheres is four (i.e., each sphere is in contact with four neighbors).

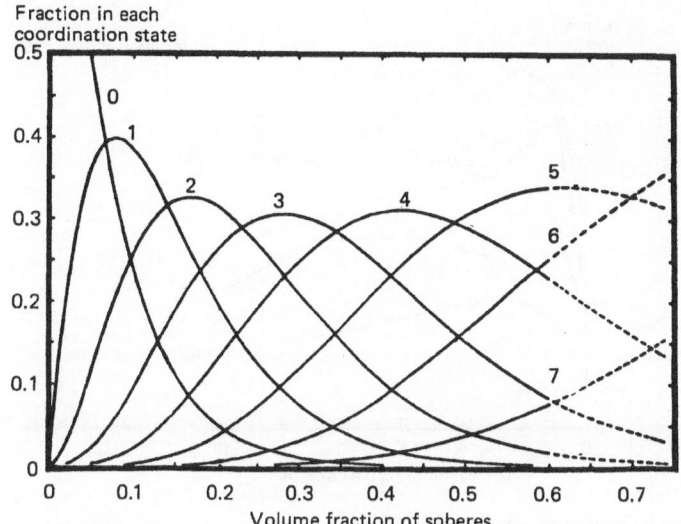

Figure 1.   Taken from G.A. More,[4] with permission of publisher.
            Figure illustrates how nearly all particles in a matrix
            are in contact with at least one other particle as the
            volume fraction of particles approaches 30% or more.

Treatment of Dysfunctional Blood Loss

     Numerous studies of menstrual blood loss and the influence
of IUDs have been reported.[5-11] An example of the effect of Lippes
Loop IUDs on menstrual blood loss, illustrated in Figure 2, is taken
from data provided to the IFRP by a research center in Cairo,
Egypt.[12] Values of menstrual blood loss plotted at time zero represent the average of two menstrual cycles before the IUDs were
inserted. Menstrual blood loss data are typically highly skewed,
as indicated by the difference between the mean and the median (2nd
quartile) values. Blood loss values depicted here are lower than
some reported in the above-cited references, but the gradual decrease in excess blood loss over time after IUD insertion is fairly
typical. Thus, if the sustained release of an antifibrinolytic
agent could counteract the excess blood loss for the first six to
eight months of IUD use, it could have a beneficial effect on
removals for bleeding. Additional benefits could result if the
duration of menstrual blood flow were also reduced.

     Successful treatment of menorrhagia with AMCA and a similar
antibleeding drug, epsilon-aminocaproic acid, has been reported.[13-15]
However, this oral treatment requires several grams of drug daily.
Sustained release of microgram quantities daily of epsilon-amino-

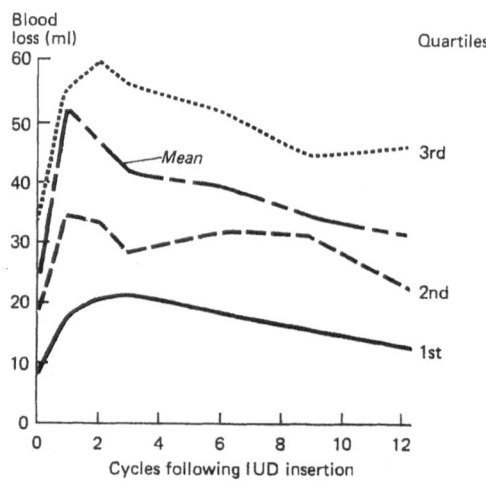

Figure 2.   The menstrual blood loss for 61 women using a Loop IUD
            for at least one year is plotted against the number of
            cycles after IUD insertion. Curves represent the first,
            second and third quartiles and the mean. The large dif-
            ference between the second quartile and the mean indicates
            a high degree of skewness in the distribution.

caproic acid from Silastic IUDs reduced menstrual blood loss of
rhesus monkeys.[16]   Tauber et al.[17] found that intrauterine instilla-
tions of either AMCA or aprotinin reduced the amount and duration
of menstrual bleeding.

DEVELOPMENT AND RESULTS

Medicated Loop Fabrication

     Although studies were conducted to determine the amount of
proteolytic enzymes to be inhibited in the endometrial secretions
and menstrual blood serum,[18] the actual design criteria for the
medicated IUD were set by the physical limitations of the system.
These criteria were, essentially, to deliver as much drug as possible for as long as possible from a stable carrier. A modified
Lippes Loop was selected as the vector for the drug because it is
(a) easily adaptable to medicament loading and (b) it is a public
sector device acceptable throughout the world with well documented
bleeding side effects. By reducing the cross-sectional dimensions
of the transverse arms of the loop, it was possible to provide a

drug reservoir with a capacity of 165 mm^3 in the annular space
without significantly changing the physical characteristics of the
device (Figure 3).

Ethylene vinyl acetate (EVA) was selected as the matrix
material because, in addition to meeting the requirements for a drug
delivery system as described above, it offered low fabrication
temperature and heavy drug-loading capacity. EVA has been shown
to be biocompatible and capable of releasing macromolecules.[3] For
our development work, Dupont 3165 EVA copolymer resin was used.

The blending of the drug, 40% by weight, into an EVA matrix
was accomplished using a hot platen laboratory press. For example,
one third of a four-gram batch of AMCA was hot pressed inside an
envelope made from six grams of EVA that had been pressed into a
sheet. The envelope was pressed between two polished stainless-
steel sheets lubricated with a thin coating of magnesium stearate.
After two such folding and pressing operations, the second portion
of AMCA was similarly blended into the EVA. After the final portion
of AMCA was added, the pressing and folding was repeated ten more
times to produce two homogenous drug-loaded sheets, 0.57 ± 0.05
mm thick.

The drug-loaded sheets were then cut into rectangles 0.8 by
2.25 cm, 0.8 by 1.75 cm, and 0.8 by 1.15 cm. Each rectangle was
formed into a split tube and pressed into a 3.2-mm diameter hole

Medicated Loop IUD

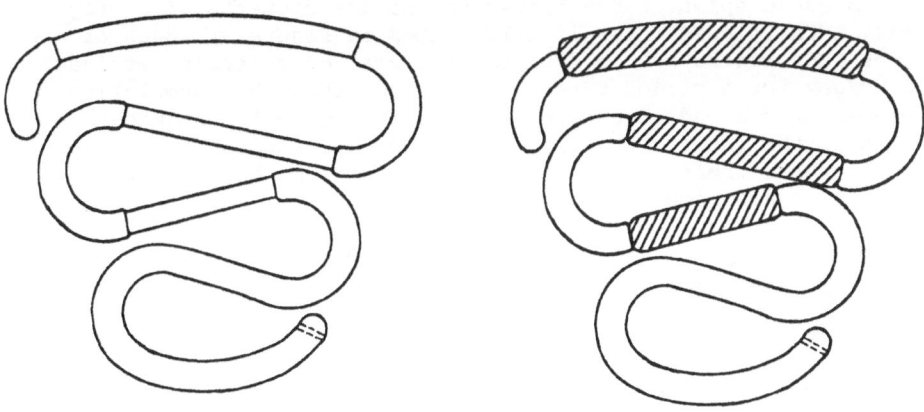

Modified Loop D   After addition of medication

Figure 3.   Schematic illustration of the Loop IUD before and after
             the addition of sustained-release medication.

in a Teflon forming block. The block was heated to 80°C to set
the sheets into split tube configurations. These sleeves were
placed over the three reduced sections of the modified Loop with
the split oriented toward the midplane. Bonding of the medicated
EVA sections to the body of the Loop was accomplished by press-
forming the assembly in a die held at 93°C for two minutes and
applying 15,000 lbs to the die for 1.5 minutes. The die was then
chilled until it could be handled with bare hands, and the medicated
loop was quenched in cold water immediately after it was removed
from the die. Total drug contained in the three medicated sections
of each Loop was 92 mg.

In Vitro Release Rates

     Three AMCA-medicated IUDs were immersed in 100 ml each of pH
7.1 buffered physiological saline held at 37°C. A fine stream of
air was bubbled throughout the solution to ensure continuous mixing.
Analyses were performed by En-Cas Analytical Laboratories, Winston-
Salem, NC. Over a one-year period of testing, the IUDs were blotted
and weighed at scheduled intervals, and the respective buffered
solutions were analyzed for AMCA and replaced with fresh solution.
A blank buffered solution was analyzed along with the test samples
to monitor for possible interferences. AMCA analysis was performed
by the Fluoram fluorometric method.[19] The weight of the blotted
devices increased by a maximum of 8% of their original weight at
126 days exposure and was 5% more than the original weight after
one year of exposure.

     A cubic spline curve fitted to the measurements of average
daily AMCA release rates is illustrated in Figure 4. Each of the
three IUDs tested met or exceeded the goal of releasing at least
50 µg/day for a period of at least six months. The cumulative
release at the end of one year, shown in Figure 5, is less than
one half the total drug load in the IUD. At the end of one year
of exposure, there appeared to be no loss in mechanical strength
or loss of adhesion of the matrix to the IUD vector.

In Vivo Tissue Reaction

     Four types of medicated devices were tested in rabbits. In
each case, one 10-mm long medicated portion of the modified Loop
was implanted in the right uterine horn of a rabbit, and a nonmedicated control section was implanted in the left uterine horn. One
type of device was medicated with 40% AMCA as described above.
Another was similarly fabricated using a 40% loading of aprotinin
(Trasylol) instead of AMCA. The third type was designed by the
Southern Research Institute (SoRI) to release AMCA through a poly-

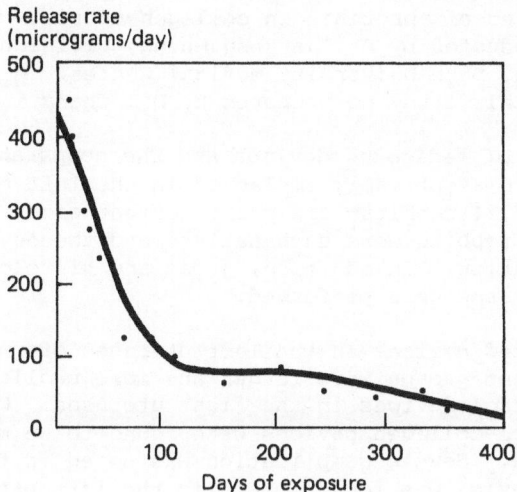

Figure 4.   Daily release rates per IUD as measured in vitro over
a one-year period.

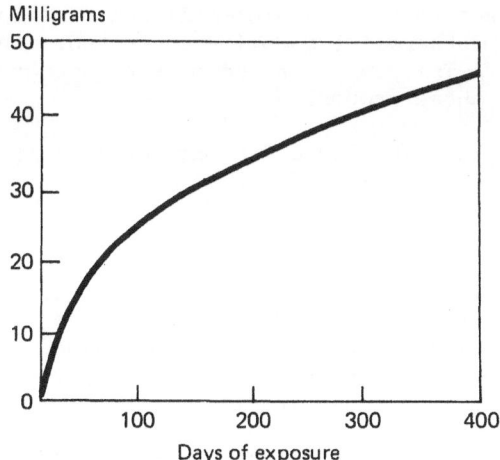

Figure 5.   Cumulative release of AMCA per IUD as measured in vitro
over a one-year period.

urethane diffusion barrier,[3] and the fourth, prepared by Dr. Milos
Chvapil, consisted of aprotinin in collagen matrix. The animal
studies were conducted by Dr. Jerjang Chang, Division of Laboratory
Animal Resources, Duke University Medical Center. A summary of
the results of this study as prepared by Dr. Chang is quoted below:

> Four kinds of medicated devices and the comparable control
> devices were aseptically implanted in the left and right
> uteruses of 24 rabbits—six per treatment group. Thirty days
> later, the rabbits were euthanatized and the devices retrieved
> for observation. In addition, gross and histologic evaluations
> of the uteruses were performed.
>
> The medicated devices in the left uteruses of rabbits in all
> the treatment groups were larger and more swollen than those
> of the control devices in the right uteruses. Of these groups,
> the trasylol-collagen devices were found to be markedly swollen
> and rounded. Severe complication was noted in this group and
> only one device was found intact in the left uterus. The
> swelling characteristics of the devices in the EVA-AMCA, SoRI-
> AMCA, and EVA-Trasylol group were similar.
>
> Tissue reactions to the implanted medicated or control devices
> were characterized by mucosal atypical hyperplasia (mucosa
> infoldings), inflammation, focal ulceration, and metaplasia
> of the endometrium. Of the four groups, SoRI-AMCA appeared
> to induce the least tissue reaction (this device released AMCA
> at a lower rate than the EVA-AMCA device). The tissue reactions
> of the uteruses to the trasylol-collagen were not significant
> despite the postsurgical complication noted. The tissue re-
> actions to EVA-Trasylol appeared more pronounced than that
> of the other three groups.
>
> A summary of the histologic findings appears in Table I.

Teratogenic Studies

Teratogenic studies of AMCA, EACA, EVA and Trasylol were done
by Dr. D. Moyer[20] utilizing Sprague-Dawley rats as experimental
animals. A simulation of the effects of sustained intrauterine
release of the materials was obtained by mixing them with Silastic
382 without catalyst and injecting the mixture into the uterine
lumen between implantation sites on the ninth day of pregnancy.
To reduce the EVA to a state fine enough to inject through a hypo-
dermic needle, it was blended in the hot press with an equal amount
of polyethylene oxide. The water-soluble polyethylene oxide was
leached away to form a felt-like sheet of EVA. The EVA felt was
then micronized in a blender in a silicone oil carrier. The micronized slurry was filtered through a wire-mesh screen. Relative

TABLE I.   SUMMARY OF GROSS AND HISTOLOGIC FINDINGS IN VIVO
STUDY OF AMCA AND TRASYLOL/MEDICATED DEVICE

Experimental Group	Rabbit No.	Left Uterus	Right Uterus
EVA-AMCA	18	Endometrial mucosa has moderate papillary pattern.	Endometrium has slight infolding.
	21	Not remarkable.	A foci of granulomatous lesion at submucosa.
	23	Chronic inflammation and focal ulceration of endometrium.	Focal mucosal infolding.
	136	Not remarkable.	Not remarkable.
	279	Focal chronic inflammation.	Not remarkable.
	276	Not remarkable.	Not remarkable.
SoRI—AMCA	17	Uterus red, edematous; chronic fibrous reaction of the serosa.	Uterus red, edmatous; chronic inflammation of the serosa.
	16	Uterus red; focal infolding of endometrial mucosa.	Not remarkable.
	864	Not remarkable.	Not remarkable.
	76	Not remarkable.	Not remarkable.
	82	Not remarkable.	Not remarkable.
	84	Not remarkable.	Not remarkable.
TRASYLOL—COLLAGEN	80	Not remarkable.	Not remarkable.
	77	Slight mucosal infolding.	Not remarkable.
	79	Not remarkable.	Not remarkable.
	19	Focal coagulatial necrosis.	Not remarkable.
	134	Uterus opened at implanted site; purulent inflammation of serosa.	Slight purulent inflammation of serosa.
	135	No necropsy.	
EVA—TRASYLOL	278	Not remarkable.	Focal chronic inflammation.
	275	Focal mucosal ulceration and necrosis.	Focal mucosal ulceration.

TABLE 1 (Continued)

Experimental Group	Rabbit No.	Left Uterus	Right Uterus
	277	Endometrial focal infolding; with inflammation.	Focal mucosal infolding.
	306	Not remarkable.	Not remarkable.
	305	Mild inflammation with slight infolding of the mucosa.	Slight inflammation, focal metaplasis of mucosa.
	307	Slight inflammation.	Not remarkable.
	24	Not remarkable.	Not remarkable.
	20	Not remarkable.	Not remarkable.
	22	Not remarkable.	Not remarkable.
	78	Not remarkable.	Not remarkable.

[a] The device was not found in the left uterus at necropsy.

[b] Died before a necropsy could be performed.

numbers of absorptions of fetuses at various dosage levels of AMCA and EVA for the control and experimental uterine horns are illustrated in Figure 6.

DISCUSSION

Contraceptive use is least prevalent in the developing world where the need is greatest, and it is there that sustained-release types of contraceptives are most likely to be acceptable. There are no sustained-release contraceptives generally available at low cost in the developing world. However, Depo-Provera, the injectable contraceptive that lasts up to three months per injection, is a relative of sustained-release contraceptives; it is popular in the developing world, primarily because of the general acceptance of injections to treat or prevent diseases and its high contraceptive efficacy without further action by the subject.[21]

Worldwide acceptance of some type of contraceptive has become essential. Starting 1.17 million years ago, one couple whose living descendants grew at the rate of 0.000017 per year would by now have populated the world at its present level. The current population growth rate is 1000 times greater than 0.000017, but world population growth must return to a value near zero sometime in the future or the earth will not be able to contain all its inhabitants.

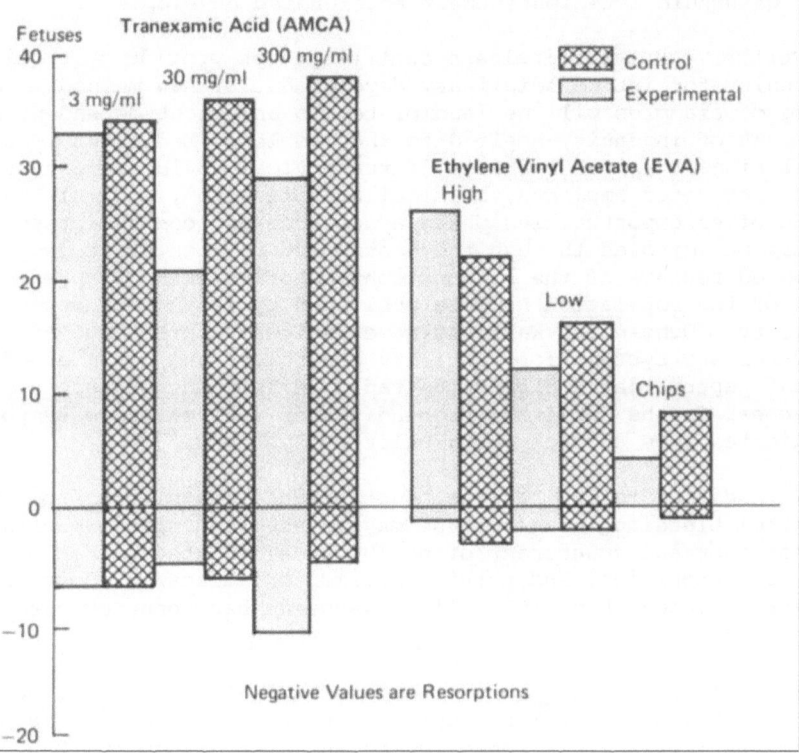

Figure 6.   Relative number of live and resorbed fetuses in the
            control and experimental uterine horns of rats exposed
            to intrauterine AMCA and EVA.[20]

        Population growth can be reduced through contraception, sexual
abstinence, sterilization, abortion, morbidity, and mortality. Morbidity currently has the largest effect on population reduction
because modern medicine has reduced mortality rates. But morbidity,
which is caused by the absence of sanitation, public health programs, education and adequate nutrition, is tragically inefficient
at controlling fertility.[22] Most societies find population stabili-
zation by high morbidity and mortality unacceptable, which gives
rise to hopes for early implementation of worldwide crash efforts
to promote the use of better alternatives (i.e., better contraceptives, better family planning programs). China, for example, has
changed its official pronatal attitude in response to the realities
of overpopulation.[23] Because sustained-release contraceptive
systems have the potential to overcome many of the disadvantages

of the contraceptive methods currently available in the developing
world, we should anticipate their accelerated development.

Further, sustained-release contraceptives provide an excellent
opportunity for interdisciplinary development of new methods. Any
listing of examples will be incomplete, to an extent dependent on
the amount of ingenuity applied to the problem. Medicated IUDs,
vaginal rings, vaginal barriers, intracervical devices, cervical
valves, medicated implants, chemical sterilization, and male barrier
methods offer opportunities where acceptance and contraceptive efficacy may be improved through the controlled release of drugs. Well
referenced reviews of the various contraceptive methods appear in
issues of the Population Reports published by the Johns Hopkins
University. Duncan and Kalkwarf have reviewed the subject of sustained-release systems for fertility control,[24] and a number of
relevant papers that indicate the rapid development of such systems
will appear in the published proceedings of the Amsterdam symposium
on Medicated IUDs and Polymeric Delivery Systems.[25]

In addition to the release of proteinase inhibitors from IUDs
to control bleeding, drug release may be used to improve contraceptive efficacy and counteract other IUD side effects such as dysmenorrhea, expulsion, and pelvic inflammatory disease. Some of
the current research on IUD delivery systems has been reviewed by
Chaudhury.[26]

Vaginal rings, which have been used to release progestins,[25]
could also be used to release prostaglandin abortafacients (Pop
Report G Series). The Proceedings of an International Workshop
on New Developments in Vaginal Contraception[27] describes much of
the current research on vaginal sustained-release systems. It is
also noteworthy that sustained-release implants may also be applicable to male contraception.[28]

CONCLUSION

There appear to be many opportunities to improve old and
develop new contraceptive methods based on the sustained release
of drugs from a biocompatible matrix material such as EVA. The
IUD example in which release of the drug is based primarily on the
connectivity between particles in the matrix represents a technology
that can transfer easily to other systems and to local manufacture
in developing countries. Sustained-release systems are being
applied beneficially to counteract food shortages and environmental
deterioration. It is highly appropriate that the same types of
systems can be and are being applied to the source of these problems: population pressure.

REFERENCES

1. D.H. Lewis, D.R. Cowsar, and M.D. Hamilton, in: "Proceedings
    5th International Symposium on Controlled Release of Bioactive
    Materials," F.E. Brinkman and J.A. Montemarano, eds., Gaithes-
    burg, Maryland (1978).
2. M.E. Tuttle and R.W. Baker, in: "Proceedings 7th International
    Symposium on Controlled Release of Bioactive Materials," D.H.
    Lewis, ed., Ft. Lauderdale (1980).
3. R. Langer and J. Folkman, Nature 263:797 (1976).
4. G.A. More, in: "Fourth International Congress for Stereology,"
    N.B.S. Spcl. Pub. 431:41 (1976).
5. J. Guillebaud and J. Bonnar, Br. J. Obstet. Gynecol. 85:707
    (1978).
6. A.J. Gallegos, R. Aznar, G. Merion, and E. Guizer, Contracep-
    tion 17(2):153 (1978).
7. P. Liedholm, G. Rybo, N.O. Sjoberg, and L. Solvell, Contra-
    ception 9(6):627 (1974).
8. R. Malmquist, L. Petersohn, and L.P. Bengtsson, Contraception
    9(6):627 (1974).
9. C.G. Nilsson, Contraception 15(4):379 (1977).
10. J. Guillebaud, J. Bonnar, J. Moregead, and A. Matthews, Lancet
    387 (1976).
11. R. Rovera, J.R. Gaitan, C.L. Navarra, J. Valles, H. Almonte,
    R. Ruiz, and A.B. Hernandez, Contraception 17(3):195 (1978).
12. F. Hefnawi, M.M. Yacout, M. Hosin, Z. El Sheika, and M. Has-
    sanein, Int. J. Gynaecol. Obstet. 15:79 (1977).
13. L. Westrom and L.P. Bengtsson, J. Reprod. Med. 5(4):41 (1970).
14. J.M. Kasonde and J. Bonnar, Br. Med. J. 4:17 (1975).
15. D.W. Nibbelink and C.D. Jakobsen, Thrombos. Diathes. Haemorrha.
    (Stag) 29:508 (1973).
16. S.T. Shaw, D.L. Moyer, and D.E. Aaronson, et al., Contraception
    11:395 (1975).
17. P.F. Tauber, A.S. Wolf, W. Herting, and L.J.D. Zoneveld, Fer-
    til. Steril. 28(12):1375 (1977).
18. F.B.G. Schumacher, personal communication, U. of Chicago School
    of Medicine (1978).
19. K.P. Wood and K. Sangduk, Nature 202(4934):794 (1964).
20. D. Moyer, communication, Teratogenicity Testing. IFRP Library
    (1980).
21. W. Rinehart and L. Winter, Population Reports, Series K 1 (1975).
22. J. Bongaarts, Science, 208:564 (1980).
23. M. Chen, Int. Fam. Plann. Perspect. 5(3):92 (1979).
24. G.W. Duncan and D.R. Kalkwarf, in: "Human Rep. Concept. and
    Contraception," Harper and Row (1973). p. 483.
25. E.S.E. Hafez and W.A.A. Van Os, in: "Proc. Int. Symp. Amsterdam,
    Martinus Nijhoff," The Hague (1979).
26. R.R. Chaudhury, Obstet. Gynecol. Surv. 35(6):333 (1980).

27. G.I. Zatuchni, A.G. Sobrero, J.J. Speidel, and J.J. Sciarra,
     in: "Vaginal Contraception," Harper and Row (1979).
28. Spec. Prog. of Res., Dev. and Res. Training, in Hum. Rep.,
     WHO 7th Ann. Rpt. (1978).

FIBROUS POLYMERS FOR THE DELIVERY OF CONTRACEPTIVE STEROIDS TO THE FEMALE REPRODUCTIVE TRACT

Richard L. Dunn and Danny H. Lewis

Southern Research Institute
2000 Ninth Avenue South
Birmingham, Alabama 35255

Lee R. Beck

Department of Obstetrics and Gynecology
University of Alabama in Birmingham
Birmingham, Alabama 35294

INTRODUCTION

Research and development on the application of controlled-release technology to fertility regulation was initiated in the late 1960s and has been accelerated in recent years.[1,2] Since sustained-release doses obviate the problem of cyclic overdosing and underdosing associated with the conventional administration of steroids, the technology, in principle, affords a means of effecting an optimum pharmacological response with a minimum dose of exogenous steroid.[3] Depending upon the half-life of the drug in plasma, the duration of the dose regimen, and the route of administration, the total dose can be reduced to 1/100 or less for continuous versus intermittant delivery.

Among the various new sustained-release systems under development for the delivery of contraceptive steroids, the most advanced are subdermal implants, vaginal rings, vaginal microcapsules, medicated IUDs, and injectable, biodegradable microcapsules.[4] All of these can be used to deliver continuous low doses of natural as well as synthetic steroids. However, only the Progestasert,® a medicated IUD which delivers 65 µg/day of progesterone directly to the uterus, has reached commercialization.

The medicated IUD represents a major advance toward achieving minimal intervention fertility control, since it is based upon local, rather than systemic, delivery of contraceptive agents. Progestogens delivered directly to the uterine lumen in low doses are believed to act mainly on the uterine mucosa to induce changes in the endometrium which prevent implantation. These effects can be obtained, supposedly, without an influence on normal ovarian function or other systemic processes.

The Progestasert, a T-shaped device designed by Alza Pharmaceutical Company to provide a constant release of progesterone through a rate-controlling polymeric membrane of ethylene vinyl acetate, has been evaluated extensively for contraceptive effectiveness, acceptability, side effects, and mechanism of contraceptive action.[5-] Less menstrual blood flow and dysmenorrhea appear to be the only advantages of the Progestasert over the conventional nonmedicated IUD; however, these advantages are significant in anemic women. A disadvantage of the Progestasert is that it has to be replaced annually. New intrauterine devices that release progesterone for three years or very low doses of levonorgestrel, a more potent synthetic progestin, for five years have been developed.[8,9]

In spite of their potential, medicated IUDs have not been widely accepted for the same reasons associated with the use of conventional IUDs: (a) difficulty with insertion; (b) expulsion soon after insertion; (c) intermenstrual bleeding; (d) pain; (e) uterine perforations; (f) unwanted pregnancies that are more likely to be ectopic; and (g) increased frequency of pelvic infection.[10-12] The purpose of the medicated IUD should be to use the medication for contraceptive effects and the device only as a carrier. In this manner, smaller, less troublesome IUDs with novel forms free of the side effects associated with conventional IUDs could be designed.

One approach to novel medicated IUDs is that of a fibrous polymer for the intrauterine delivery of contraceptive steroids. Hollow fibers loaded with a progestogen which released at a constant rate over several years would afford several advantages over current medicated IUDs. The smaller size and greater flexibility of the fibers would improve the ease of insertion and decrease the pressure of the IUD against the uterine wall. The decreased pressure would lower the chances for uterine perforations and diminish the pain associated with the wearing of an IUD. The flexibility of the fibers would allow them to be arranged into almost any configuration so as to provide greater comfort with less expulsion. Fibers would also provide a greater surface area for release of the progestogen and subsequent interaction with the endometrium. In addition, fibers loaded with an active progestogen could be produced with good uniformity and at extremely low cost compared to current medicated IUDs.

METHODS AND MATERIALS

Essentially three methods are available for producing fibers from polymers. These are called wet-, dry-, and melt-spinning processes. Wet spinning involves the extrusion of a solution of a polymer through an orifice into a nonsolvent, thus coagulating the polymer into a strong filament. In the dry-spinning process, a solution of a polymer is again forced through an orifice, but the solution is fed into a heated column which allows evaporation of the solvent and consequent formation of a fiber. The melt-spinning process is somewhat simpler and the process most often used commercially. Solid polymer is heated above its melting point and extruded through an orifice and cooled to afford a filament. In each process, the molten polymer or polymer solution is forced through small holes called spinnerets. In practice, one filament or several thousand filaments may be spun at a time, depending upon how many holes are in the spinneret base plate. In these experiments the melt-spinning process was used to prepare all of the steroid-loaded fibers.

Two types of diffusion-controlled systems can be obtained from the combination of a steroid with a polymer to produce a fiber (Figure 1). Fibers in which the steroid is dissolved or dispersed throughout the polymer matrix yield a monolithic system. The release of steroid from this system is first order and the release rate decreases with time. Hollow fibers containing steroid within the lumen constitute reservoir systems in which the release of steroid is constant (zero order) over a prolonged period. These systems can be prepared by the filling of hollow fibers with steroid or by coaxial spinning in which the steroid-loaded core of the fiber is spun at the same time as the rate-controlling sheath or outer membrane.

Monolithic Fibers

In these studies, a melt rheometer was used to prepare the monolithic fibers. The melt rheometer was preheated to the desired temperature and then loaded with the polymer-drug mixture. An extrusion ram with weights attached was placed in the heated barrel, and the mixture was allowed to heat to the spinning temperature before it was extruded. As the molten material was extruded through the spinneret, it cooled and formed a fiber which was collected in loose coils. Various extrusion temperatures and ram weights were used to provide uniform fibers.

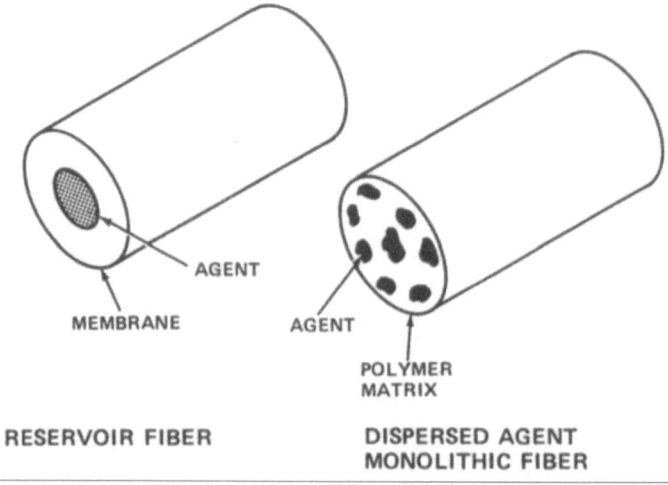

Figure 1. Diffusion-controlled fiber.

Reservoir Fibers

Reservoir or coaxial fibers were prepared by three different methods. In the first system, the steroid mixed with a viscous polymer was added to the center (core) feed section in the barrel of a ram extruder. The wall polymer was added to the outside (sheath) feed section located in another barrel of the same ram extruder. Both sheath and core materials were heated to the same temperature, and then pistons were pressed down through the two feed sections to extrude both the sheath polymer and the core mixture through a spinneret containing two concentric orifices (Figure 2). There were two major problems with this method: (a) since the core mixture had to be heated to approximately the same temperature as the sheath polymer, it often degraded or became so fluid that it flowed out of the spinneret with no control; and (b) the ratio of core material to sheath material that comprised the fiber could be changed only by changing the spinneret.

In the second method of coaxial fiber preparation, the steroid was suspended or dissolved in a suitable lumen fluid. This lumen fluid was then pumped from an outside source into the coaxial-fiber spinneret with a metering pump. This method eliminated the requirement to heat the drug-core fluid to high temperatures, and it permitted a change in the ratio of core material to sheath material by varying the speed of the metering pump. This method however, gave problems with either separation of the drug from the lumen fluid during the metering operation or inadequate metering of the lumen fluid because of high viscosities.

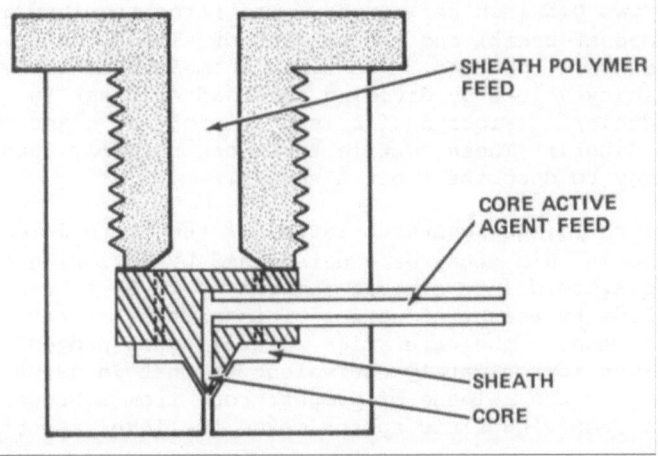

Figure 2.   Coaxial-fiber spinneret.

        The optimum method for coaxial-fiber production was identical
to the second method described above except that the outside reservoir was heated and a melt pump was included.   This system allowed
the core material to be heated to its melting temperature and pumped
to the spinneret where it encountered the molten sheath polymer.
The sheath polymer had been heated to its optimum spinning temperature in the barrel of the ram extruder.   The separation of heating
chambers permitted better control of the spinning process, and the
individual control of the feed rates of the core and sheath materials
resulted in greater flexibility in the preparation of fibers with
various core-to-sheath ratios.

        The polymers used for fiber formation comprised both biodegrad-
able and nonbiodegradable materials.   The biodegradable aliphatic
polyesters were prepared by established procedures from commercially
available monomers.   The nonbiodegradable polypropylene and polyethylene were obtained from industrial sources.

In Vitro Characterization

        For intrauterine applications, it was necessary that the steroid-
loaded fibers possess sufficient strength and flexibility before
and after release of the steroid.   Therefore, the mechanical properties of the fibers were determined initially and after in vitro
or in vivo exposure.   Five three-inch samples were cut from each
type of fiber, and the samples were placed in the Instron Tensile
Tester set at a gauge length of one inch.   The rate of separation

of the clamps was 0.5 inch per minute. The force required to break
the fibers (load at break) and the percent of elongation of the
fibers at break were recorded. The strength measurements were converted to tenacity values by dividing the load at break in grams
by the fiber denier. (Fiber denier is the weight in grams of 9000
meters of the fiber.) These textile terms are normally used in
fiber technology to describe fiber strength.

The in vitro release characteristics of the steroid-loaded
fibers prepared in this study were determined by following the
release of the steroid into a media comprising 27.5% by weight of
ethanol and 72.5% by weight of water. This particular receiving
fluid was used because the saturation solubility of progesterone
in this media was approximately equivalent to that in serum. In
addition, the in vitro release of progesterone from a Progestasert
device in this receiving fluid approximated the level reported for
the in vivo release.

The amount of fibers used in each experiment was that calculated to increase the concentration of progesterone in the receiving
fluid by at least 0.06 µg per ml per day. The monolithic fibers
were simply cut to the required lengths and immersed in the receiving fluids. The reservoir fibers were cut to the required lengths,
but the ends of the fibers were sealed with either molten sheath
polymer or poly(methyl methacrylate) from a solventless two-compo-
nent denture-base resin which cured at room temperature. The sealed
fibers were incubated in vials containing 50 ml of the 27.5% aqueous
ethanol at 37°C in a shaker bath. Three-ml aliquots of receiving
fluid were removed periodically and assayed for progesterone by
measuring the absorption peak at 247 nm on a UV spectrophotometer.
A 3-ml aliquot of fresh receiving fluid was then added to the vial.

In Vivo Evaluations in Baboons

For the in vivo studies of the fibrous system, the baboon
primate model established by the Human Reproductive Biology Laboratory at the University of Alabama in Birmingham for the evaluation
of controlled-release systems, particularly for progestational
agents, was selected. The primate studies were designed to determine the level and duration of progestational effects upon the
baboon endometrium after placement of the medicated fibers in the
uterus.

In the first series of experiments, a coaxial fiber with a
sheath of polyethylene and a core of polyethylene/progesterone
(50/50) was cut to various lengths based upon its in vitro release
rate of 0.8 µg/cm/day to give doses of 25, 50, 75, 100, and 125
µg of progesterone per day. Fiber lengths corresponding to these

five doses were sealed at the ends, coiled into approximate 3-cm diameter circles, secured with nylon sewing thread, and inserted into the uteri of normally cycling adult female baboons with the aid of a Cu-7(TM) inserter. A nonmedicated polyethylene fiber of 156 cm in length was inserted into one baboon as a control.

All six animals were permitted to go through one menstrual period and were biopsied on Day 12 of the subsequent perineal cycle. The biopsies were separated into two parts for fixation in neutral buffered formalin for light microscopy and 2.5% of glutaraldehyde for scanning electron microscopy. After about 300 days, the fibrous coils which had not been expelled were removed from the baboons, and the residual progesterone was extracted to determine the in vivo rate of release.

In a second series of experiments, baboons with nonmedicated control fibers and medicated fibers at dosage levels of 5, 12.5, and 25 μg/day of progesterone were mated to determine the efficacy of the fibrous contraceptive system.

RESULTS AND DISCUSSION

Monolithic fibers were prepared from nylon 4, nylon 6, nylon 6-12, polyethylene, polypropylene, polycaprolactone, and poly(DL-lactide) with 10-30% by weight of progesterone. The nylon polymers required temperatures greater than 200°C for satisfactory melt spinning. These higher temperatures caused some slight decomposition of either progesterone or the polymer as evidenced by the yellow color of the fibers. The other polymers were all spun at temperatures less than 200°C and no discoloration of the fibers were noted. Spinning performance was satisfactory for all polymer/drug combinations including those with the higher loadings.

Reservoir or coaxial fibers were prepared with both nonbiodegradable and biodegradable polymers as rate-controlling membranes. The nonbiodegradable polymers were polypropylene and polyethylene with several different molecular weights of polyethylene resin being evaluated to obtain optimum mechanical properties. The biodegradable polymers were poly(DL-lactide), poly(L-lactide), a 75/25 copolymer of DL-lactide and glycolide, and polycaprolactone. The higher-molecular-weight polyethylene, polypropylene, and polycaprolactone gave the best spinning performance and yielded fibers with greater uniformity, better mechanical strength, and higher flexibility.

Various mixtures of progesterone with polymers were used as the core for the coaxial fibers. The level of progesterone in the fiber cores ranged from 25 to 100% of progesterone. Polymers used as the core matrix for progesterone included polyethylene, polypropylene, nylon 6, silicone oil, polyethylene glycol (400 M.W.), polyethylene glycol (20,000 M.W.), and polycaprolactone. Fibers with cores of 100% progesterone were stiffer and weaker than the other fibers. Metering the progesterone to the spinneret was also difficult because progesterone went from a very low viscosity liquid at the melt to a crystalline solid upon cooling, and problems with plugging of the feed line and nonuniformity of feed control were often encountered. The liquid polymers containing progesterone, e.g. silicone oil, and polyethylene glycol-400 gave similar problems. Polyethylene, polypropylene, and nylon-6 yielded higher melt viscosities with better metering control, but progesterone tended to separate from these polymers at the higher temperatures required for spinning. Polyethylene glycol-20,000 when mixed with progesterone and heated to its melting point gave a stable homogenous mixture with a level of viscosity just sufficient for melt-pumping. However, the polyethylene glycol core contributed very little to the strength of the coaxial fiber. The optimum core matrix for progesterone was found to be polycaprolactone. This polymer melts at a lower temperature than progesterone, yet mixtures of the two materials above the melting point of progesterone are both homogenous and highly viscous. The higher melt viscosity allowed easy control of the metering process. In addition, polycaprolactone containing progesterone formed a strong and flexible fiber.

The strength and flexibility of the coaxial fibers loaded with progesterone were found to depend upon several factors. These included the polymeric sheath, the polymeric core matrix, the sheath-to-core ratio, and the extent of fiber orientation as determined by its draw ratio. These effects are shown in Tables I-III. The higher-molecular-weight polyethylene, Hostalen GM 5010, yielded fibers with properties similar to those obtained with polypropylene. Polycaprolactone produced the strongest biodegradable fibers. As shown in Table II, the strength of the polyethylene coaxial fibers increased as the progesterone in the core was replaced with higher-molecular-weight polymer. A similar effect is shown in Table III where the fibers with a larger proportion of sheath polymer have better mechanical properties. The drawn or oriented fibers gave higher tenacity values with lower elongations at break, as expected from data on commercial fibers.

It is important in a nonbiodegradable fibrous delivery system that the mechanical properties do not deteriorate significantly upon release of the drug. To test this effect, several polypropylene coaxial fibers were removed after 78 days in vitro exposure, and one progesterone-loaded polyethylene fiber was recovered after 171 days in the uterus of a baboon. The mechanical properties of the recovered fibers when compared to those of the initial fibers showed an improvement in strength and elongation (Table IV). This result can be explained by the method in which fiber tenacity is

TABLE I. EFFECT OF SHEATH POLYMER ON MECHANICAL
PROPERTIES OF COAXIAL FIBERS[a]

| Sheath Polymer | Mechanical Properties | | |
	Tenacity, g/d	Elongation at Break, %	Tensile Factor
Polyethylene, Exxon LD-600	0.07	210	1
Polyethylene, Hostalen GM 5010	0.30	1800	14
Polypropylene	0.30	1500	13
Poly(DL-lactide)	0.26	5	0.6
Poly(L-lactide)	0.30	0	0
75/25 Poly(DL-lactide-co-glycolide)	0.23	14	0.9
Polycaprolactone	0.17	1005	5.4

[a] All cores were 75/25 progesterone/polyethylene glycol-20,000.

TABLE II. EFFECT OF CORE MATRIX ON MECHANICAL
PROPERTIES OF COAXIAL FIBERS[a]

| Core Matrix | Mechanical Properties | | |
	Tenacity, g/d	Elongation at Break, %	Tensile Factor
100% P_4[b]	0.03	35	0.2
75/25 P_4/PEG[c]	0.07	210	1.0
50/50 P_4/P.E.[d]	0.16	65	1.3
100% P.E.	0.14	725	3.8

[a] All sheath polymers were Exxon LD-600 polyethylene.

[b] P_4 = progesterone.

[c] PEG = polyethylene glycol (20,000 M.W.).

[d] P.E. = polyethylene (Exxon LD-600).

TABLE III.   EFFECTS OF SHEATH THICKNESS AND FIBER
ORIENTATION ON MECHANICAL PROPERTIES OF COAXIAL FIBERS[a]

Sheath:Core Ratio	Draw Ratio	Mechanical Properties		
		Tenacity, g/d	Elongation at Break, %	Tensile Factor
3.3	2.7	1.2	610	30
1.7	2.7	0.9	400	15
4.5	5.3	2.8	50	19
1.8	5.3	1.9	30	11

[a] Polypropylene sheath, 75/25 progesterone/polycaprolactone core.

TABLE IV.   RETENTION OF FIBER PROPERTIES AFTER RELEASE
OF PROGESTERONE

Sample 9893-9[a]	Tenacity, g/d Before	After	Elongation at Break, % Before	After	Tensile Factor Before	After
5	0.6	1.0	235	335	9	18
6	0.9	1.4	150	280	10	23
7	1.2	2.4	80	125	11	27
8	1.7	4.3	55	55	12	31
b	0.2	0.2	65	95	1	2

[a] Polypropylene fiber, in vitro exposure.

[b] Polyethylene fiber, in vivo exposure.

determined. (Fiber tenacity is the breaking load (grams) of the fiber divided by its denier, which is the weight in grams of 9000 meters of the fiber.) Removal of the crystalline drug reduces the denier or weight of the fiber, and since the strength of the fiber is obtained primarily from the polymeric sheath the division of approximately the same breaking load by a lower denier gives the resultant higher tenacity. The removal of the crystalline drug also allows the fiber to be elongated further before breakage occurs.

Both the monolithic and reservoir fibers were tested for in vitro release of progesterone. Release profiles for 30%-loaded polypropylene, polyethylene, and nylon-6 as given in Figures 3-5, respectively, demonstrate typical first-order release kinetics. It is also apparent from the figures that the release of progesterone from these materials increases with the polarity and hydrophilicity of the polymers.

The observed release profiles of the monolithic fibers can be described mathematically by Fick's Law of diffusion for devices with cylindrical geometry:[13,14]

$$\frac{dM_t/M\infty}{dt} = \frac{-4\ DC_s}{r_o^2\ C_o} \ln(1-M_t/M\infty)$$

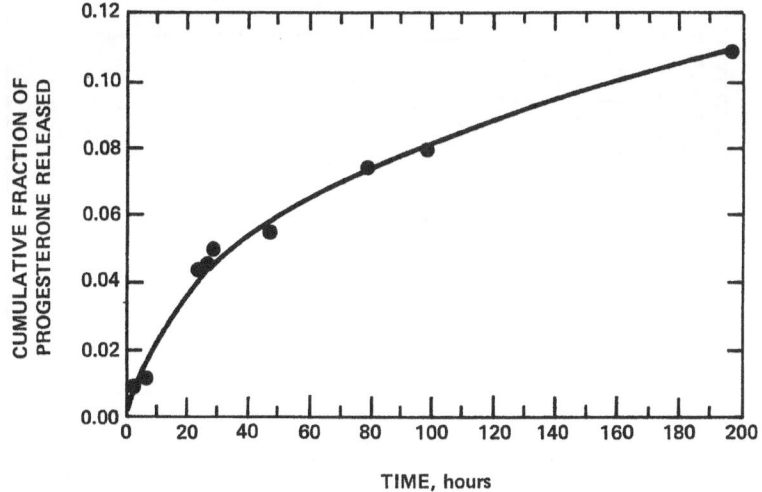

Figure 3. In vitro release of progesterone from 30%-loaded polypropylene fibers.

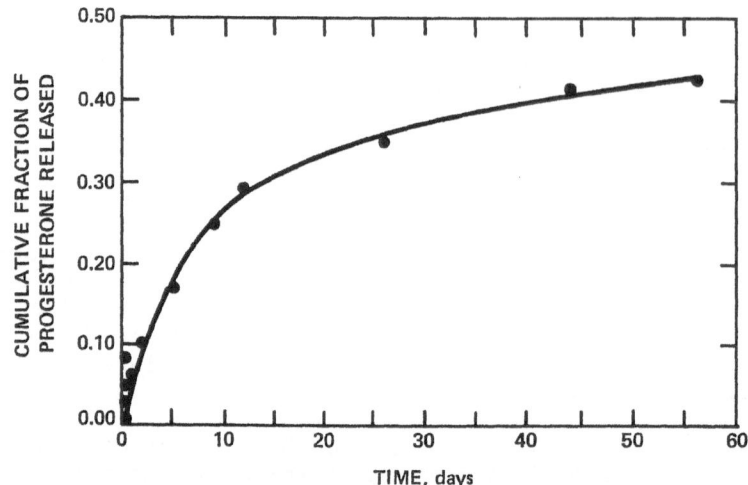

Figure 4. In vitro release of progesterone from 30%-loaded
           polyethylene fibers.

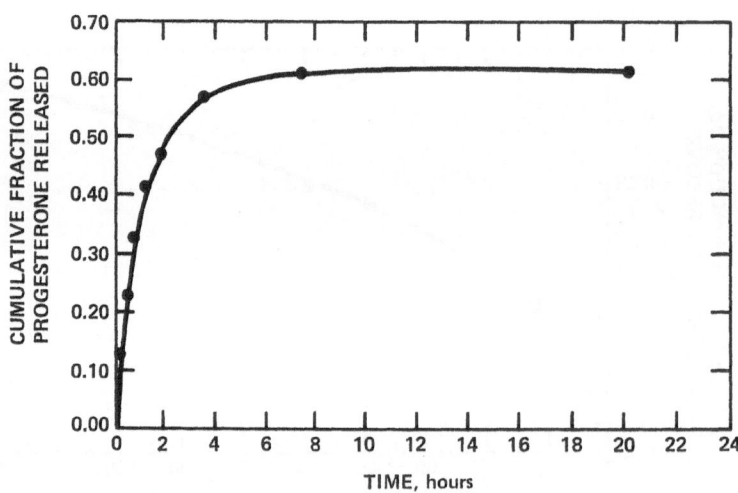

Figure 5. In vitro release of progesterone from 30%-loaded
           nylon 6 fibers.

where $\dfrac{dM_t/M\infty}{dt}$ = fractional rate of release of drug

D = diffusion coefficient of the drug in the polymer, cm^2/sec

C_s = saturation solubility, g/cm^3

r_o = radius of the cylinder, cm

C_o = drug loading in g/cm^3

$M_t/M\infty$ = fraction of initial mass released at time t

The product of the diffusion coefficient and the saturation solubility yields the permeability product, $D \cdot C_s$, which expresses the
ability of an agent to permeate a particular polymer membrane.

Integration of the above equation and rearrangement of the
terms gives the following expression:

$$\frac{C_o r_o^2}{4} \cdot [1-M_t/M\infty] \; [\ln(1-M_t/M\infty)] + M_t/M\infty = D \cdot C_s \cdot t$$

A plot of the terms on the left side of the equation versus time
in seconds yields a straight line whose slope is the desired permeability product, $D \cdot C_s$; These calculations when performed for the
progesterone-loaded monolithic fibers gave the values of $D \cdot C_s$ shown
in Table V.   Based upon these values, the slower-releasing polyethylene and polypropylene materials were required for long-term
delivery of progesterone for contraceptive action.

TABLE V.   VALUES OF $D \cdot C_s$ FOR PROGESTERONE
IN CANDIDATE POLYMERS

Fiber-Forming Polymer	$D \cdot C_s$, $g \; cm^{-1} \; sec^{-r}$
Nylon 6	3.7×10^{-10}
Nylon 6-12	1.6×10^{-10}
Polycaprolactone	7.0×10^{-12}
Polyethylene	1.2×10^{-12}
Poly(DL-lactide)	6.4×10^{-13}
Polypropylene	3.3×10^{-13}

The in vitro release profiles of the reservoir or coaxial
fibers were also determined. In general, all of the coaxial fibers
exhibited constant or zero-order release of progesterone as illustrated by the mass released being a linear function of time. The
most linear release profiles as shown in Figures 6-9 were obtained
with polyethylene as the sheath material. Each graph has been normalized to show the mass of progesterone released per cm of fiber;
thus the slope of the graph is the release rate in μg of progesterone per cm per day.

The polyethylene coaxial fibers also showed a good correlation
of release rate with sheath thickness. This correlation is shown
in Figure 10. As predicted, the release rate increased with a
decrease in the thickness of the fiber sheath or rate-controlling
membrane.

Essentially zero-order kinetics were also followed by the polypropylene coaxial fibers in the release of progesterone; however,
a slight burst or acceleration in release rate was observed during
the first two to three weeks of in vitro release (Figure 11). The

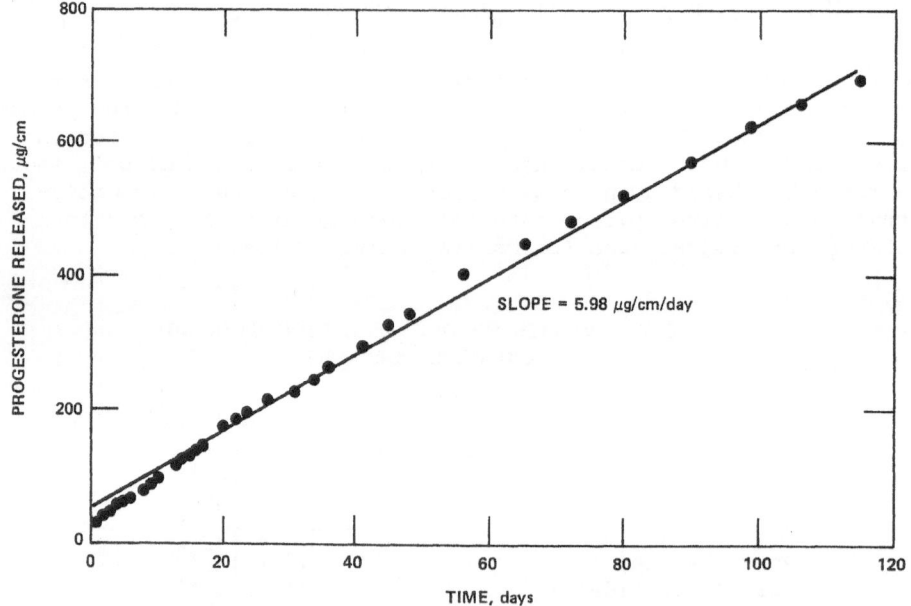

Figure 6.   Release of progesterone from fibers: polyethylene
           sheath, 100% P₄ core, ends sealed with P.E.

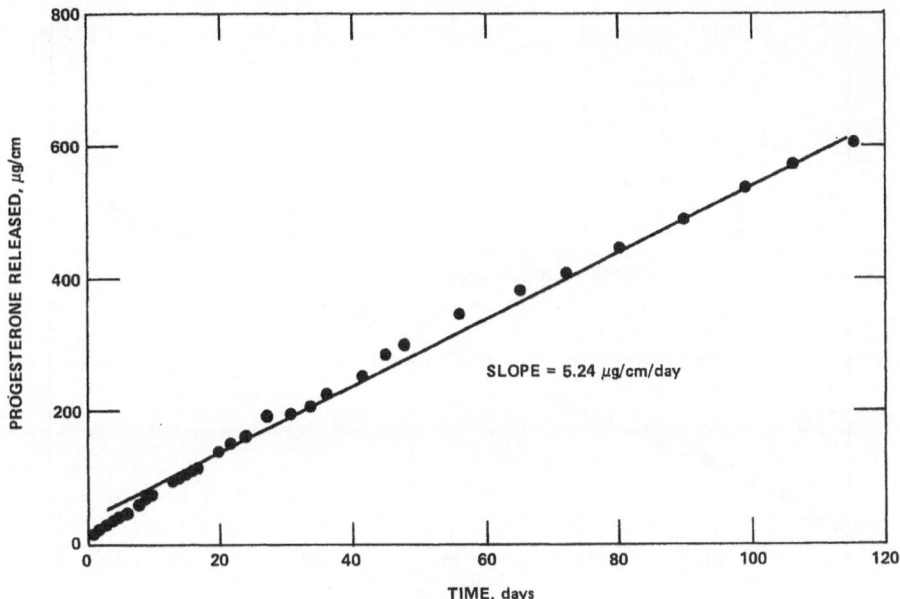

Figure 7.   Release of progesterone from fibers; polyethylene sheath, 100% P_4 core, ends sealed with MMA.

burst is suspected to be caused by migration of the progesterone to the fiber surface during the spinning and drawing processes. As soon as this excess of progesterone is released, a steady-state equilibrium is obtained in which the further release of progesterone is constant. Drawn fibers have a slower release of progesterone than the undrawn sample. Apparently the higher orientation and crystallinity produced by drawing of the fiber decreased its permeability to progesterone.

The biodegradable coaxial fibers yielded rather interesting data for the release of progesterone. Poly(L-lactide) was extremely impermeable to progesterone and gave no release until the ends of the fiber were cut to expose the steroid. The nonpermeability of poly(L-lactide) to progesterone was attributed to its highly crystalline structure. Polycaprolactone was quite permeable to progesterone and released the entire drug loading in less than one day. Apparently progesterone has a high saturation solubility in polycaprolactone, as indicated by other researchers. The release rates of the poly(DL-lactide) and the 75/25 poly(lactide-co-glycolide) coaxial fibers were relatively high, approximately four times the predicted rates. In addition, these fibers showed a burst effect

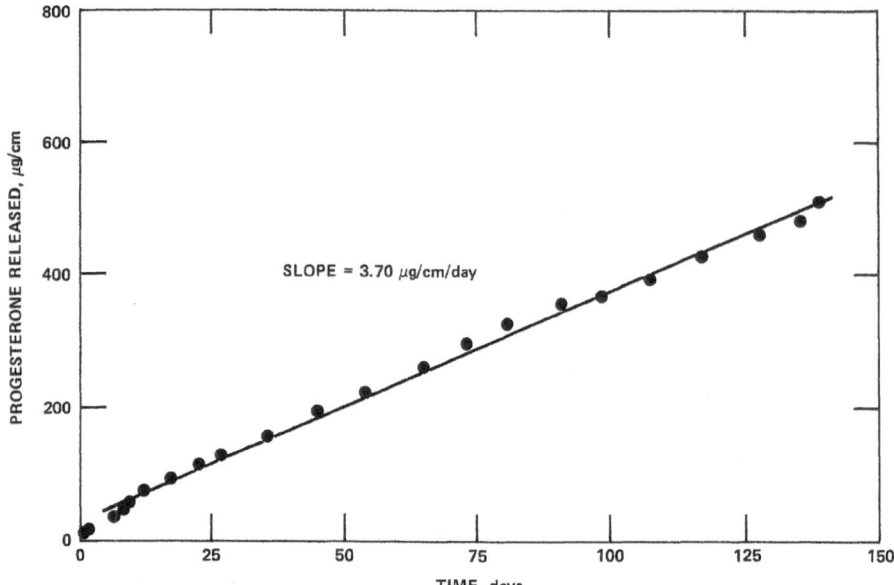

Figure 8.   Release of progesterone from fibers; polyethylene
            sheath, 75/25 P₄/PEG core, ends sealed with P.E.

after approximately 12 days with almost complete depletion of the
drug in 20 days. This high burst was attributed to the plasticizing
action of the aqueous ethanol receiving fluid on the polymers as
the fibers became soft and tacky in a short time.

    The results of the in vivo experiments with the fibrous coils
in baboons were in good agreement with those predicted from the
in vitro data. Biopsies obtained from the baboon uteri showed that
the progesterone-releasing fibrous coils had a pronounced effect
upon the endometrium that was not observed with control fibers.
The higher the dosage level of the fibrous coils, the greater was
the effect upon endometrium. The glandular and surface epithelium
of the biopsies from baboons with medicated fibers were flattened,
and there was hypertrophic decidualization of the stroma cells.
A periodic acid-Schiff stain showed that the hypertrophic stroma
cells were filled with glycogen and glycoprotein, a response usually
associated with pregnancy.

    Scanning electron micrographs of the surface epithelium showed
that the fibers with no progesterone had no effect. But those
medicated fibrous coils which remained in the uterus showed a pronounced flattening of the surface epithelium with the higher doses

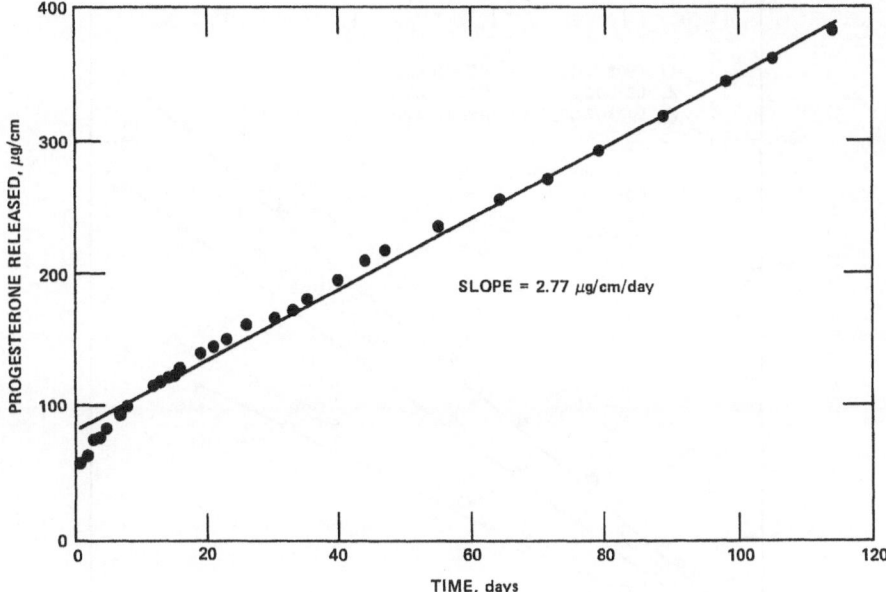

Figure 9.   Release of progesterone from fibers: polyethylene
            sheath, 75/25 P$_4$/PEG core, ends sealed with MMA.

(100 and 125 µg/day), causing epithelial denudation with resultant
bleeding.   These results indicated that the amount of progesterone
released from the fibers in the 50-125 µg range was too high.

    In addition to the effects of the dosage level on the endome-
trium, the retention of the fibrous coils in the uterus was also
affected by the amount of progesterone released.   Fibrous coils
with no progesterone, as well as those coils releasing only 25 and
50 µg/day of progesterone, were expelled within a short period from
the uterus of the baboons.   The fibrous coil with the 75-µg/day
dose was borderline and tended to drop down into the vagina.   However, the larger fibrous coils releasing 100 and 125 µg/day of
progesterone were retained in the uterus for approximately nine
months.   Apparently the progesterone released from the fibrous coils
with the larger dosage suppressed the uterine contractions which
would have normally expelled the fibers.

    The fibrous coils were removed from the baboons after approxi-
mately nine months and the residual progesterone extracted to determine the in vivo release rate.   The results of these studies given
in Table VI show the close agreement between the in vitro and the
in vivo release rates of the fibers.

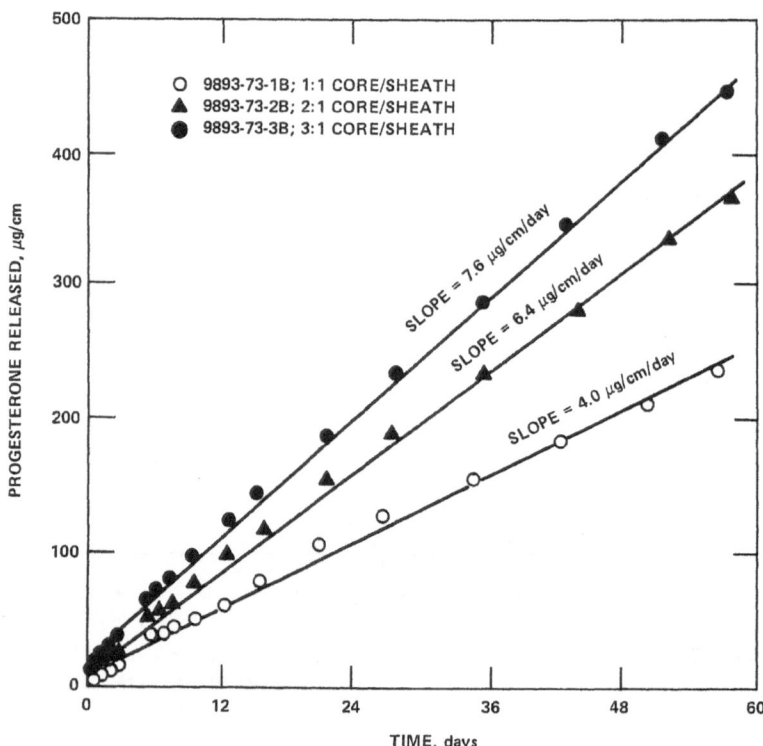

Figure 10. Release of progesterone from fibers: polyethylene
            sheath, 75/25 P /PEG core.

TABLE VI.   RESIDUAL PROGESTERONE IN SAMPLES RECOVERED FROM
            IN VIVO TESTS IN BABOONS

Theoretical Dose µg/day	Elapsed Time Days	Residual Progesterone, µg	Release Rate, µg/cm/day	
			In Vivo	In Vitro
125	295	1350	0.71	0.78
100	276	1260	0.76	0.78
75	288	88	0.73	0.78

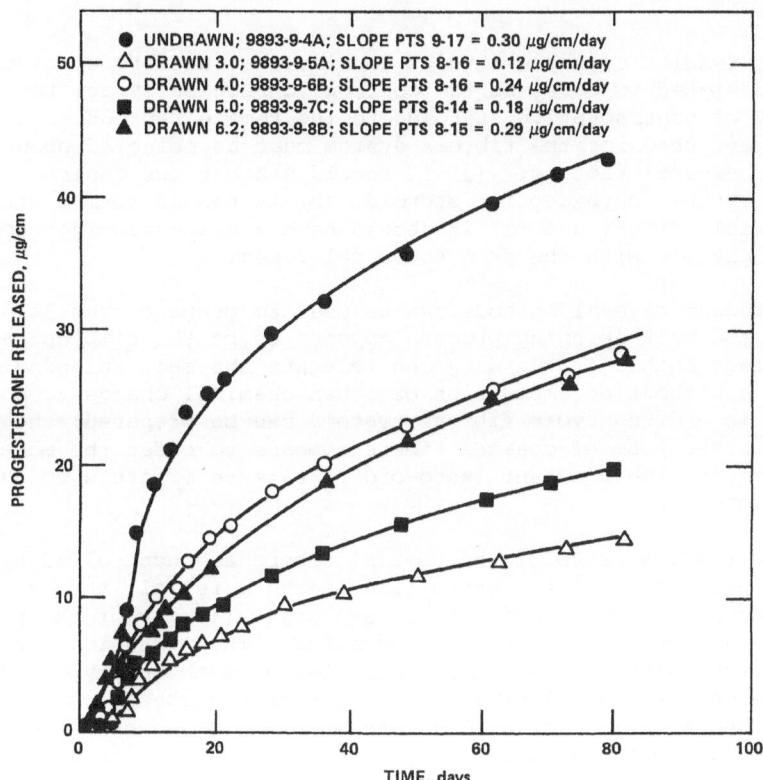

Figure 11. Release of progesterone from fibers: polyethylene
            sheath, 75/25 P_4/PEG core.

     Because of the pronounced effects of the progesterone-releasing
fibers upon the endometrium, fibrous coils with lower dosage levels
of progesterone and smaller coil diameters were used for the fertility tests. Although considerable difficulty was experienced
in retaining medicated and nonmedicated fibrous coils in the baboon
uteri, twelve matings were obtained. Eight matings were with four
animals with control fibers, three matings were with two animals
with fibrous coils releasing 12.5 µg/day of progesterone, and one
mating was with an animal treated with a fibrous coil releasing
25 µg/day of progesterone. No pregnancies resulted from any of
the matings, suggesting that the control fiber itself may be an
effective contraceptive. When the fibrous coils were removed, the
animal immediately became pregnant upon the next mating cycle,
indicating no residual effects of the fibrous contraceptive system.

CONCLUSIONS

The results of these studies confirm that a fibrous polymer can be designed to serve as the controlled-release system for the delivery of contraceptive steroids to the female reproductive tract. The polymer used for the fibrous system must be selected upon the basis of several factors: (a) it should exhibit the desired permeability to the contraceptive steroid; (b) it should form a strong and flexible fiber; and (c) it should have a melt-spinning temperature compatible with the drug to be delivered.

Although several methods can be used to prepare drug-loaded fibers, the melt-spinning process appears to be the simplest and most direct method if the drug can tolerate the melt-spinning temperatures without decomposition or other chemical changes. Both monolithic and reservoir fibrous systems can be prepared; the latter system in the form of coaxial fibers appears to offer the most potential for the constant (zero-order) release of drugs to the action site.

The release rates of the coaxial fibers are controlled by the polymer used as the rate-controlling sheath material, the thickness of the sheath, and the orientation and crystallinity of the polymeric sheath as effected by fiber drawing. The mechanical properties of the coaxial fibers are controlled by both the type and molecular weight of the polymers used as either the sheath or core matrix, the drug loading of the core matrix, the sheath thickness, and the fiber orientation.

In these studies, coaxial fibers with a core of progesterone and polycaprolactone surrounded by a sheath of either polypropylene or high-molecular-weight polyethylene were found to exhibit satisfactory mechanical properties and release rates for the long-term delivery of progesterone to the female reproductive tract. The in vivo release rates of fibers placed in the uteri of baboons were found to correlate closely with those determined by in vitro measurements in an ethanolic solution. The release of progesterone in the baboon uterus appeared to have a pronounced effect upon the endometrium. Subsequent fertility trials with the fibrous system demonstrated the contraceptive efficacy of both the medicated and nonmedicated fibers. The fertility studies also indicated the problems associated with retention of the fibrous system in the baboon uterus without the release of large doses of progesterone to suppress uterine contractions. New designs of the fibrous system other than the simple coil used in the initial studies are needed (Figure 12). These designs, fabricated from progesterone-loaded coaxial fibers spun to give the proper release of progesterone for about five years, should yield a novel and improved medicated IUD without the problems associated with current IUDs.

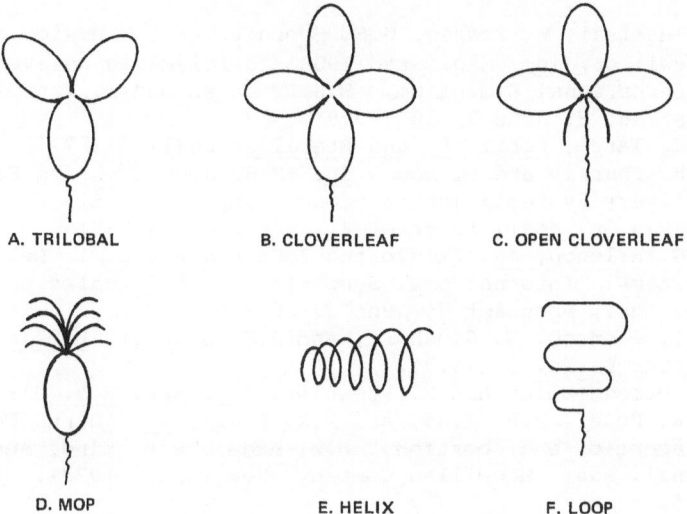

Figure 12. Fibrous IUD designs.

ACKNOWLEDGEMENTS

     We are grateful to Ms. Valerie Z. Pope, Ms. Melody D. Hamilton,
Ms. Brenda H. Perkins, Mr. W. Curtis Stoner, and Dr. Donald R. Cowsar
for their assistance in this work. We also wish to acknowledge
the Program For Applied Research on Fertility Regulation (PARFR)
for their financial support under Contract No. 206SRI with special
thanks to Dr. Gerald I. Zatuchni.

REFERENCES

1.   G.W. Duncan and D.R. Kalkwarf, in: "Human Reproduction: Concep-
     tion and Contraception," E.S.E. Hafez and T.N. Evans, eds.,
     Harper and Row, New York, (1975). pp. 483-503.
2.   H.L. Gabelnick, ed., "Drug Delivery Systems," Workshop Sponsored
     by NICHD, Bethesda, Maryland, August 2-3, (1976).
3.   D.R. Cowsar, in: "Controlled Release of Biologically Active
     Agents," A.C. Tanquary and R.E. Lacey, eds., Plenum Press,
     New York, (1974). pp. 1-13.
4.   L.R. Beck, D.R. Cowsar, and V.Z. Pope, Research Frontiers in
     Fertility Regulation 1(1):1 (1980).
5.   J. Newton and J. McEwan, Fertil. Contracept. 1:35 (1977).

6. M. Haefeli, W. Zodraw, U.S. Spornitz, K.S. Ludwig, and A.
    Wetwillor, in: "Medicated IUDs and Polymeric Delivery Ststems:
    International Symposium," E.S.E. Hafez and W. Van Os, eds.,
    Abstract 3, June 27-30 (1979).
7. H.J. Tatum, Fertility and Sterility 28(1):3 (1977).
8. B.B. Pharris and P. Rowe, in: "Medicated IUDs and Polymeric
    Delivery Systems: International Symposium," E.S.E. Hafez and
    W. Van Os, eds., Abstract 4, June 27-30 (1979).
9. C.G. Nilsson, in: "Medicated IUDs and Polymeric Delivery
    Systems: International Symposium," E.S.E. Hafez and W. Van
    Os, eds., Abstract 7, June 27-30 (1979).
10. P.T. Piotrow, W. Rinehart, and J.C. Schmidt, Population Reports,
    Series B, No. 3 (1979).
11. W. Droegemuller and R. Bressler, Ann. Rev. Med. 31:329 (1980).
12. H.W. Rudel, F.A. Kind, and M.R. Henzl, in: "Birth Control-Con-
    traception and Abortion," H.W. Rudel, F.A. Kind, and M.R.
    Henzl, eds., Macmillan Company, New York, (1973). pp. 154-
    185.
13. R.W. Baker and H.K. Lonsdale, in: "Controlled Release of Bio-
    logically Active Agents," A.C. Tanuqary and R.E. Lacey, eds.,
    Plenum Press, New York (1975). pp. 15-71.
14. D.H. Lewis and D.R. Cowsar, in: "Controlled Release Pesticides,"
    H.B. Scher, ed., American Chemical Society. ACS Symposium
    Series, No. 53 (1977). pp. 1-16.

CONTROLLED RELEASE OF METRIBUZIN, 2,4-D, AND MODEL AROMATIC AMINES FROM POLYSACCHARIDES AND POLY(VINYL ALCOHOL)

C.L. McCormick, K.W. Anderson,
J.A. Pelezo, and D.K. Lichatowich

Department of Polymer Science
University of Southern Mississippi
Hattiesburg, MS 39401

INTRODUCTION

In our continuing investigations of polymeric controlled-release herbicides,[1-5] we report preliminary results on biodegradable polysaccharides and poly(vinyl alcohol) with pendent herbicides or model amines joined via carbamate or ester bonds. Studies of similar systems with polysaccharides or poly(vinyl alcohol) with pendent carboxy-functional herbicides have been reported.[6-9] Additionally Gebelein[10] has reviewed the reactions of poly(vinyl alcohol), including the reaction with phenyl isocyanate.

EXPERIMENTAL

Synthesis

The syntheses of polymeric herbicides from polysaccharides or from poly(vinyl alcohol) under homogeneous reaction conditions have been reported previously.[2,3,5] Polysaccharides included cellulose, chitin, amylose, and amylopectin. Reactive herbicide derivatives were the acid chloride of 2,4-dichlorophenoxyacetic acid (2,4-D) and the isocyanate derivative of 4-amino-6-tert-butyl-3-(methylthio)-as-triazin-5(4H)one (metribuzin).

$$(1)$$

$$(2)$$

The poly(vinyl alcohol) models with pendent carbamate bonds were prepared by first dissolving PVA while stirring at 70°C. After the solutions were cooled to room temperature, the model isocyanates were then added dropwise under nitrogen. A three-fold molar excess of isocyanate/hydroxyl groups was used to favor substitution. The reaction mixtures were stirred at ambient temperature for four hours to allow complete reaction. The resulting polymers were precipitated twice from suitable solvents (depending upon the derivative) and then dried under vacuum.

$$(3)$$

Characterization

The characterization data[2,3,5] for the synthesized polymers were obtained through a variety of techniques including infrared spectroscopy, membrane osmometry, and solution viscometry. Infrared spectra confirmed the existence of carbamate (1700-1707 cm^{-1}) or ester (1725-1730 cm^{-1}) linkage. Reduced viscosities, $\eta_{sp/c}$, at a concentration of 0.25 g/dl were determined in N,N-dimethylacet-amide/LiCl solutions.[3] Degrees of substitution were determined by an exhaustive hydrolysis method;[11] the weight percentage herbicide present in each polymer was then calculated. These values and reduced viscosities are reported in Table I.

Release Studies

Hydrolysis studies were conducted by placing 0.1 g of polymer in 50 ml of distilled water. At designated intervals, aliquots were withdrawn for analysis by high-pressure liquid chromatography. The column used was a Waters μ-Bondapak® C-18 reverse phase column and the mobile phase was 60/40 v/v acetonitrile/water. Dual ultraviolet detectors were used to measure absorbances; peak heights were compared to calibration curves to determine concentration of released compound. The apparent concentration of the herbicide or the model amine in the aqueous phase was plotted as a function of time for each of the polymers listed in Table I.

TABLE I.   PHYSICAL DATA FOR POLYMERIC CONTROLLED RELEASE HERBICIDES

Compound #	Structure	DS^a	$wt\%^b$	Reduced^c Viscosity	Release Figure
82 L15	CEL–OCR$_2$	0.7	49	0.32	1
90 L13	CHI–OCR$_2$	1.1	54	0.59	2
84 L17	AM–OCR$_2$	0.7	49	0.37	3
85 L23	AMP–OCR$_2$	1.2	61	0.58	4
100L8	AM–OCNHR$_1$	1.2	57	0.58	5
103L3	CHI–OCNHR$_1$	1.0	47	0.52	6
106L4	CHI–OCNHX$_1$NHCNHR$_1$	0.7	28	0.62	7
77–21c	PVA–OCNHR$_4$	0.5	51	–	8
77–21b	PVA–OCNHR$_3$	0.8	55	–	9

[a] degree of substitution = # pendent groups/ repeating unit
[b] weight percentage of herbicide or aromatic amine
[c] η_{sp}/c at 0.25 g/dl

CEL– cellulose
CHI – chitin
AM – amylose
AMP –amylopectin

RESULTS AND DISCUSSION

The polymers used in synthesis of the controlled-release systems listed in Table I exhibit a wide range of physical properties, despite the fact that each possesses hydroxyl functionality used for preparation of carbamate or ester derivatives. It can be assumed that the homogeneous solutions methods[3] (N,N-dimethylacetamide/LiCl) employed during synthesis should lead to more uniform substitution along the backbone than would heterogeneous methods. Degrees of substitution for the polymers range from 0.5 to 1.2 and the weight percentages of herbicides from 28 to 61%.

Interactions of the unmodified polymers with water should be noted prior to discussion of release rates. The beta 1→4 glycoside linkages in cellulose and chitin yield extended chain structures which form hydrogen bonds. Water is strongly adsorbed but apparently fails to penetrate the unmodified structure. Amylose and amylopectin, which possess alpha 1→4 glycoside linkages, swell in water, the latter being partially soluble because of branching. Poly(vinyl alcohol), prepared from hydrolysis of poly(vinyl acetate) has water solubility which is a function of degree of saponification and molecular weight.

Release profiles, showing measured cumulative concentration of released species with time, are given in Figures 1 through 9 for each of the polymeric herbicides; these are normalized for sample weight. A number of qualitative arguments based on physicochemical processes may be made to support each of the release profiles. Quantitative measurements, however, are complicated by side reactions, differential swelling, particle size, concentration factors, diffusion effects, surface effects, etc. Two competing reactions involving release of the pendent herbicide and its subsequent hydrolysis are obviously occurring in some systems.

Figures 1 through 4 show concentration profiles for cumulative release of 2,4-D from cellulose, chitin, amylose, and amylopectin, respectively. The herbicide is attached through ester linkages as shown in equation (1). Two general trends are observed. For the cellulose and chitin derivatives, the cumulative concentration of 2,4-D passes through a maximum, because of simultaneous processes. First, the surface groups are hydrolyzed, leaving behind the original, non-swellable, structures of cellulose and chitin. As the surface concentration is reduced, the underlying pendent groups become less accessible. Second, the released herbicide then decomposes, and the concentration of the herbicide in solution decreases.

In the cases of amylose and amylopectin derivatives, the polymers become more water-swellable as hydrolysis proceeds; more groups

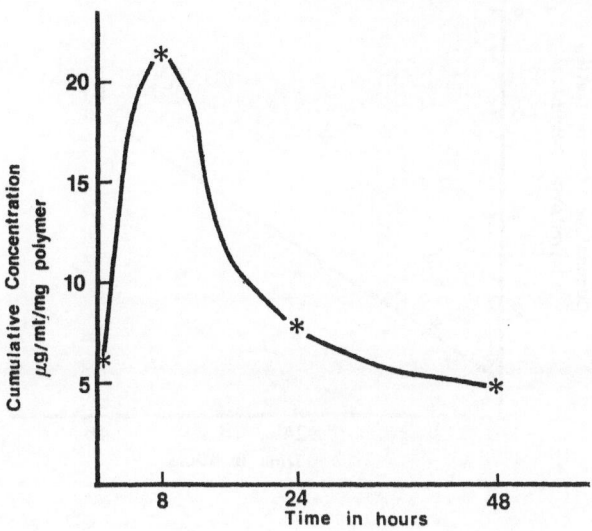

Figure 1.   Release of 2,4-D from CEL–O$\overset{\text{O}}{\overset{\|}{\text{C}}}R_2$

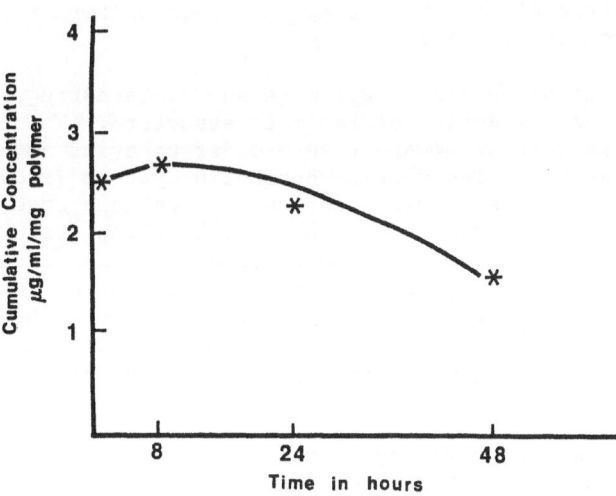

Figure 2.   Release of 2,4-D from CHI–O$\overset{\text{O}}{\overset{\|}{\text{C}}}R_2$

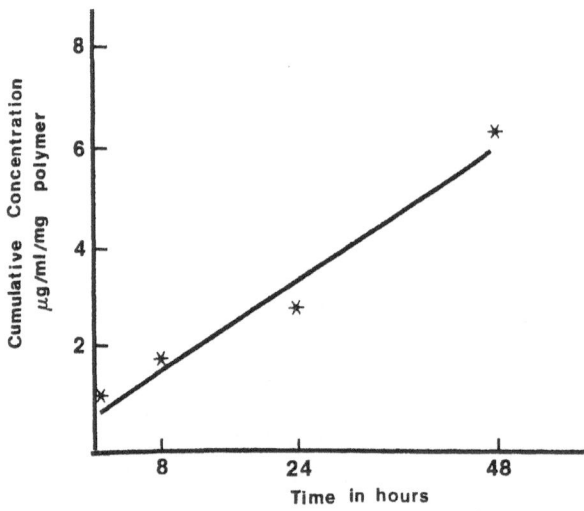

Figure 3.   Release of 2,4-D from AM-OCR$_2$ (with $\overset{O}{\overset{\|}{C}}$)

on the interior become accessible. Such phenomena could even lead
to autoacceleration. Apparently, released herbicide degradation
negates the latter effect, resulting in rather uniform release re-
sembling zero-order kinetics.

The metribuzin-containing polymers show interesting profiles
(Figures 5, 6, and 7) again relatable to structure. The amylose-
metribuzin polymer shows apparent zero-order behavior as did the
amylose-2,4-D system. The chitin-metribuzin systems (Figures 6
and 7) show pseudo first-order kinetics with release rate faster
than that of herbicide decomposition. The leveling effect observed·
is, however, consistent with the model of decreasing surface concentration and accessibility. From Figures 6 and 7 it may be assumed
that metribuzin degradation by hydrolysis is low over the time frame
of the study. It would be expected that for a longer time an
eventual downturn in the observed solution concentration would be
observed.

Model systems of poly(vinyl alcohol) have been prepared to
measure the effects of substituents on hydrolysis rate. Figures 8
and 9 are profiles for the release of p-chloroaniline and p-toluidine
from PVA carbamate systems. These polymers, prepared as shown by
equation (3), show almost constant rates over the period of study.
These closely resemble the behavior of the amylose-metribuzin polymer—a result expected due to the similar solubility characteristics
of PVA and amylose in water.

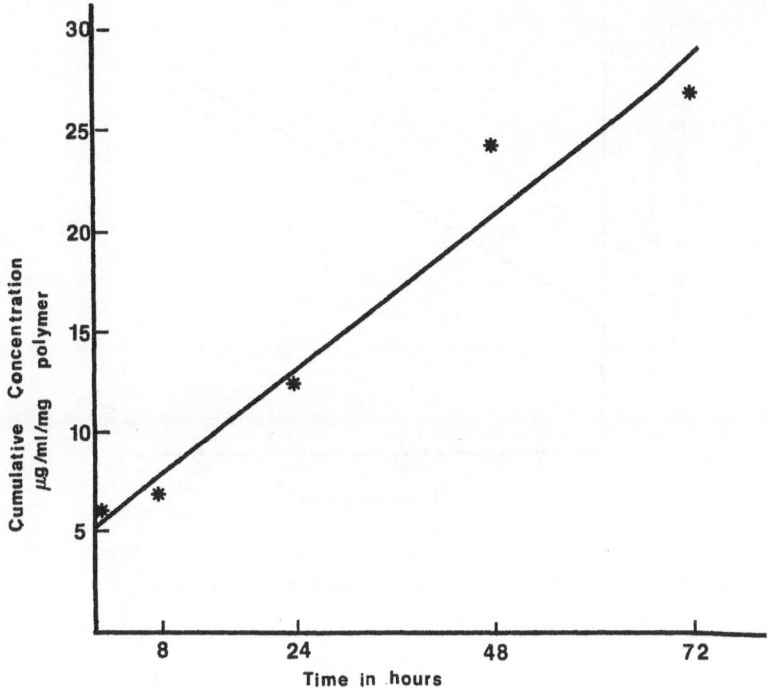

Figure 4.   Release of 2,4-D from AMP-OĊR$_2$ (with O double-bonded above C)

An attempt to predict cumulative release profiles can be made based on two competing processes as outlined in equation (4).

$$\text{P-H} \xrightarrow{k_1} \text{P} + \text{H} \xrightarrow{k_2} \text{DECOMPOSITION PRODUCTS} \qquad (4)$$

P-H represents the polymeric herbicide, H the released herbicide, k_1 and k_2 the rate constants for release and decomposition of the herbicide, respectively. If we assume pseudo first-order rates of release and decomposition (likely with large concentrations of water), then the ratio of the cumulative concentration of herbicide in solution, C_H, to the original concentration of pendent groups, $C_{\text{P-H}_O}$ at time t is given by equation (5).

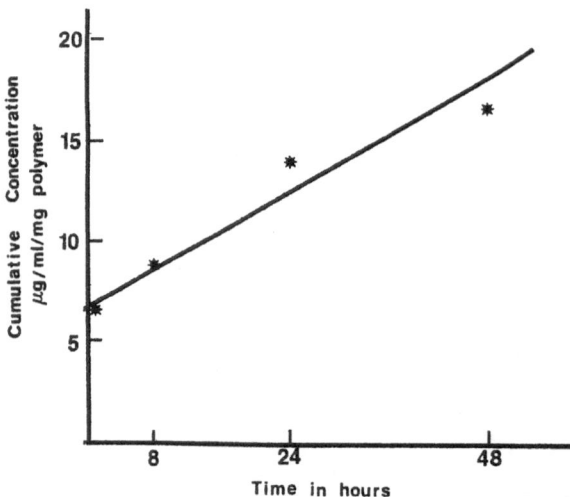

Figure 5.   Release of metribuzin from AM–OCNHR$_1$

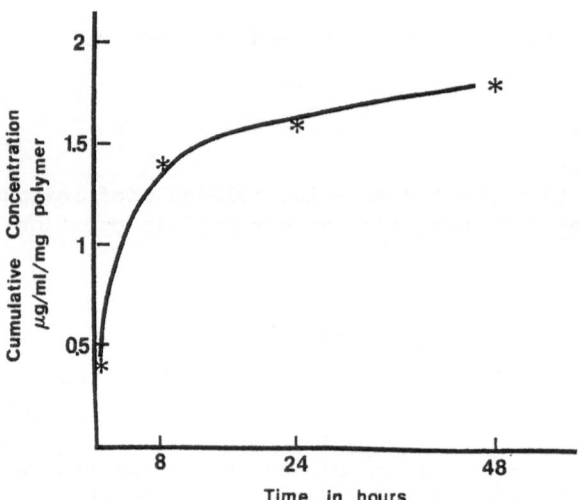

Figure 6.   Release of metribuzin from CHI–OCNHR$_1$

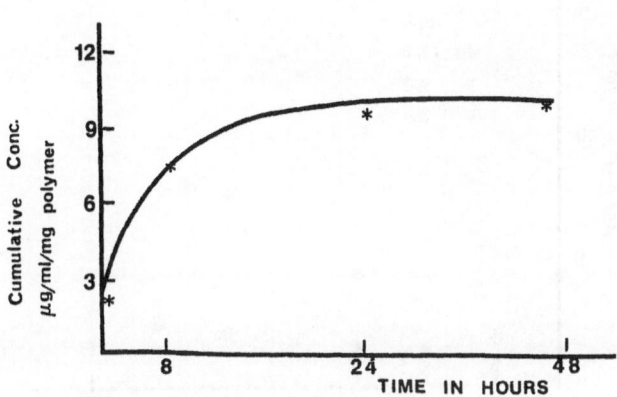

Figure 7.   Release of metribuzin from $CHI-O-\overset{O}{\overset{\|}{C}}-NH-X_1-NH-\overset{O}{\overset{\|}{C}}-NHR_1$

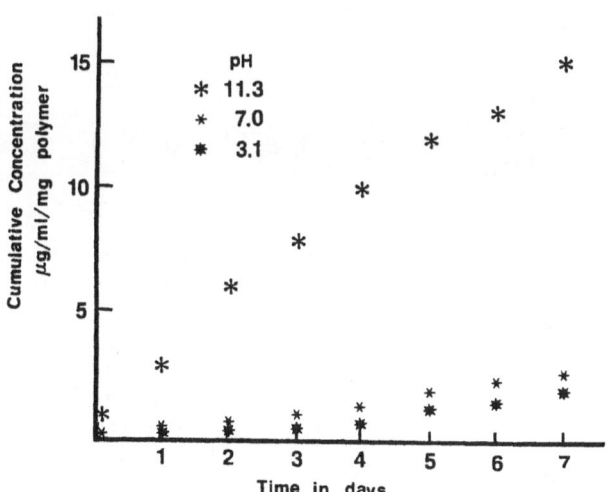

Figure 8.   Release of p-chloraniline from $PVA-O\overset{O}{\overset{\|}{C}}NHR_4$

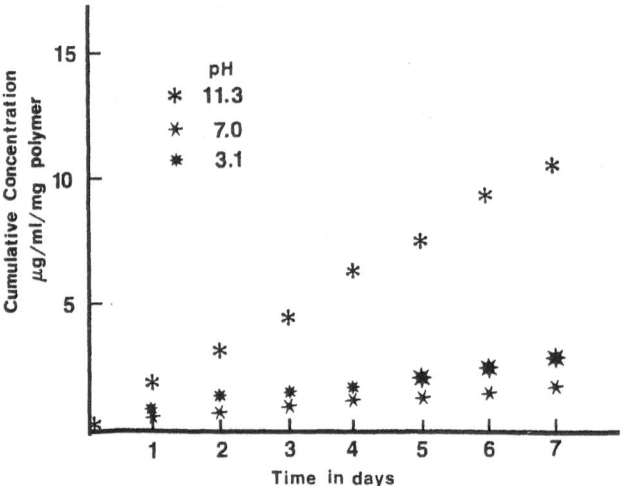

Figure 9.   Release of p-toluidine from PVA-OCNHR₃

$$\frac{C_H}{C_{PH_0}} = \frac{k_1}{k_2 - k_1} \left[e^{-k_1 t} - e^{-k_2 t} \right]$$

(5)

If $k_1 \gg k_2$, the herbicide concentration observed in solution will depend mainly upon the release; if $k_2 > k_1$, then very little herbicide can accumulate. Figure 10 illustrates theoretical curves based on k_2/k_1 values ranging from 0 to 10 for the plot of C_H/C_{p-H_0} vs $k_1 t$. For short time periods and large values of k_1 relative to k_2 ($k_2/k_1 \approx 0$), a relatively linear portion of the curve would be seen. At longer times for ($k_2/k_1 \approx 0$), a leveling effect would be observed. For ($k_2/k_1 = 0.1$) a decrease in the cumulative concentration is observed at extended times. Finally, as k_2 becomes large relative to k_1 an abrupt shift in the curve occurs, leading to a distinct maximum followed by a slow decrease in concentration with time.

Each model polymer system synthesized for this work shows a release profile which can be predicted theoretically by equation

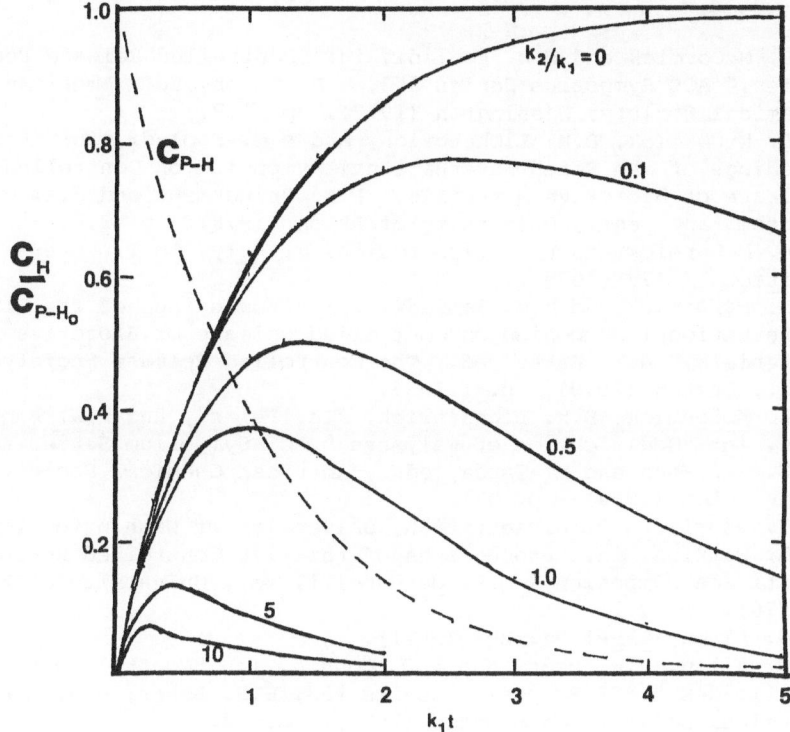

Figure 10.   Concentration profiles for H from equation (5) using
various values of k_2/k_1.

(5).   Such predictions would likely be inaccurate because of local
concentration effects at the reaction site brought about by solubility changes in the polymer.   In some systems, first-order
kinetics would not hold.   Additionally, factors such as diffusion,
neighboring groups effects, etc. must be considered in each instance.
Further studies of this type (on carefully prepared model systems)
are underway in our laboratories.

ACKNOWLEDGEMENTS

        Support for portions of the above research by the NOAA Sea
Grant Program and Hopkins Agricultural Chemical Company is gratefully acknowledged.

REFERENCES

1. C.L. McCormick and M.M. Fooladi, in: "Controlled Release Pesti-
    cides," ACS Symposium Series #53, H.B. Scher, Ed., American
    Chemical Society, Washington (1977). p. 112.
2. C.L. McCormick, D.K. Lichatowich, and M.M. Fooladi, in: "Pro-
    ceedings of the Fifth International Symposium on Controlled-
    Release of Bioactive Materials," F.E. Brinckmann and J.A.
    Montemarano, eds., University of Akron (1978). p. 3.6.
3. C.L. McCormick and D.K. Lichatowich, J. Poly. Sci. Letters
    Edition 17:479 (1979).
4. C.L. McCormick and M.M. Fooladi, in: "Proceedings of the Sixth
    International Symposium on Controlled Release of Bioactive
    Materials," R.W. Baker, ed., The Controlled Release Society,
    Inc., Dayton (1979). p. III-27.
5. C.L. McCormick, D.K. Lichatowich, J.A. Pelezo, and K.W. Ander-
    son, in: "Modification of Polymers," ACS Symposium Series #121,
    C.E. Carraher and M. Tsuda, eds., American Chemical Society,
    Washington (1980). p. 371.
6. A.N. Neogi, Ph.D. Dissertation, University of Washington (1970).
7. R.M. Wilkins, in: "Proceedings of the 1976 Controlled Release
    Pesticide Symposium," N.F. Cardarelli, ed., University of Akron
    (1976). p. 7.1.
8. G.G. Allan, TAPPI 54:1293 (1971).
9. G.G. Allan, J.W. Beer, and M.J. Cousin, in: "Controlled Release
    Pecticides," ACS Symposium Series #53, H.B. Scher, ed., American
    Chemical Society, Washington (1977). p. 94.
10. C.G. Gebelein and K.E. Burnfield, in: "Modification of
    Polymers," ACS Symposium Series #131, C.E. Carraher and M.
    Tsuda, eds., American Chemical Society, Washington (1980).
    p. 83.
11. J.A. Pelezo, Ph.D. Dissertation, University of Southern Mis-
    sissippi, (1979).
12. O. Levenspiel, in: "Chemical Reaction Engineering," 2nd ed.,
    John Wiley and Sons, New York (1972). pp. 58-62, 177-178.

SYNTHESIS AND PROPERTIES OF UREA FORMALDEHYDE

RESINS GENERATING 2,6-DICHLOROBENZONITRILE

Etienne H. Schacht, Guido E. Desmarets,
and Eric J. Goethals

State University of Gent
Laboratory of Organic Chemistry
Krijgslaan 271 (S-4), B-9000
Gent, Belgium

INTRODUCTION

One approach to the design of pesticide formulations with controlled-release properties is the combination of the biocide with polymers. This concept has been discussed in detail in various review articles. A large variety of polymers has been used for this purpose, among them urea formaldehyde resins.[1-3] The urea formaldehyde resins have certain benefits as carrier systems for biocides. Besides the relatively low cost, they are known to degrade slowly when applied to the soil[4] and so have been proposed as slow-release nutrients for horticultural crops.[5] The urea-formaldehyde prepolymer contains reactive groups and consequently, apart from physical combinations, chemical combinations with pesticides having appropriate functional groups may be prepared as well.

We have been using urea formaldehyde systems for the preparation of formulations generating 2,6-dichlorobenzonitrile (I).

2,6-dichlorobenzonitrile
"dichlobenil"
(I)

2,6-dichlorothiobenzamide
"chlorthiamid"
(II)

(N-methylol)-2,6-dichloro-
thiobenzamide
(III)

2,6-Dichlorobenzonitrile, ordinarily called "dichlobenil", is a
herbicidal compound having a high control effect[6] to many annual
weeds and some perennial weeds and is widely applied. Dichlobenil,
however, is highly volatile and has a high mobility in the soil,
which involves risk of phytotoxicity. Application to paddy fields
is hardly applied because of strong phytotoxic effects when used
in quantities sufficient to provide an effective concentration for
killing weeds. In order to overcome these defects "prodrugs" of
dichlobenil have been developed. 2,6-Dichlorothiobenzamide (II,
called "chlorthiamide")[7] and its N-methylol derivative (III)[8] are
advantageously used as dichlobenil generators, but these compounds
too have similar defects as described before with respect to dichlobenil.

We considered that the above mentioned defects could be reduced
or eventually eliminated if an appropriate controlled-release formulation could be prepared. Urea formaldehyde resin was selected
as the carrier system for reasons mentioned before. The obtained
formulations were subjected to release experiments in laboratory
assays as well as to biological evaluations in greenhouse tests.

RESULTS AND DISCUSSION

The formulations were made by suspending the finely powdered
pesticide into a concentrated urea formaldehyde prepolymer, subsequent acidification with orthophosphoric acid, and curing for
two days at 50°C at reduced pressure. The resulting reaction product was ground and divided into fractions of different size range
by sieving. The content of active ingredient in the finally obtained formulation was determined by chlorine analysis. Concentrations up to 30% could be prepared.

It was found that the content of the effective ingredient is
influenced by the sieving procedure. More specifically it was observed by electron microscopy (Figures 1 and 2) that dichlobenil
particles adhering to the surface of the powdered product were removed under violent vibration, resulting in a reduction of the
content of the reactive ingredient. This finding has to be taken
into account in preparing reproducable samples.

In order to gain information about the release characteristics
of the various formulations, samples of known particle size were
immersed in distilled water (pH = 6,8), and the amount of herbicide
released was determined spectrophotometrically. The results for
a set of dichlobenil formulations of different particle size are
given in Figure 3. It is evident from these data that the release
rate, from urea formaldehyde formulations, is lower than that for
the commercial dichlobenil granula and decreases with increasing

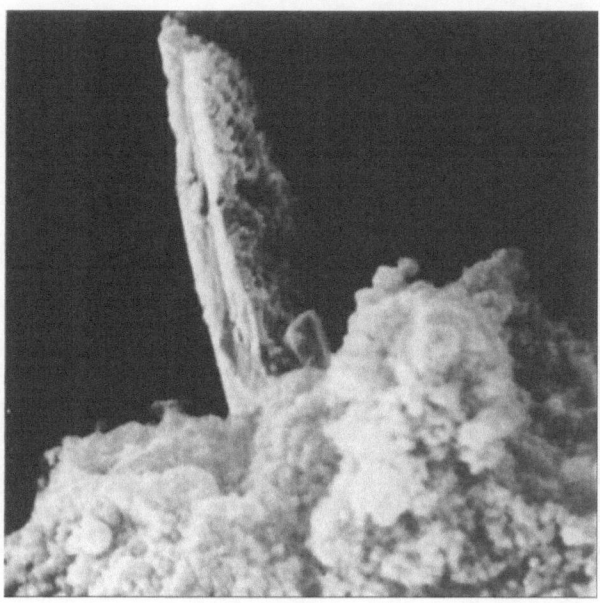

Figure 1.   Electron micrograph (X5750) of an urea formaldehyde
            formulation of dichlobenil, before sieving, showing a
            dichlobenil particle adhering to the surface.

particle size. Similar laboratory assays were carried out for the
urea formaldehyde formulations of II and III. The results are shown
on Figure 4. The rate at which the dichlobenil generators are released is considerably lower than that for dichlobenil.

     In the case of dichlobenil the linkage with the urea formal-
dehyde polymer is only physical, whereas for chlorthiamid and its
methylol derivative chemical linkage is likely to occur and may
account for the slower rate of release. It is generally accepted
that the condensation reactions of the urea formaldehyde prepolymer,
which consists of methylolurea derivatives, when occurring in acidic
medium, are bimolecular reactions between hydroxymethyl groups and
an amide group with formation of methylene linkages:

$$\sim\!\!\overset{\displaystyle O}{\overset{\|}{C}}\!-NH-CH_2OH \;+\; H_2N-\overset{\displaystyle O}{\overset{\|}{C}}\!\!\sim \quad\xrightarrow[-H_2O]{H^+}\quad \sim\!\!\overset{\displaystyle O}{\overset{\|}{C}}\!-NH-CH_2-NH-\overset{\displaystyle O}{\overset{\|}{C}}\!\!\sim$$

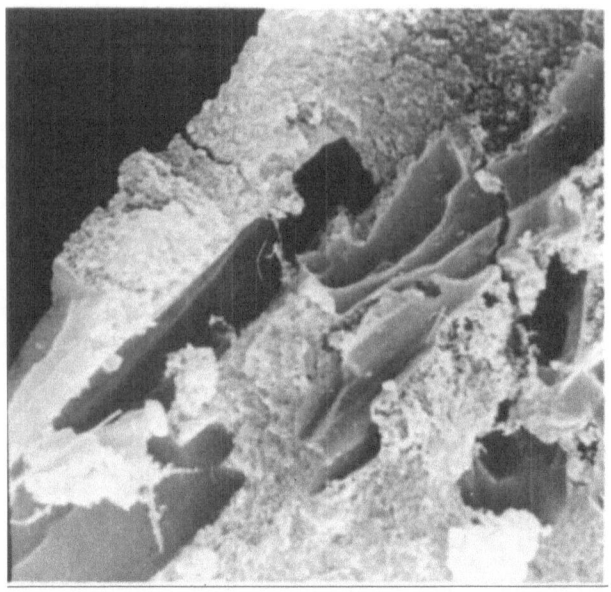

Figure 2.   A typical electron micrograph (X1200) of a urea
            formaldehyde formulation of dichlobenil after seaving.
            Note the holes in outer surface due to removal of
            dichlobenil particles under violent vibration.

Therefore it is most likely that in this medium the thioamid function of II as well as the methylol group of III can get involved,
leading to covalent binding of the pesticide into the resin.

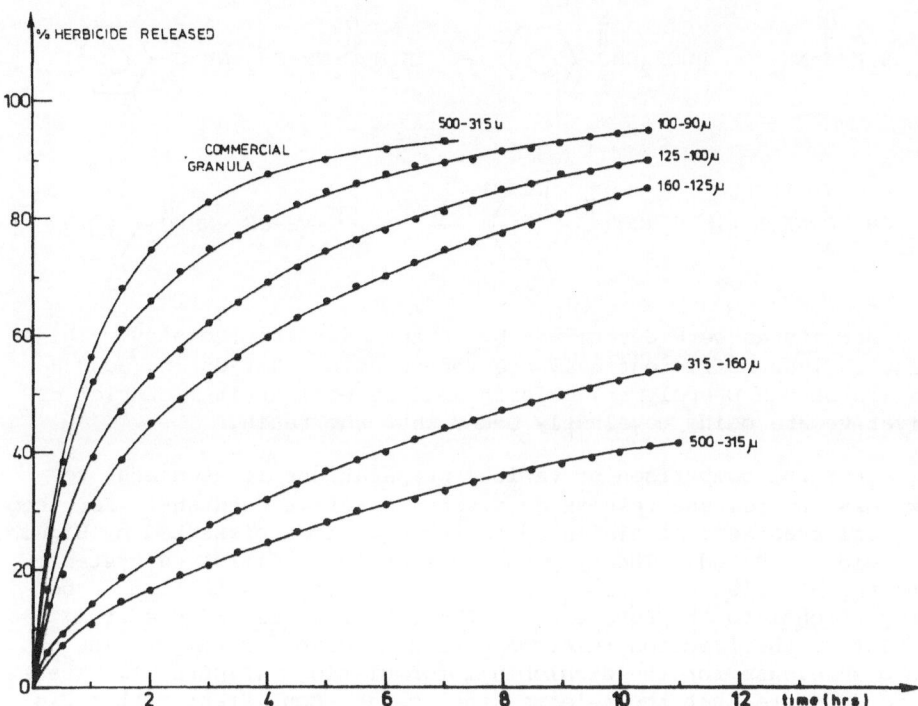

Figure 3.   Time-release curves for dichlobenil-urea formaldehyde
            formulations of varying particle size, obtained in
            water at 25°C.

        It was found that by continuous extraction of formulations
of II and III only part of the active ingredient could be recovered.
The amount extracted depends on the initial ratio formaldehyde:
urea, the time and temperature of the condensation reaction, and
the curing procedure; e.g.: for the formulations P-UF and MP-UF
mentioned in Figure 4, 80%, respectively, less than 1% could be
recovered by extraction. In addition, on reaction of urea with
III and of N-methylol acetamide with II in acidic aqueous medium
the expected condensation product was isolated as the main reaction
product:

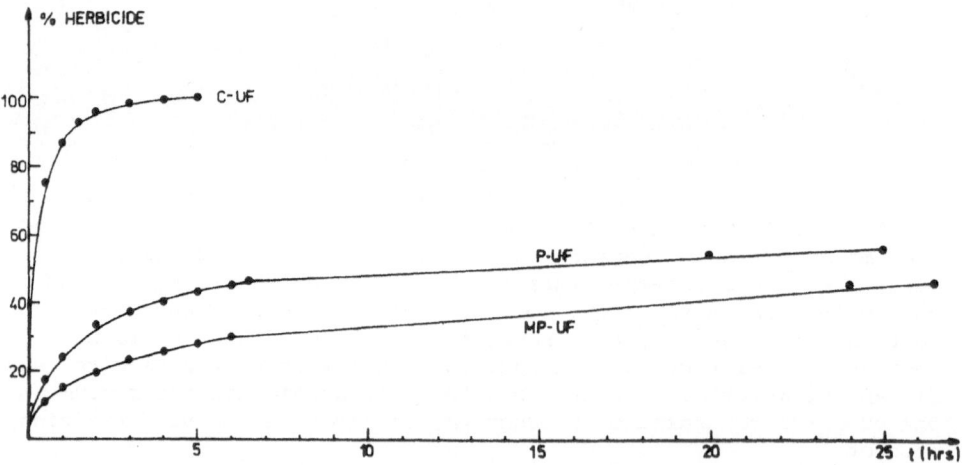

The structures were determined by IR and mass spectrometry. This result gives sufficient evidence for assuming that during condensation of the prepolymer, chlorthiamid as well as its methylol derivative are being covalently bound into the resin.

For the comparison of various preparations it is useful to express the release results by a representative constant. For theoretical treatment of similar data the equations presented by Higuchi are widely quoted. Theory predicts that for a dissolved system the amount released would increase exponentially with time or be proportional to the square root of time for a dispersed system. A plot of the fraction released versus t gave a straight line up to 50% release for the dichlobenil formulations (Figure 5). These data indicate that the release kinetics are consistent with a dispersed monolithic-type release system.

Figure 4.   Comparison of the rate of release of dichlobenil (C-UF), chlorthiamid (P-UF), and its methylol derivative (MP-UF) from urea formaldehyde resins (63-90 μ) in water at 60°C.

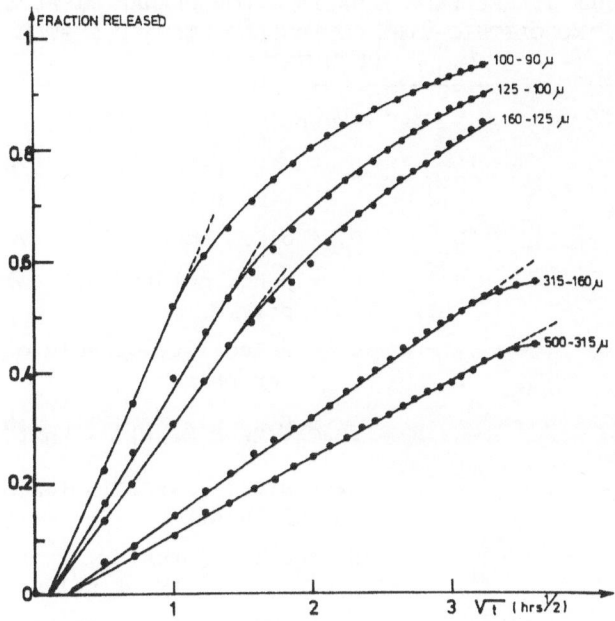

Figure 5. Plot of the fraction released versus $t^{\frac{1}{2}}$ for release experiments of dichlobenil-urea formaldehyde formulations (15 weight % active ingredient) of varying particle size in water at 25°C.

Higuchi derived equations[10] describing the release from monolithic delivery systems for several shapes including planar, cylindrical, and spherical. For each device the membrane may be either non-porous, the rate being controlled by diffusion of the solute through the polymer matrix, or porous, the rate being controlled by the solubility of the active ingredient in the leaching solvent. The equations for cylindrical as well as for spherical devices are extremely complex. For simplicity the equations derived for planar systems were taken as good approximation. The corresponding equations for planar systems are as shown in Table I. The influence of solvent strength on the release characteristics has been used before by Noren et al.[3] (on ureaform microcapsules) as a criterion to distinguish porous from non-porous structures.

Release experiments were carried out on dichlobenil formulations in various methanol-water systems. It was found that an increase of the methanol content in the solvent system results in an increase in the rate of release (Table II), because of the increased solubility of dichlobenil in the solvent systems with increasing concentration of methanol. The dependence of the rate

TABLE I.   RELEASE EQUATIONS FOR PLANAR DISPERSION
MONOLITHIC-TYPE CONTROLLED-RELEASE SYSTEM
(T. HIGUCHI)

Non-Porous

$$Q = [D_m C_p (2A - C_p) t]^{\frac{1}{2}} = k_H' \, t^{\frac{1}{2}}$$

Q = tot. release/unit area at time t

D_m = diff. coeff. in polymer

A = conc. solute/unit volume in polymer matrix

C_p = solubility of solute in polymer phase

Porous:

$$Q = [D_f C_s \frac{\varepsilon}{\tau} (2A - \varepsilon \, C_s) t]^{\frac{1}{2}} = k_H \, t^{\frac{1}{2}}$$

D_f = diff. coeff. in leaching solvent

ε and τ = porosity, resp. tortuosity of polymer matrix

C_s = solubility in solvent

TABLE II.   COMPARISON OF THE HIGUCHI CONSTANTS (k)
OF DICHLOBENIL FORMULATIONS WITH PARTICLE SIZE
AND SOLUBILITY IN WATER/METHANOL SYSTEMS AT 25°C

Particle Size (μ)	$k_{(H)}$ [a] (hrs $^{-\frac{1}{2}}$)	% Water	Solubility (g/l)
90-100	0.56		
100-125	0.41		
125-160	0.34	100	0.033
160-315	0.18		
	0.14		
	0.28	75	0.12
	0.45	50	0.59
315-500	0.98	25	3.82
	1.44	15	6.88
	3.90	0	22.93

[a] $k_{(H)}$ is the slope of the linear stage of a plot of the fraction - released versus $\sqrt{t}$ (linearity up to ±50%).

of release on solvent indicates that the dichlobenil formulations produced in our work have a porous structure. The release data obtained for the formulations of chlorthiamid and its methylol derivative did not fit the Higuchi equations. For those preparations chemical reactions are involved in the release mechanism and complicate the overall release behavior.

Evaluation of the Pesticidal Activity

The presently described formulations were subjected to greenhouse screenings. In order to evaluate the residual activity in the soil a conventional bioassay was set up. Radish seeds were sown, at a rate of 15 seeds per pot, some immediately and others 10 days, 18 days or 28 days after application of the herbicide. When 20 days had passed from sowing, above-ground parts of radish were cut down and the fresh weight was measured and compared to that obtained in untreated control area. For comparison a commercial wettable powder of the non-formulated herbicide was tested in the same manner. The results are shown in Table III.

TABLE III.   RESIDUAL ACTIVITY IN SOIL

Herbicidal[a]		Dosage (kg/ha)	Fresh Weight %[b]			
			0 days[c]	10 days	18 days	28 days
Dichlobenil	U.F.	1	7,3	44,0	55,3	75,8
		3	0	12,5	26,4	50,4
	W.P.	1	8,0	83,8	100	100
		3	0	32,4	53,7	69,5
Chlorthiamid	U.F.	1	4,0	26,0	36,9	70,0
		3	0	0	5,5	15,9
	W.P.	1	8	83,8	100	100
		3	0	32,4	53,7	69,5
N-Methylol derivative	U.F.	1	12,7	44,8	83,8	100
		3	1,3	28,6	50,2	65,5

[a] U.F. = urea formaldehyde formulation (100-200 μ); W.P. = wettable powder.

[b] Fresh weight of above ground parts of radish 20 days after sowing, compared with untreated check.

[c] Sowing occurred resp. 0, 10, 18, or 28 days after treatment.

As seen from these results, the urea formaldehyde formulations of dichlobenil and of chlorthiamid have an improved residual activity when compared with the conventional wettable powder. The formulations of the methylol derivative, however, gave rather poor results, which may be explained by a too slow rate of release. It should be pointed out that, in the formulations used in this test, the amount of active ingredient being chemically fixed to the resin was 80% for chlorthiamid (II) and 100% for the methylol derivative (III). Additional tests of the dichlobenil formulations on artemisia (wormwood) showed a prolonged residual effect. In contrast with treatment with dichlobenil granulas, no regrowth was observed even 40 days after treatment (Table IV).

In using wettable powders of dichlobenil as comparative herbicide in paddy fields, considerable phytotoxicity to rice plants was already observed at a dosage not sufficient to bring about complete kill of the weeds. However, as evidenced by the results reported in Table V with urea formaldehyde formulations, weeds can be controlled completely with no phytotoxicity.

CONCLUSION

Incorporation of dichlobenil into urea formaldehyde resins leads to formulations with prolonged residual activity. The rate of release can be varied by changing the particle size. Combination of the dichlobenil generators chlorthiamid and its methylol

TABLE IV. CONTROLLING EFFECT ON WORMWOOD

Herbicide	Dosage (kg/ha)	Control Effect	
		17th day	40th day
Dichlobenil-U.F.	1.5	9	9.5
	3	10	10
Dichlobenil granule (6,7%)	1.5	8	6 regrowth
	3	9	7

Practical experiment:

- Wormwood sterns of 4-cm length planted:
- after growing for 33 days: above ground parts cut off;
- 3 days later: + formulation;
- regrowth evaluated on 17th and 40th day.   0 = no effect
                                            10 = complete
                                                 kill

TABLE V.   PHOTOTOXICITY TO RICE PLANTS

| Herbicide | Dosage (kg/ha) | Control Effect | | | Phytotoxicity to Rice Plant |
		Sagittaria pygmaea	Bulrush	Barnyard Grass	
DBN-U.F.	0.3	10	10	10	0
	1	10	10	10	0
DBN-W.P.	0.3	3	6	8	1.5
	1	9.5	9	9.5	3

- soil containing seeds of bulrush and barnyard grass placed on fertilizer incorporated soil.
- 2 leaved stage seedlings of rice plant and tubers of Sagittaria pygmaea transplanted.
- soil irrigated in water (4 cm depth).
- suspension of pesticide added.
- evaluation 25 days after treatment: 0 = no effect
                                          10 = total kill

derivative with urea formaldehyde polymers shows an even more re-tarded release. Greenhouse experiments confirmed the laboratory evaluations and demonstrated a reduced phytotoxicity of the urea formaldehyde formulations towards rice plants.

EXPERIMENTAL

Materials

    Dichlobenil and chlorthiamid were obtained as analytical grade products from the Duphar Company (The Netherlands). The methylol derivative of chlorthiamid was prepared as described by Wyma et al.[11]

Synthesis of the Urea Formaldehyde Formulations

    As an example the urea formaldehyde formulations of dichlobenil were prepared as follows: a 500-ml 2-neck flask equipped with a stirrer and a condensor was charged with 30 g (0.5 mole) of urea and 65 g (0.7 mole) of a 38% aqueous solution of formaldehyde in which the pH value was adjusted to 7.5 by addition of sodium hy-droxide. The mixture was refluxed under agitation for two hours, and 15 ml of water was removed by distillation under reduced pres-sure. Then 20 g (0.12 mol) of finely powdered dichlobenil was added to the obtained viscous syrup at 60°C and 1.5 ml of 05% phosphoric acid was added. The resulting gel was isolated and further heated for 48 hours at 50°C under reduced pressure. The dried resin was pulverized and sieved.

Release Experiments

In 400 ml of water was dispersed 10 mg of the formulation, and the dispersion was stirred at a constant speed of 200 rpm. The dispersion was sampled at predetermined intervals and filtered. The amount of herbicide release was determined by U.V.

ACKNOWLEDGEMENT

The authors thank Nissan Chemical Industries Ltd. for performing the bioassays of the formulations.

REFERENCES

1. R.J. Geary, U.S. Patent 3,223,513; 3,074,845 (1965).
2. G. Matson, U.S. Patent 3,516,941 (1970).
3. .G. Noren, G. Korpi, G. England, J. Appl. Pol. Sci. 24:2369 (1979).
4. S. Katz and C. Fassbender, J. Agr. Food. Chem. 14:336 (1966).
5. D. Maynard and O. Lorenz, Vegetable Crops Series 196 (1978).
6. H. Koopman and J. Daams, Nature (London) 186:89 (1960).
7. Shell Research Letd., Belg. Pat. 612,252 (1962), C.A. 58:3362 (1963).
8. J. van Daalen, J. Daams, H. Koopman, and A. Tempel, Rec. Trav. Chim. 86(11):1159 (1967).
9. J. de Jong and J. de Jonge, Rec. Trav. Chim. 72:139 (1953).
10. T. Higuchi, J. Pharm. Sci. 52:1145 (1963).
11. J. Wyma, J. van Daalen, N. Daams, and F. van Deursen, J. Agr. Food Chem. 18(4):674 (1970).

POLYMERS CONTAINING PENDENT INSECTICIDES

William E. Meyers and Danny H. Lewis

Southern Research Institute
2000 Ninth Avenue South
Birmingham, Alabama 35255

Robert K. Vander Meer and Clifford S. Lofgren

USDA-SEA/AR
Gainesville, Florida 32604

INTRODUCTION

The Fire Ant Problem

The fire ants <u>Solenopis invicta</u> and <u>Solenopsis richteri</u>, were accidentally imported into the United States from South America through the port of Mobile, Alabama. Present evidence indicates that <u>richteri</u> was introduced about 1918, and its spread has been only moderately successful during the succeeding 62 years. At the present time, <u>richteri</u> infestation is limited to a small region of northern Alabama and Mississippi. In contrast to this, <u>Solenopsis invicta</u> has been extremely successful at establishing itself in the southeastern United States. Since its introduction in the mid 1940s, this species has expanded its range to nine southern states encompassing more than 50-million hectares of land.[1] This phenomenal rate of spread is accounted for by two factors. The natural spread of the ants via mating flights is ideally suited to avoid inhibition by natural and man-made barriers.[2-4] Mating takes place in swarms which have a minimum altitude of 500 feet above the ground. Following mating, a queen may alight miles from her home nest. A second major factor in the rapid spread of the ants has been the influence of transport by man. Commercial movements of nursery stock and sod during the 1940s and 1950s, prior

to the institution of quarantine procedures, greatly aided the
introduction of the ants into uninfested regions.

The spread of the fire ant has been slowed somewhat by the
natural limitations of its present environment. In those regions
where the ants have met desert conditions or cold winters, extreme
environmental conditions have clearly slowed their advance. However, considering how well the South American ant has adapted to
the southern United States and the lack of competition from indige-
nous species, the ants may well overcome these limitations. Theoretical models derived from the present rate of spread of the ants
across Texas have predicted that the ant could reach California
in as little as six years.[6] This model did not consider the potential for accidental introduction of the ant into the Pacific coast
states.

At present, the northern movement of the ants has been mostly
along the temperate regions of the Atlantic coast in the Carolinas,
and no clear evidence of adaptations to colder climates has been
presented. Failure to hibernate results in significant depletion
of ant numbers during the winter months, and a cyclic pattern of
expansion and contraction of ant numbers is observed even in Florida.
This pattern correlates with the severity of the winter conditions
in that state.[7] However, modifying its behavior or mound structure
or taking advantage of nesting sites near or within man-made structures could conceivably allow the ant to expand into colder regions.

Attempts to blunt the invasion of fire ants have taken two
forms: eradication programs designed to eliminate the pest in infested areas and quarantine regulations directed at limiting the
spread of fire ants beyond their present habitat. The eradication
program has been fraught with problems since its inception. The
primary obstacle to this effort has been in identifying an environmentally acceptable approach to fire ant control. At times this
work has been near abandonment.[8] Early approaches relied on hep-
tachlor and dieldrin as the primary toxicants, but with the dis-
covery of kepone and later mirex[9,10] in the late 1950s, the eradication effort appeared promising. Several effective formulations
employing mirex were tested.[10-20] Many of these employed a soybean
oil bait to encourage ingestion by the ant.[14,18,19,21] Ultimately,
however, mirex and its analogs were found to be environmentally
unacceptable.[22-32] The registration of mirex was revoked in 1971
with limited exceptions.[33] Since this time, the fire ant eradication efforts have been mainly limited to identifying and testing
compounds to replace mirex in the program. To date, the USDA Gainesville laboratory (USDA-SEAAR) has assayed over 5000 formulations
for potential use in the eradication effort with limited success.
Only a few agents have shown acceptability in the laboratory tests,
but with the exception of several now being field tested[34] all have
been unacceptable for use in large-scale control programs.[35-39]

The fire ant quarantine was instituted in 1956. It basically
consists of controls imposed on suppliers who ship soil, agricultural products, nursery stock, or sod from areas designated as
infested to other regions of the country.[22] Like the eradication
program, the quarantine has experienced difficulty in the availability of effective toxicants. Dieldrin and aldrin have been used
in the past as agents for this purpose. In recent years the quarantine has relied on the chlorinated cyclodienes, chlordane and hep-
tachlor, with adequate success. However, since 1975, the EPA has
sought to restrict the use of these compounds. The use of chlordane
and heptachor was terminated in December of 1979.

The efforts to control the spread of the fire ant arise mainly
as a consequence of two considerations: the economic effect of
fire ant infestations in crop land and the health hazard posed by
the presence of the ant in populated regions.

Agricultural damage arising from fire ant infestation is difficult to assess due to the diverse nature of the losses. Fire ants
are reported to feed on seedlings, germinating seed, and flowers,
and they sting livestock and agricultural personnel. Particularly
vulnerable to fire ant predation are ground-nesting birds, newborn
livestock, and beneficial arthropods. Damage to farm machinery
is encountered when the equipment strikes the mounds. This results
in frequent cleaning and repairs as well as increasing the likelihood that workers will be stung while performing these operations.[1,4,41-43] A significant loss of productivity of hay and grazing
land is associated with heavy infestations. Farm laborors often
demand higher wages to work heavily infested fields, and in some
cases they refuse to enter the fields at all.[44] Numerous other
accounts of damage attributable to fire ants have been recorded
without adequate substantiation.

There have been instances reported in which fire ants are
reputed to have beneficial effects such as their predation upon
sugar cane borers, boll weevils, and lone star ticks.[45,46] It is
difficult to determine if the fire ants are filling a role that
had not been performed by other predatory species prior to the
introduction of the fire ant. Most of the data concern pest populations in infested areas with or without the application of pesticides employed to combat the fire ant. It is to be expected that
many beneficial predators were already displaced from these regions
by the fire ant. There is substantial evidence that this type of
displacement occurs when fire ants enter a new region.[47,48] While
it is difficult to place a dollar figure on fire ant damage in the
agricultural arena, at least one survey (commissioned by Allied
Chemical) placed that figure at $48 million in 1972 and further
estimated the net loss in land value at that time to be $500
million.[1]

The difficulties encountered in controlling the imported fire ant stem from the social characteristics of the species coupled with its exceptionally high rate of spread. The primary social characteristic which contributes to the difficulty of chemical control is the method of food distribution found in the colony. All food encountered by the foraging members of the colony is distributed to the other members by trophyllaxis. The food is passed by regurgitation through a chain of intermediates to the queen and brood. Ants showing abnormal behavior patterns or signs of toxicity are effectively excluded from the chain. Since rapid-acting pesticides never reach the queen, they cannot effectively destroy the reproductive capacity of the nest. Other factors contributing to the difficulty of control are the following:

The mode and frequency of infestation by mating flights.

The rapid development of the colonies.

The absence of effective competitors.

The omnivorous nature of the species.

The ability of a solitary queen to regenerate a complete colony within a single season.

The high mobility of the colonies (making it possible to reestablish if their immediate environment becomes unsuitable).

The magnitude and economics of the eradication program prevent the delivery of toxicant to the nonforaging members of the colony by direct means. The use of toxic baits which are efficiently incorporated into the food chain of the colonies by the foraging workers is the method of choice. Many researchers have shown that a complex pattern of food distribution exists within the fire ant colony.[1,40,49-51] The exact pattern of distribution, however, may depend on the physical and chemical nature of the nutrient (carbohydrate, protein, lipid, etc).[51,52] Lipid-containing baits, especially soybean oil, have been found to be extremely effective in promoting the entrance of chemicals into the food chain.[14,9,21,54,55] This finding is limited, of course, to the case where the formulation is neither repulsive nor immediately toxic to the ants. At present, soybean oil toxicants are most efficiently employed when incorporated onto the surface of corn cob grits prior to dispersal.[18]

In consideration of these findings, the requirements for an effective bait toxicant have been summarized as follows:

(1) The toxicant must be compatible with soybean oil.

(2) The toxicant must display delayed toxicity such that no
     more than 15% of ants ingesting this material are killed
     in the first 24 hours.

(3) The toxicant must display this delayed toxicity over a
     10- to 100-fold concentration range.

(4) The toxicant must be environmentally acceptable.

    While many toxicants are compatible with soybean oil, only
mirex and its analogs have been shown to fulfill requirements two
and three; however, these toxicants have been judged environmentally
unsafe. This is not unexpected since requirements two and three
are often incompatible with the present definition of environmental
acceptability. One common mechanism by which a toxicant can show
delayed action is by requiring a slow metabolic alternation to yield
the active agent as is the case with mirex. Such compounds are
usually slowly degraded, if at all, in the environment, and they
accumulate in nontarget organisms. This accumulation presents a
potential environmental hazard.

    At present, few compounds available have the potential for
meeting the stringent requirements listed above. The application
of controlled-release technology may offer one means of meeting
this goal because this technique offers a means of obtaining delayed
toxicity from environmentally acceptable toxicants. At least two
controlled-release approaches are applicable to this problem: the
encapsulation of toxicant within rate-controlling excipients and
chemical attachment of toxicants to polymers by hydrolytically reversible linkages. While both approaches will yield toxicants with
delayed action, preliminary findings with microcapsules suggested
the polymeric approach to be more promising.

Previous Controlled-Release Approaches for Control of the Fire Ant

    Controlled release and particularly microencapsulation are
not new to the fire ant problem. In 1971 Markins and Hill[55,57]
reported the use of microencapsulated mirex-oil baits. The objective of that work was not to obtain delayed action, since this was
inherent with mirex baits, but to extend the field life of the toxicant and limit its dissipation into the environment. The microcapsules were not designed to be ingested by the ants but rather
to be carried to the nest and broken open. These and subsequent
studies[58,59] showed that the microcapsules prepared with gelatin
and "plastic" wall materials did achieve the desired effect.

    The use of microencapsulation to delay toxicity became more
attractive when mirex was withdrawn from the eradication program.
At that time the evidence suggested that microcapsules less than
10 microns in diameter could be ingested by the fire ants and re-
gurgitated during trophyllaxis. The slow release of toxicant from

the microcapsules was then expected to yield delayed toxicity. Several formulations based on this approach were tested by the USDA.

In general, all microcapsule preparations tested by the USDA have failed to delay the toxic effects of their incorporated toxicants. A further complication has arisen in subsequent studies of the feeding habits of the fire ant.[52] Researchers of the USDA have observed that while the ants are capable of ingesting 5-micron particles, they have been observed to separate dye-labeled microcapsules from the bait medium and direct them into the buccal pocket. The contents of this pocket are later discarded with the possible result that the microcapsules would not enter the food chain. The reason for this behavior may be obligatory for particles in the micron size range or may be determined either by the chemical nature of the wall material or by detection of the presence of toxicant through a taste mechanism. Contents of the buccal pocket have been observed to be discharged onto larvae with the ultimate consequence that they enter the food chain by this route. This has been shown to be the case with large dry protein particles.[53]

Thus, a microcapsule bait system cannot be completely ruled out; however, the likelihood of success remains in question. Such a system could not be adequately tested by the simple cup screening procedure, and whole-colony tests would be required. The application of microcapsules to a bait toxicant seem inappropriate until further basic studies have been completed.

Another approach, structure modification, has been studied with regard to its application to toxicity delay for fire ant control. This technique is not fully controlled release and is best described as controlled activation. Toxicants are chemically modified to yield nontoxic products which are returned to their active state by digestive or metabolic processes. While these compounds are not stabilized to environmental degradation, they can display delayed toxicity since the time required to activate sufficient quantities of the protoxicant to yield a lethal dose may be several days. The majority of the work in this area has been performed by USDA researchers[60,61] employing esters of either trichlorfon (Dylox) or the highly toxic monofluoronated two-carbon acids and alcohols. Some success has been obtained with the monofluoronated esters, but the trichlorfon esters show little toxicity at low concentration and insufficient delay at high concentration. The toxicity observed with high concentrations of trichlorfon esters is probably a property of the protoxicant form since no delay is observed; thus, the active concentration range of these compounds will be very small. The monofluoroesters are probably too toxic for general application.

Polymeric toxicants are a combination of controlled release and the protoxicant approach. The significant difference is that the high-molecular-weight toxicant species cannot pass into the metabolic machinery due to the inability of the target insect to transport such materials across biological membranes. Only after the toxicant is released from the polymer does the compound display toxicity. In addition to delaying the activity of the toxicant, other properties may be advantageously altered such as solubility and taste. A proper choice of the polymer backbone can affect the solubility of the toxicant in a bait medium, and a high-molecular-weight polymeric form may be expected to elicit a diminished gustatory response.

Unlike microencapsulated toxicants, polymeric insecticides would not be expected to show greatly enhanced stability to environmental conditions since the pendent toxicants are still exposed to chemical and photolytic degradation. Another advantage gained in addition to those cited above is the reduced mobility of the high-molecular-weight formulation. This would diminish the extent to which the toxicant is leached out of the area of application into the surrounding environment.

POLYMERS WITH PENDENT TRICHLORFON

The pesticide trichlorfon (Dylox) has long been known to be toxic to fire ants. However, due to its rapid action it is not effective as an agent for control of the species. The structure of trichlorfon is shown below:

$$(CH_3O)_2P-CH-CCl_3$$

with the P bearing a O (double bond) and the CH bearing an OH group.

It is one of the few approved insecticides which exhibits a functional group useful in forming covalent linkages which are hydrolytically unstable. The hydroxyl group of trichlorfon is useful for the formation of ester linkages to polymer carriers. An example of this type of compound is shown below as the ester of trichlorfon with poly(acrylic acid).

$$-[CH_2-CH]_N-$$

with the CH bearing $C=O$, then O, then $(CH_3O)_2P-CH-CCl_3$ (the P bearing a double-bonded O).

The preparation of esters of trichlorfon was explored using most of the conventional methods for ester formation. Among these methods were reaction with acyl chlorides and anhydrides, and the use of acyl activators such as carbodiimides, carbonyldiimidazole, and n-hydroxysuccinimide. All methods explored were ineffective when considering the economic constraints of industrial-scale synthesis. The use of acylation catalysts such as N,N-dimethylamino-pyridine was also ineffective. With the exception of reaction with anhydrides of fluoronated acids, such as trifluoroacetic acid and perfluorosuccinic anhydride, no simple ester synthesis seemed feasible. The problem was the reduced reactivity of the secondary hydroxyl of the trichlorfon molecule. This group is hindered by the presence of the nearby trichloromethyl moiety and is apparently hydrogen bonded to the nearby phosphoryl oxygen. Further complicating the chemistry was the inherent instability of the compound itself. Under basic conditions or at temperatures exceeding 40°C, trichlorfon exhibits a high propensity to dehydrohalogenate and rearrange to yield a compound with much diminished toxicity which is incapable of ester formation. Thus, all attempts to improve the yields of various synthesis resulted in significant degradation of the pesticide.

Dr. Melvin Look of the USDA reported the synthesis of esters of trichlorfon with lauric acid.[60] The method employed was the dehydration of the free acid in the presence of trichlorfon chloro-sulfonic acid. He reported that good yields could be obtained by heating the reactants at 40°C for one hour. We repeated his work with similar success.

We at first attempted to employ Look's procedure with various acrylic monomers but were unsuccessful due to apparent sulfonation of the double bond under the reaction conditions employed. We then turned to direct coupling of trichlorfon to preformed polymers with pendent acid functionality. Although most such polymers were insoluble in chloroform, several were found to dissolve when sufficient chlorosulfonic acid was present. Using this procedure, we successfully prepared the acrylic product mentioned previously in satisfactory yield. However, the polymeric toxicant displayed limited toxicity in tests with the fire ant and showed only limited (15%) substitution.

Several lines of evidence suggested that the limited toxicity was a reflection of the limited loading and a too-slow hydrolysis of the pesticide from the polymer backbone. It was proposed that both of these problems could be eliminated by the use of a spacer group between the pesticide and the polymer backbone. Such a polymer is shown schematically in Figure 1.

POLYMERIC TOXICANT

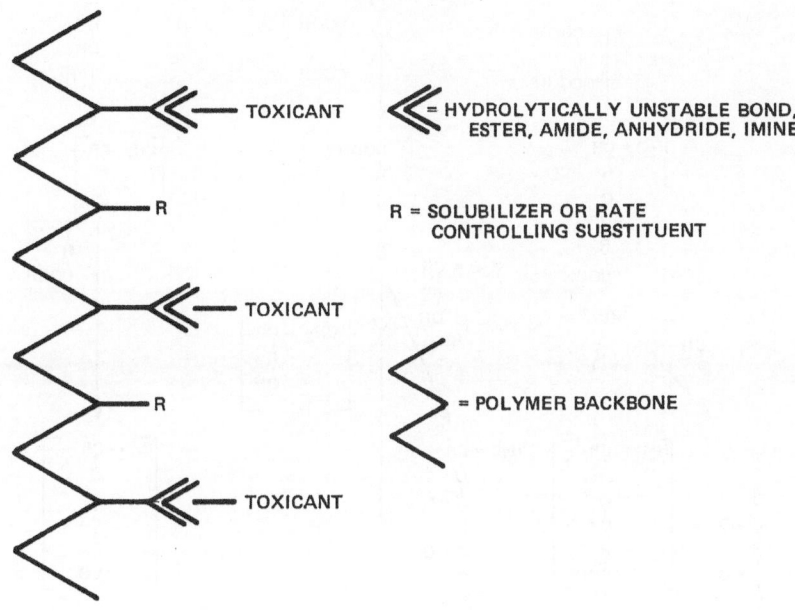

Figure 1. Polymeric pendent pesticide with a spacer group.

We chose to attempt the synthesis of several such polymers using a hydroxyl-containing polymer, a diacid spacer, and trichlorfon. The diacid spacers chosen were those shown below.

$$HO\overset{O}{\overset{\|}{C}}-(CH_2)_2-\overset{O}{\overset{\|}{C}}OH \qquad \text{succinic acid}$$

$$HO\overset{O}{\overset{\|}{C}}-CH=CH-\overset{O}{\overset{\|}{C}}OH \qquad \text{maleic acid}$$

$$HO\overset{O}{\overset{\|}{C}}-(CF_2)_2-\overset{O}{\overset{\|}{C}}OH \qquad \text{perfluorosuccinic acid}$$

Figure 2 shows the various routes which can be employed to prepare a polymer of the type desired. The five possible routes begin with one of three starting points.

One synthesis begins with preparation of a polymer with pendent hydroxyl groups as shown at the far right of Figure 2. Onto this polymer one can attach the diacid spacer by treating the polymer with the cyclic anhydride of one of the diacids shown above.

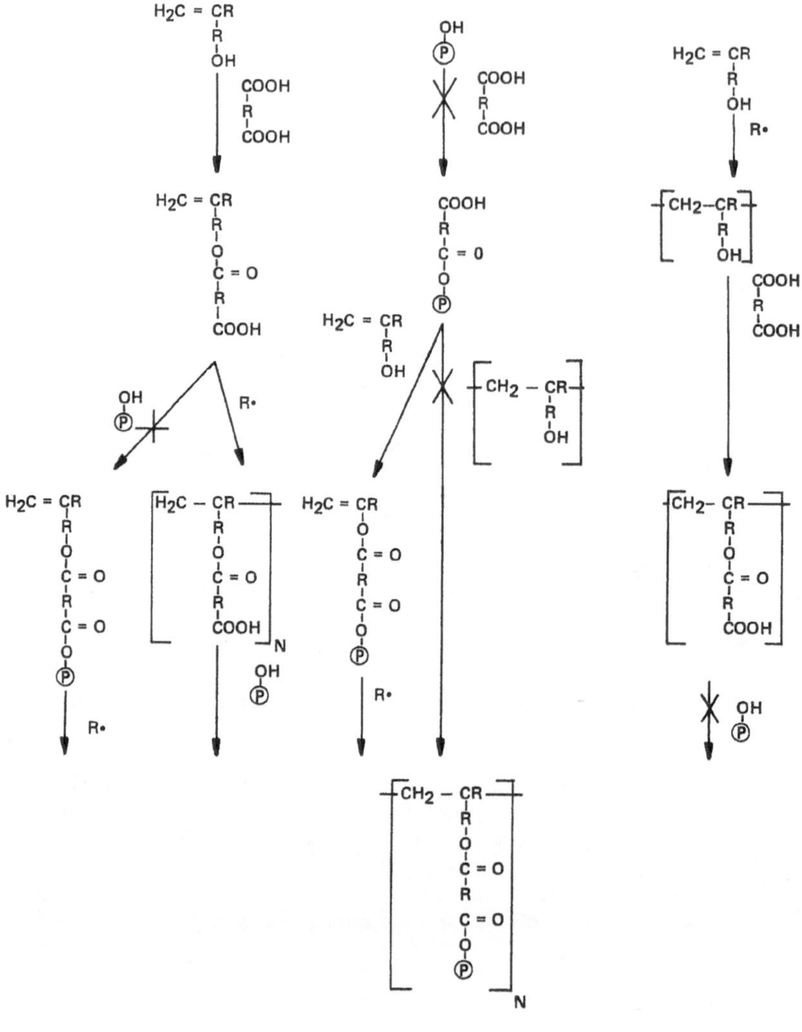

Figure 2. Synthetic routes to polymers with pendent trichlorfon.

    The use of cyclic anhydrides is necessitated by the importance
of avoiding polymer crosslinking during this step. However, substitution of diacids onto a preformed polymer is never 100% efficient,
and our greatest success was 80% of substitution. This is not of
itself a problem, but it led to significant difficulties during
the subsequent step. The dehydration to attach trichlorfon also
resulted in substantial crosslinking of the polymer which arose

when the remaining unsubstituted hydroxyls of the polymer formed
esters with the pendent acid functions. Polymers produced by this
approach were amorphous, insoluble masses.

The center scheme shown in Figure 2 may be completed by two
alternative routes. The procedure begins with the coupling of the
diacid spacer to the hydroxyl-containing pesticide. Preferably,
this would be done by employing the cyclic anhydride. However,
only perfluorosuccinic anhydride was reactive with trichlorfon.
Monoester formation with straight-chain aliphatic diesters was attempted with adipic acid, but only the chlorosulfonic acid coupling
was effective, and the cleanup and isolation proved economically
unfeasible.

However, the highly reactive perfluorosuccinic acid ester of
trichlorfon was carried to the second stage of this scheme. The
right-hand branch of this scheme requires the coupling of the
product monoester to a preformed hydroxyl-containing polymer. We
studied dextran, poly(vinyl alcohol), and poly(2-hydroxyethyl methacrylate). Again, we employed the chlorosulfonic acid procedure
for ester formation to avoid destruction of the trichlorfon. The
result was unsatisfactory. The product polymers showed evidence
by IR of ester formation but the presence of very little trichlorfon.
Apparently, as soon as the pendent groups became coupled, a remaining free hydroxyl on the polymer would attack the labile trichlorfon-
perfluorosuccinic acid linkage to release the trichlorfon and form
an intramolecular crosslink.

The left-hand branch of this scheme, which employs the monomer
instead of the preformed polymer, was attempted to avoid the problem
just described. However, we were unable to implement the chlorosulfonic acid coupling procedure due to its propensity to sulfonate
the acrylic moiety of the monomer. A carbodiimide coupling was
partially successful, but we were unable to isolate a sufficient
quantity of pure product to prepare polymer for testing. Use of
an unpurified product yielded a polymer which apparently suffered
the same limitations as the derivatives prepared with the preformed
polymer.

The scheme at the left of Figure 2 was then studied. The
acrylic monomer was prepared by reaction of the cyclic anhydrides
of the three diacids employed, and the product was purified by re-
crystallization. The left-hand branch, wherein the monomer is
reacted with trichlorfon prior to polymerization, was deemed un-
workable since the chlorosulfonic acid coupling could not be employed in the presence of the acrylic function. No other coupling
procedure seemed economically feasible. Thus, we were left with
the right-hand branch of this scheme wherein the monomer is purified
and polymerized, the polymer is purified, and this is followed by

coupling of the trichlorfon by chlorosulfonic acid dehydration. This procedure was successfully used in the preparation of the three desired polymers (Figure 3).

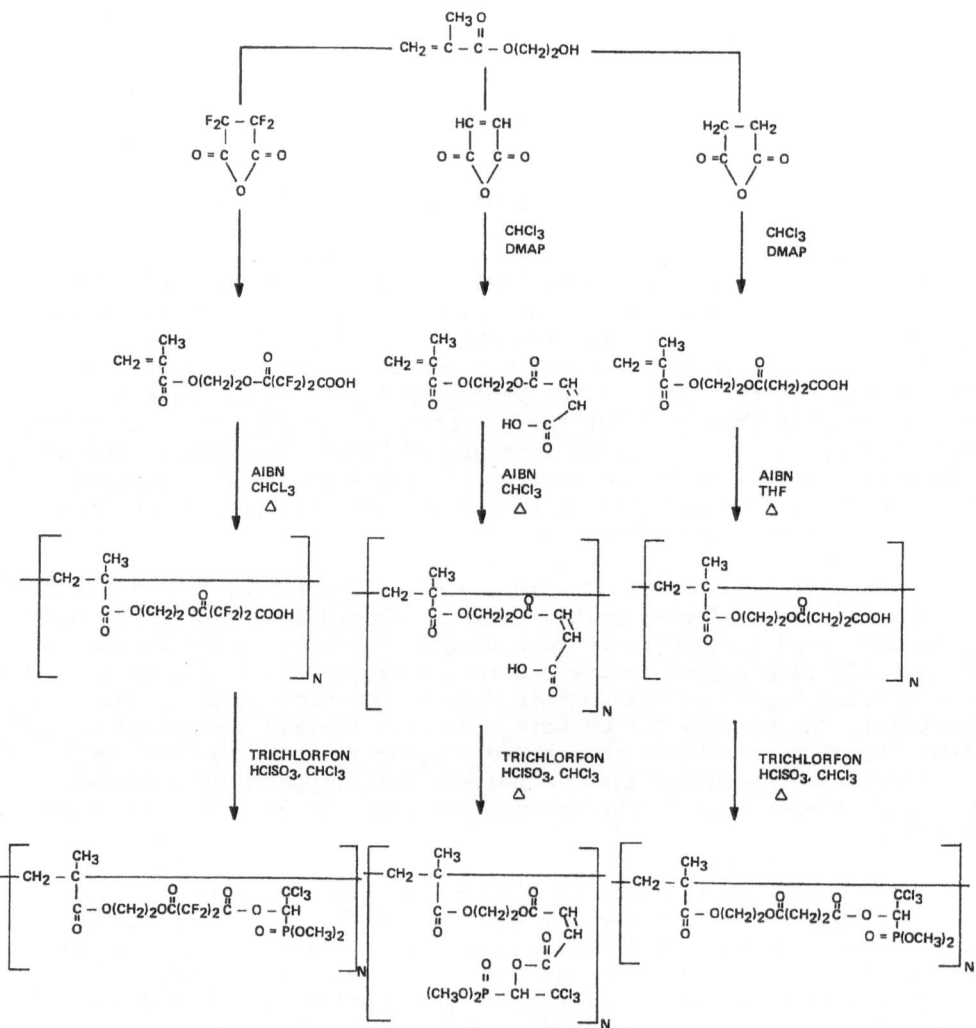

Figure 3.   Synthesis of HEMA/trichlorfon polymers with diacid spacers.

PREPARATION AND TESTING OF POLYMERS WITH PENDENT TRICHLORFON

Figure 3 depicts the synthesis of the three polymers with diacid spacers. The hydroxyl-containing monomer employed was 2-hydroxyethyl methacrylate (HEMA) and was chosen more for convenience than for special properties desirable in the final product. This monomer, however, does offer the benefits of extended chain length and an additional ester linkage which would add slightly to the rate of release. The succinic and maleic condensation reactions were performed in chloroform and required dimethylaminopyridine as a catalyst. It was necessary to reflux the reaction mixture to achieve reaction, and we anticipated that the HEMA might poly-merize during the refluxing step. We first employed a quinone inhibitor to avoid polymerization, but we later found it unnecessary and deleted it. An excess of HEMA was employed, and following the reaction, the unreacted monomer and solvent were removed under vacuum leaving a viscous oil which crystallized after several days at 4°C.

The reaction with perfluorosuccinic anhydride (PSA) was per-formed neat at room temperature without the need for a catalyst or radical scavenger. An excess of PSA was employed and was easily removed under vacuum.

Following the coupling of the diacid spacer to the monomer, each product was polymerized. Azobisisobutyronitrile (AIBN) was employed as a free-radical initiator in each case. The solvent for the PSA and maleic products was chloroform, and tetrahydrofuran was used with the succinic product. The choice of solvent was dictated by the desire that the polymer spontaneously separate from solution. Though the product polymers were insoluble in chloroform, adequate solubility was obtained when chlorosulfonic acid was added. A slight molar excess of trichlorfon was added to each reaction mixture, and the stirred solution was heated to 40°C. After 4 hours at 40°C, the polymers separated, and the solvent was decanted. The product polymers were dried under vacuum for 24 hours, and each appeared as a glassy amorphous film.

To compare the release rates of these polymeric pesticides with the ester prepared with poly(acrylic acid), we synthesized the PAA compound by direct reaction of poly(acrylic acid) (molecular weight 50,000) with trichlorfon using chlorosulfonic acid in chloro-form. Again, the unsubstituted polymer was insoluble in chloroform, but it dissolved after the addition of chlorosulfonic acid. The product remained soluble. The chlorosulfonic acid was neutralized with sodium bicarbonate, and the sodium sulfate was removed by filtration. The polymer remained in solution in chloroform and was precipitated by the addition of diethyl ether. The polymer was reprecipitated three times from chloroform with ether.

Figure 4 shows schematically the method employed to determine
the rate of hydrolysis of these polymers. Ten milliliters of distilled water was placed in a 12-ml, screw-cap tube. Each polymer
(200 mg) was weighed under dry conditions into a small-diameter
dialysis bag sealed at one end. Approximately 2 ml of water from
the screw-cap tubes was transferred into the dialysis bag, and the
other end was quickly sealed. After the bags were dropped into
their respective tubes, the tubes were closed and placed in a device
which rotated them end over end at 25°C.

At selected intervals a 5-ml sample was removed from each tube
and stored for analysis. The 5-ml of water was replaced, and the
rotation was continued. At the end of the experiment, the entire
sample from the tube was removed. The volume external to the bag
was separated and stored, and the contents of each bag were removed
and stored for analysis. Prior to the analysis, the water was
removed with heating under a gentle stream of nitrogen. The polymer
carriers were still observable in the samples extracted from the
dialysis bags. Control samples were also run including: free
trichlorfon, each polymer treated with chlorosulfonic acid but
without trichlorfon, and dialysis bags containing only water.

Analysis was by the modified Fisk-Subbarow colorimetric
procedure.[62] This analysis is sensitive to total phosphate rather
than trichlorfon. While insufficient sample was available to employ
chromatographic separation, all previously examined polymeric

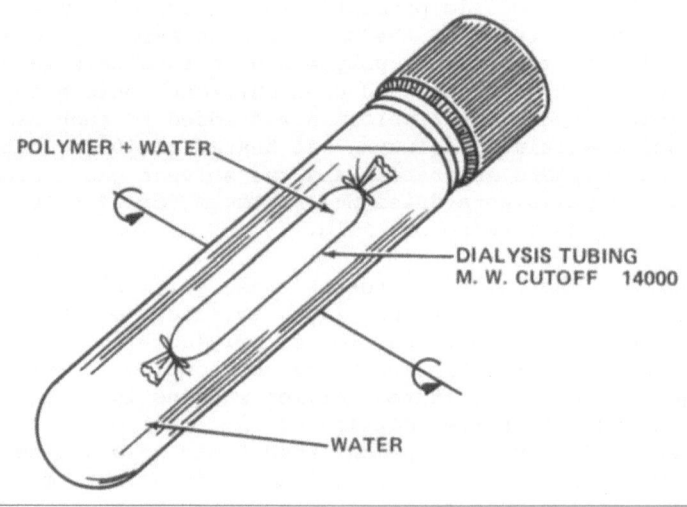

POLYMER + WATER

DIALYSIS TUBING
M. W. CUTOFF   14000

WATER

Figure 4.   Apparatus for determining release rates for pendent-
polymeric toxicants.

derivatives showed only trichlorfon as a discernable hydrolysis
product by TLC. While it is not inconceivable that some of the
product from the polymers with diacid spacers may have been the
diacid monoester of trichlorfon, the spacers were originally chosen
such that under conditions of the ant's digestive tract the mono-
esters would be autocatalytically cleaved to yield free trichlorfon.

RESULTS AND DISCUSSION

     Figure 5 shows the early-time release of trichlorfon from the
poly(acrylic acid) product. The half-life for release was approximately 14 hours. This result was substantially less than the half-
life expected. This finding has forced us to re-examine our
rational for the lack of toxicity for the PAA polymer. It appears
likely that the ants are able to rapidly detoxify or eliminate
trichlorfon, and dosages administered slowly over a period as short
as 14 hours cannot be considered cumulative. It would still be
expected that faster releasing polymers would be more toxic, but
half-lives shorter than 14 hours could never be expected to yield
delayed toxicities of 24 hours or greater.

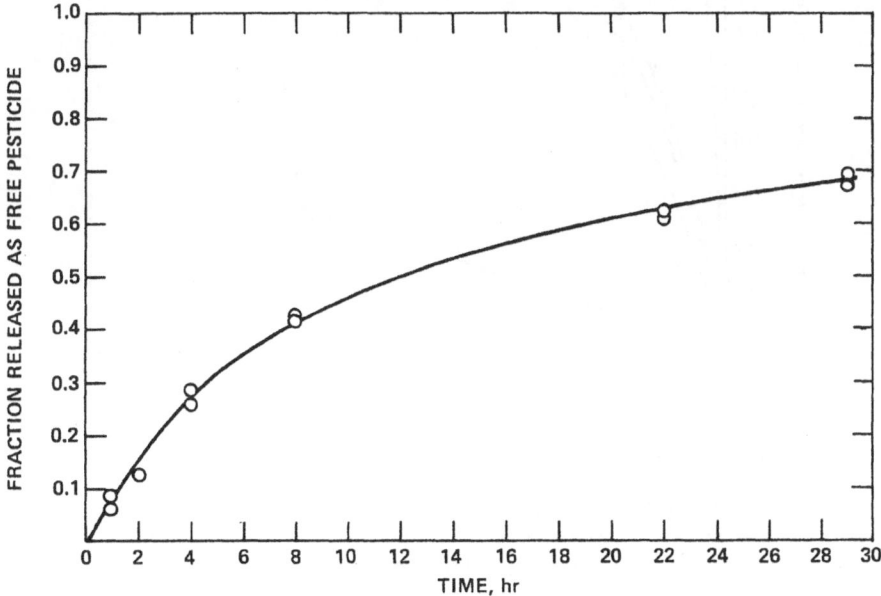

Figure 5.   Release of trichlorfon from poly(acryloyl trichlorofon).

Figure 6 shows the release data for all of the polymers tested.
The hydrolysis of trichlorfon from the three polymers with diacid
spacers was significantly more rapid than that from the poly(acrylic
acid) product. Little difference can be seen among the diacid-con-
taining polymers when compared to the poly(acrylic acid) product.
However, the order of these three is in opposition to the rates
that would be expected based on the stability of the ester formed
with each diacid. On these grounds, we would have expected that
the polymer containing perfluorosuccinic acid would have been the
fastest, followed by the polymer containing maleic acid. In fact,
the maleic acid polymer was fastest, and the perfluorosuccinic
polymer was slightly slower even than the succinic product. It
is possible that despite the lability of the bond, the fluorocarbon
nature of the bridging diacid was sufficient to exclude water from
the region of the ester linkage.

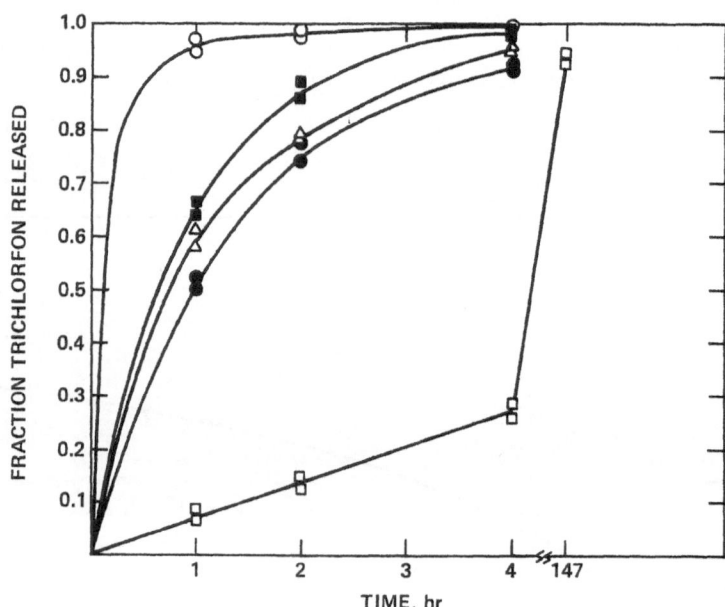

O   FREE TRICHLORFON
■   HEMA/TRICHLORFON, MALEIC ACID SPACER
△   HEMA/TRICHLORFON, SUCCINIC ACID SPACER
●   HEMA/TRICHLORFON, PERFLUOROSUCCINIC ACID SPACER
□   ACRYLIC ACID/TRICHLORFON

Figure 6.   Release rates for trichlorfon-containing polymers.

This figure also shows the observed release of free trichlorfon from the dialysis bag. Clearly, the observed delay of release for the polymeric forms cannot be accounted for as simply the time required for trichlorofon to diffuse through the dialysis membrane. A break in the time axis was employed to show that the poly(acrylic acid) product did indeed release all of its active content.

Table I shows the pertinent data for each of the polymers. The percent of substitution represents the percent of available polymer sites that had trichlorfon attached. There was significant improvement with the polymers having diacid spacers. This was probably due to reduced steric hinderance for attachment at a greater distance from the polymer backbone. When the mass of the bridging diacid is considered, however, the increased loading becomes less significant. The percent by weight of trichlorfon for each polymer is nearly equivalent for all preparations. The observed half-life of each polymer is also shown in Table I.

Further work with the trichlorfon polymer does not appear to be justified at this point for two primary reasons: (1) the apparent detoxification capacity of the fire ant toward trichlorfon greatly diminishes the likelihood of success, and (2) trichlorfon is now suspected of being a possible pollution hazard by the EPA. This should not be construed to mean that research on the use of polymeric pesticides should be abandoned however. In fact, our success in this preparation evidences the potential for this approach when employed with other pesticides.

ACKNOWLEDGEMENTS

We wish to acknowledge the laboratory efforts of Mr. Raphael J. Thornton, Mrs. Linda W. Young, and Ms. Garnette D. Draper. Also, we are grateful for the technical assistance of Dr. Donald R. Cowsar. We are appreciative of the support provided by the United States Department of Agriculture Animals and Plant Health Inspection Service.

REFERENCES

1. C.S. Lofgren, W.A. Banks, and B.M. Glancy, Annual Review of Entomology 20:1 (1975).
2. G.P. Markin, J.H. Dillier, S.O. Hill, M.S. Blum, and H.R. Hermann, J. Ga. Etomol. Soc. 6:145 (1971).
3. W.C. Rhoades and D.R. Davis, J. Econ. Entomol. 60:554 (1967).
4. H.B. Green, Miss. State Univ. Exp. Sta. Bull. 737:23 (1967).
5. G.H. Culpepper, US Dep. Agr. Agr. Res Serv. 867:8 (1953).

TABLE I. PROPERTIES OF POLYMERS WITH PENDENT TRICHLORFON

Sample Number	Polymer	Group	Substitution, %	Weight Percent Toxicant	Half Life in H_2O, hr
A-146-70-3	Poly(Acrylic Acid)	--	15.8	37.4	14.00
A-146-72-1	Poly(Hydroxyethyl methacrylate)	Succinic acid	52.6	40.7	0.85
A-146-70-5	Poly(Hydroxyethyl methacrylate)	Maleic acid	51.1	41.2	0.77
A-146-72-3	Poly(Hydroxyethyl methacrylate)	Perfluoro- Succinic acid	73.9	46.5	0.95

6. H.B. Mills, Chairman, Report of committee on imported fire
    ant, National Academy of Sciences, to administrator, Agr. Res.
    Serv., US Dept. Agr. 15 (1967).
7. O.F. Francke, Paper delivered at Imported Fire Ant Workshop,
    May (1979).
8. C.S. Lofgren, C.E. Stringer, and F.J. Barlett, J. Econ. Entomol.
    55:405 (1962).
9. W.A. Banks, J. Econ. Entomol. 66:785 (1973).
10. W.A. Banks, C.S. Lofgren, D.P. Jouvenaz, D.P. Wojcik, and J.W.
    Summerlin, Environ Entomol 2:182 (1973).
11. W.A. Banks, D.P. Jouvenaz, C.S. Lofgren, and D.M. Hicks, J.
    Econ. Entomol. 66:241 (1973).
12. W.A. Banks, G.P. Markin, J.W. Summerlin, and C.S. Lofgren,
    J. Econ. Entomol 65:1468 (1972).
13. C.S. Lofgren, F.J. Bartlett, C.E. Stringer, Jr., and W.A.
    Banks, J. Econ. Entomol 57:695 (1964).
14. E.S. Raun and R.D. Jackson, J. Econ. Entomol. 59:620 (1966).
15. M.V. Fogle, Croplife (1968). Feb. 1968, 22, 27, 28, 30.
16. G.P. Markin and S.O. Hill, J. Econ. Entomol. 64:193 (1971).
17. C.E. Stringer, Jr., C.S. Lofgren, and F.J. Barlett, J. Econ.
    Entomol. 57:941 (1964).
18. C.S. Lofgren, F. J. Bartlett, and C.E. Stringer, J. Econ.
    Entomol. 57:62 (1963).
19. W.A. Banks, C.E. Stringer, and N.W. Pierce, J. Ga. Entomol.
    Soc. 6:205 (1971).
20. C.S. Lofgren, C.E. Stringer, and F.J. Barlett, J. Econ. Entomol.
    54:1096 (1961).
21. United States Department of Agriculture, Animal and Plant
    Health Inspection Service, Plant Protection Quarantine Manual,
    301.81.
22. H.L. Collins, J.R. Davis, and G.P. Markin, Bull. Environ.
    Contam. Toxicol. 10:73 (1973).
23. G.W. Ware and E.E. Good, Toxicol. Appl. Pharmacol. 10:54 (1967).
24. C.C. VanValin, E.K. Andrews, and L.L. Eller, Trans. Am. Fish.
    Cult. 97:185 (1968).
25. J.C. Oberheu, Pestic. Monit. J. 6:41 (1972).
26. P.W. Borthwich, Pestic. Monit. J. 7:6 (1973).
27. E.C. Naber and G.W. Ware, Poultry Sci. 44:875 (1965).
28. C.G. Bookhout, A.J. Wilson, Jr., T.W. Duke, and J.I. Lowe,
    Water, Soil, Air Pollut. 1:165 (1972).
29. T.B. Gaines and R.D. Kimbrough, Arch. Environ. Health 21:7
    (1970).
30. K.P. Baetcke, J.D. Cain, and W.E. Poe, Pestic. Monit. J. 6:14
    (1972).
31. J.L. Ludke, M.T. Finley, and L. Lusk, Bull. Environ. Contam.
    & Toxicol. 6:89 (1971).
32. W.D. Ruckelshaus, Fed. Register 37(130):299 (1972).
33. R.K. Vander Meer. Paper delivered at Imported Fire Ant Work-
    shop, May 1979.

34. Quarterly Report of Research and Methods Improvement for the Imported Fire Ant. Report No. 74(1), U.S.D.A.

35. Quarterly Report of Research and Methods Improvement for the Imported Fire Ant. Report No. 77(2), U.S.D.A.

36. Quarterly Report of Research and Methods Improvement for the Imported Fire Ant. Report No. 77(3), U.S.D.A.

37. Quarterly Report of Research and Methods Improvement for the Imported Fire Ant. Report No. 77(4), U.S.D.A.

38. R.K. Vander Meer, C.S. Lofgren, D.H. Lewis, and W.E. Meyers, in: "Proceedings 6th International Symposium on Controlled Release Bioactive Materials," R.W. Baker, ed., New Orleans (1979).

39. J. O'Neal and G.P. Markin, J. Ga. Entomol. Soc. 8:294 (1973).

40. D.J. Wojcik, Paper delivered at Imported Fire Ant Workshop, May (1979).

41. A.D. Oliver, J. Econ. Entomol. 53:646 (1960).

42. J.H. Crance, Progr. Fish Cult. 27:91 (1965).

43. H.G. Adkins, Assoc. Am. Georgraphy 60:578 (1970).

44. Personal Communication, Aubrey Station USDA-APHIS, Shelby County, Alabama.

45. T.E. Reagan, G. Coburn, and S.D. Hensley, Environ. Entomol 1:588 (1972).

46. W.G. Harris and E.C. Burns, Environ. Entomol 1:362 (1972).

47. R.A. Roe, MS thesis, Univ. of Arkansas, Fayetteville (1973).

48. W.H. Whitcomb, H.A. Denmark, A.P. Bhatkar, and G.L. Greene, Fla. Entomol 55:129 (1972).

49. E.O. Wilson, Cambridge, Mass.: Belknap Press of Harvard Univ. Press (1971) 548.

50. S.B. Vinson, J. Econ. Entomol. 61:712 (1968).

51. B.M. Glancey, C.E. Stringer, Jr., C.H. Craig, P.M. Bishop, and B.B. Martin, Ann. Entomol Soc. Am. 66:233 (1973).

52. R.K. Vander Meer, Personal communication USDA-ARS,

53. A.A. Sorensen, Paper delivered by S.B. Vinson, Imported Fire Ant Workshop, May 1979.

54. C.S. Lofgren, F.J. Bartlett, and C.E. Stringer, J. Econ. Entomol. 54:1096 (1961).

55. C.S. Lofgren, F.J. Bartlett, and C.E. Stringer, J. Econ. Entomol. 57:601 (1964).

56. G.P. Maukin and S.O. Hill, J. Econ. Entomol. 64:193 (1971).

57. G.P. Markin, J.A. Henderson, and H.L. Collins, Agr. Aviat. 14:70 (1972).

58. G.P. Markin, H.L. Collins, and J. O'Neal, J. Econ. Entomol. 68:711 (1975).

59. G.P. Markin, J. O'Neal, and H.L. Collins, J. Georgia Entomol. Soc. 10:281 (1975).

60. M. Look and L.R. White, in preparation.

61. J.P. Kochansky, W.E. Robbins, C.S. Lofgren, and D.F. Williams, J. Econ. Entomol., in press.

62. C.H. Fiske and Y. Subbarow, J. Biol. Chem. 66:375 (1925).

ANTIFOULING POLYMERS:

ROOM-TEMPERATURE-CURING ORGANOTIN POLYMERS

R.V. Subramanian and K.N. Somasekharan

Department of Materials Science and Engineering
Washington State University
Pullman, Washington 99164

We have reported extensively on antifouling formulations in which tributyltin carboxylate groups are chemically anchored to the polymer chain.[1-3] In these controlled-release formulations, the prepolymers were prepared by partial esterification by bis(tri-n-butyltin) oxide (TBTO) of linear polymers carrying carboxylic acid or anhydride groups. The free carboxylic acid or anhydride groups were than reacted with diepoxides to form thermoset organotin-epoxy polymers. Many variations of this scheme were investigated, including one which provided for simultaneous vinyl polymerization and carboxyl-epoxide reactions. Curing was accomplished at high temperatures (about 150°C) in all these reactions.

The degree of esterification of the base polymers, the structure of the epoxy monomers, and the type of catalyst used were varied in these synthetic schemes to effect changes in the average separation between TBT groups and the length of epoxy crosslinks. Resultant changes in the measured strength, fracture toughness, and dynamic mechanical behavior of the polymer systems were correlated with the structural variables employed. Toughening by carboxyl-terminated liquid elastomers was also studied and the improvement in fracture toughness correlated with the average particle size of the dispersed elastomer phase. Of the various catalysts studied, uranyl nitrate caused the highest degree of crosslinking. The formation of domains in the matrix with independent glass transitions was studied by observing variations in loss moduli; this also reflected the structural effects of the bulky TBT group and the different epoxy monomers.[1]

191

New organotin-epoxy systems curable at room temperature have been developed and characterized:[4] diglycidyl ether of bisphenol-A (DGEBA) was first modified by reacting with the TBT esters of ω-amino acids; the resulting prepolymers were then cured with diethylenetriamine (DETA) at room temperature.

Antifouling coatings that can be cured at room temperature are needed. Results on the incorporation of organotin groups into room-temperature cured urethanes, aziridines, and polyesters are reported here.

CONTROLLED RELEASE

Laboratory studies on biotoxicity[5] and performance tests in marine environments[3,6] reveal that the resistance to fouling is influenced by matrix characteristics. Laboratory tests indicate that only a very small fraction of the available tin is released during the service life of the coating.[7] Matrix hydrophilicity and permeability seem to be the factors determining the duration of fouling resistance.

Antifouling performance of these organotin carboxylate polymers indicates that their mode of action corresponds to the bulk abiotic bond cleavage model.[8] We have carefully considered all the controlling factors, viz., diffusion of water (and possibly chloride) into the polymer matrix from sea water, hydrolysis of TBT carboxylates to produce TBTO (or TBTCl), diffusion of the mobile species produced from the matrix to the surface, phase transfer of the organotin species and its migration across the boundary layer.[7,9]

The TBT group is found to undergo fast chemical exchange,[10] and hence a hydrolytic equilibrium is rapidly established between TBT carboxylates and TBTO. Laboratory determination of the release rate, under laminar flow conditions, shows that the phase transfer and migration across the boundary layer are also relatively fast.[7] Thus we have come to the conclusion that diffusion of the organotin species produced, from the matrix to the surface, controls the rate of release in epoxy systems.[7] The permeability of the matrix for the diffusion of the organotin species becomes a controlling factor.

As the mobile species produced diffuses out, the hydrolysis is expected to proceed at a concentration-dependent rate. The rate of release of tin (in g/cm^2/sec) from the surface then becomes:[9,11]

$$dq/dt = C_m D^{0.5} K^{0.5} \left[\mathrm{erf}(K^{0.5} t^{0.5}) + \frac{\exp(-Kt)}{(\pi Kt)^{0.5}} \right] \qquad (1)$$

where C_m =   the concentration of the mobile species in g/cm^3

        D =   the effective diffusivity in the matrix in cm^2/sec

        K =   the concentration-dependent hydrolysis rate in sec^{-1}

        t =   the time in sec

The most salient feature of this relation is that when Kt becomes
large, the error function erf (Kt)$^{0.5}$ approaches unity, and the
rate becomes independent of time. This zero-order rate is the
coveted characteristic of controlled-release systems. However,
we have not been able to realize this ideal behavior in the epoxy
systems.[7] This may be due partly to the tight matrix in these epoxy
systems. Past systems have only considered TBT carboxylates closely
bound to the backbone of the polymer. By varying the length of
the chain holding the TBT moiety, greater mobility of the TBT group
is to be expected. A lower glass transition temperature (T_g) is
actually observed as this chain is extended,[4,12] which means lower
activation energy for this motion. The decrease in matrix constraints allowing this motion may also result in decreased resistance to the diffusion of TBTO. The synthesis and mechanical characterization[12] of these systems have been the first steps in
pursuing the idealized controlled release from epoxy systems.

There is evidence in the literature to imply that vinyl and
urethane polymers would release organotin at a greater rate.[13] This
implication is in accordance with the current understanding of mass
transport in polymer matrices; diffusivity in the matrix is expected
to be high when the free volumes and segmental mobilities are high
and T_g's low.[14]

Organotin urethanes and organotin polyesters are also attractive from the point of view of their greater hydrophilicity. Equation (1) predicts greater rate of release when C_m is higher; the
concentration of the mobile species is expected to be higher in
hydrophilic matrices.

URETHANES

TBT ester of tartaric acid was synthesized from TBTO and
tartaric acid. TBT tartrate (a dihydroxy monomer) was then reacted
with excess tolylene-2,4-diisocyanate (TDI) to produce the NCO-
terminated prepolymers. The prepolymers were cured by crosslinking
with castor oil (a trihydroxy compound). This approach guaranteed
the completion of the reaction between TBT tartrate and TDI, en-
suring a more complete incorporation of the organotin moiety into
the crosslinked structure. The cured polymers were flexible.

Trialkyltin groups can be expected to catalyze the urethane reaction. The isocyanate group can coordinate with tin, becoming more polarized and exposing the isocyanate carbon for nucleophilic attack by hydroxyl oxygen. This catalytic activity was observed in this work. Thus, when castor oil and TDI were mixed in equivalent quantities, the mixture cured to a nontacky solid only after standing for over 24 hours at room temperature. By contrast, a similar mixture cured completely in less than two hours in the presence of TBT tartrate. Similarly, the reaction between hexamethylenediisocyanate and alcohols like proponal and butanol is significantly accelerated in the presence of TBT acetate. The reaction between TDI and polyols like glycerol (dried), Isonol-93 (Upjohn Co.), and 2-ethyl-2-(hydroxymethyl)-1,3-propanediol (Aldrich, analyzed) proceed with evolution of heat and frothing in presence of TBT carboxylates. Castor oil and isocyanate react without frothing in the presence of TBT carboxylates.

Preparation of TBT Tartrate

Tartaric acid (Mallinckrodt, AR), 75 g (0.5 mole), 298 g (0.5 mole TBTO (M & T), and 250 ml of dry benzene were taken in a 1-liter flask. The flask was fitted with a Dean-Stark adapter and condenser, and heated in an oil bath at about 100°C. Water, 9.2 ml, was collected in the Dean-Stark adapter (theoretical, 9.0 ml). The solvent was removed at a rotary evaporator. The residue was used, without further purification, in the preparation of the prepolymers.

Part of the residue was recrystallized from hexane. The recrystallized sample was analyzed for tin, by treating 1-gram quantities with concentrated sulfuric acid and drops of concentrated nitric acid to destroy organic matter, subsequently heating in a muffle furnace at 600°C, and weighing as SnO_2. The Sn content was 31.99% (theoretical, 32.60).

Preparation of Prepolymers

NCO-terminated prepolymers of three different compositions were prepared:

1. 3.83 g (44 milliequivalents) of TDI (Aldrich, 97%) was taken in a beaker, and 1.46 g (4 milliequivalents) of TBT tartrate was slowly added to that with stirring. Reaction was fast and was catalyzed by tributyltin. This product was allowed to stand for one day in a desiccator.

2. 2.91 g (8 milliequivalents) of TBT tartrate was added slowly with stirring to 4.18 g (48 milliequivalents) of TDI. This product was allowed to stand for one day in a desiccator.

3.   4.37 g (12 milliequivalents) of TBT tartrate and 4.53 g (52
milliequivalents) of TDI were mixed as before, and let stand for
one day in a desiccator. The reaction scheme is presented in Figure 1.

Curing

Each of the above NCO-terminated prepolymers was mixed with
14.31 g (40 milliequivalents) of castor oil (Kellog, CP & USP).
The reaction was fast, and the mixes turned nontacky within two
hours at room temperature. However, a mixture of 3.48 g (40 milliequivalents) of TDI and 14.31 g (40 milliequivalents) of castor
oil took more than one day to set to a nontacky solid. The catalytic effect of tributyltin on the urethane reaction was evident.
The reaction scheme is presented in Figure 2.

Characterization

The crosslinked polymers possessed elastomeric properties.
About 10 g each of the above three urethane compositions containing
tin were sliced into small pieces. They were subjected to soxhlet
extraction with a 1:1 mixture of benzene (b.p. 80.1°C) and 2-butanone
(b.p. 79.6°C). The systems were guarded with calcium chloride tubes.

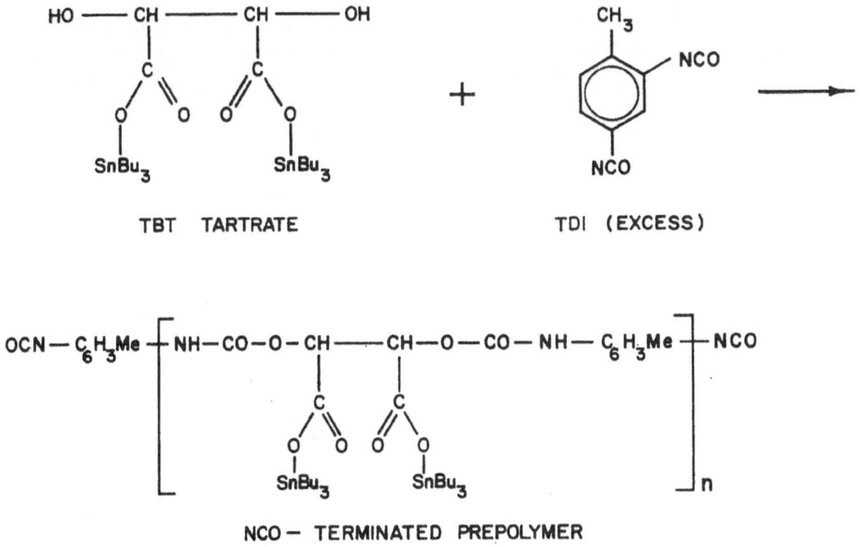

Figure 1.   Synthesis of organotin urethane prepolymer.

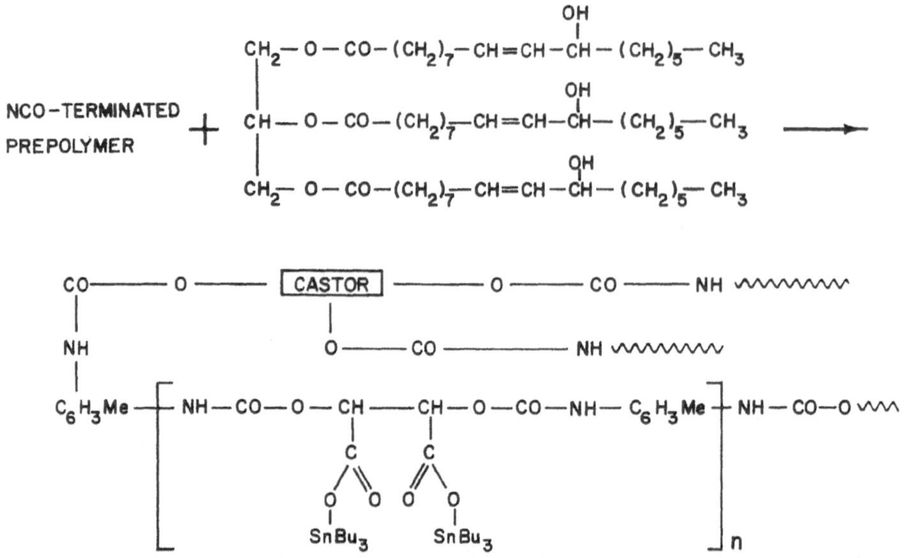

Figure 2.   Crosslinking of NCO-terminated prepolymer by castor oil.

The extraction was stopped after 50 hours. The solvents had caused
substantial swelling. The samples were dried to constant weight
by keeping them in vacuum at room temperature.

    The cured polymers and the residues after extraction were
analyzed for tin. The results are given in Table I. The sol fraction was less than 7%, and more than 90% tin was bonded to the
crosslinked structure. In contrast, when the synthetic sequence
was repeated with TBT 4-hydroxybutanoate (in place of TBT tartrate),
the bulk of the tin was found in the sol fraction; a dihydroxy
compound is required to produce the NCO-terminated prepolymer.

TABLE I.   ORGANOTIN URETHANE POLYMERS

| Composition, Equiv. | | | | Wt% Sn in | | |
TBT Tartrate	TDI	Castor Oil	Extractables, Wt%	Original Polymer	Residue	Extract[a]
4	44	40	7.1	2.39	2.33	3.08
8	48	40	6.0	4.36	4.32	4.96
12	52	40	4.8	6.04	5.70	12.80

[a] The wt% Sn in extract was calculated from wt% extractables, and
Sn in original polymer and residue.

AZIRIDINES

Poly(styrene-co-maleic acid) was prepared from commercially available poly(styrene-co-maleic anhydride) and then partially esterified by reacting with TBTO. The free-acid groups of these partial esters were found to react with a polyfunctional aziridine (XAMA-2), curing to a nontacky solid at room temperature.

Preparation of Prepolymers and Curing

Three different compositions were prepared:

1. 20.2 g (100 milliequivalents) of poly(styrene-co-maleic anhydride) (SMA-1000, ARCO Chemical Co.) and 200 ml of benzene were taken in a 500-ml flask. The theoretical amount of water to hydrolyze 50% of the anhydride groups (0.9 ml) was also added. The flask was then fitted with a reflux condenser and heated in an oil bath at about 100°C. Refluxing was continued for one day. After cooling, 29.8 g of TBTO was added. After refluxing for one hour, the solvent was removed at room temperature on a rotary evaporator. 15.9 g XMA-2 (Cordova Chemical Co.; azridine functionality 2.67 and aziridine content 6.29 milliequivalents/g) was added to the residue and mixed well. The mixture was cured in an oven at 80°C.

2. 60%-TBT Ester. 20.2 g SMA-1000 in 200 ml of benzene was refluxed with enough water to hydrolyze 40% of the anhydride groups. 35.8 g TBTO was then reacted with it. The solvent was removed at room temperature and 12.7 g XAMA-2 mixed with the residue. The mixture was cured in an oven at 80°C for one day.

3. 70%-TBT Ester. 30% of the anhydride groups in 20.2 g SMA-1000 was hydrolyzed, as above. 41.7 g TBTO was then reacted with it. After removal of the solvent, the residue was mixed with 9.5 g XAMA-2 and cured as above.

Characterization

The above crosslinked polymers were subjected to soxhlet extraction with a 1:1 mixture of benzene and 2-butanone under anhydrous conditions. The residues were dried in a vacuum oven at 80°C.

The crosslinked polymers and residues after extraction were analyzed for tin. The results are summarized in Table II. It can be seen that heavy loading of tin is possible in these polymers; up to 20% Sn loading, the sol fraction and the loss of tin on soxhlet extraction are low. Even though the TBT group undergoes exchange[10] and hence gets distributed uniformly in the prepolymers,

TABLE II.   ORGANOTIN AZIRIDINE POLYMERS

% Carboxylic Acid Groups Esterified by TBTO[a]	Extractables, Wt%	Wt% Sn in		
		Crosslinked Polymer	Residue	Extract[b]
50	6.10	17.50	17.43	18.51
60	10.11	20.20	19.86	23.18
70	19.23	22.80	18.66	39.33

[a] Fraction of carboxylic acid groups contained in poly(styrene-co-maleic acid) esterified by TBTO.

[b] The wt% of Sn in extract calculated from wt% extractables, and wt% of Sn in crosslinked polymer and residue.

because of the low molecular weight of SMA-1000 (M_n = 1600) some of the prepolymer molecules might not become part of the crosslinked structure when the percentage of esterification is very high, which partly accounts for the high sol fraction and high tin content in the sol fraction.

POLYESTERS

Organotin vinyl monomers, such as TBT methacrylate and TBT acrylates, were mixed with unsaturated polyesters and cured with a free-radical initiator. The mixtures cure at room temperature to hard, nontacky solids. Gel time can be controlled, by controlling the addition of accelerators like cobalt naphthenate and dimethylaniline.

Preparation of TBT Methacrylate

TBTO, 298 g, was taken in a beaker at room temperature (24°C). To this was added, slowly and with constant stirring, 86 g of methacrylic acid (Aldrich, 98.5%). The methacryclic acid contained 1000 ppm of hydroquinone and 250 ppm of hydroquinone monomethyl ether. The addition took about 30 minutes for completion, and the temperature never rose above 28°C. The pale yellow, cloudy liquid that resulted was kept at 3 mm of vacuum for 30 minutes. The resulting liquid was clear. The loss of weight was 9.5 g, as against the expected loss of 9.0 g. Hence, the beaker and contents were kept under vacuum for 12 hours more; no further loss in weight was observed. IR spectrum of the product showed no free carboxylic acid groups. Ten grams of the TBT methacrylate was added to 50 ml

of methanol; there was no significant cloudiness. The product was
crystallized from hexane; the recrystallized product had a freezing
point of 17–16°C.

Preparation of TBT Acrylate

TBTO, 298 g, and 250 g of hexane were taken in a 1-liter flask
fitted with a Dean-Stark adapter, condenser and addition funnel.
Acrylic acid, 75 g, (Aldrich, 99%) was added slowly, with stirring,
from the funnel. The acrylic acid contained 200 ppm of hydroquinone
monomethyl ether. At the end of the addition, the flask was heated
in an oil bath at about 80°C; 9.2 ml of water was collected in the
Dean-Stark adapter. The crystals of TBT acrylate were collected
from the cooled reaction mixture; m.p. 73.5–74.5°C.

Curing

Paraplex P-43 (Rohm and Haas) is one of the most widely used
commercial polyester resins. TBT methacrylate dissolves in this
unsaturated polyester resin up to 40%, at which point the Sn loading
is about 25%. Paraplex P-43 and TBT methacrylate were mixed in
various ratios. Twenty-five-gram quantities of these mixtures were
taken in polyethylene vials and mixed with 0.25 g of dimethylaniline;
0.5 g of benzoyl peroxide in 5 ml of benzene was added to each and
mixed well. A thermocouple was positioned at the center of the
reaction mixture and the output of the thermocouple measured as
a function of time. The gel time and peak exothermic temperature
were always about 2.5 minutes and 85°C.

WEP-661P (Ashland) is another unsaturated polyester containing
about 60% styrene. The resin is water-extendable. Both TBT methacrylate and TBT acrylate could be dissolved in the resin. Benzoyl
peroxide and methyl ethyl ketone peroxide were capable of curing
the mixture with the aid of dimethylaniline or cobalt naphthenate
or both. However, the organotin group was found to interfere with
the activity of cobalt naphthenate. If cobalt naphthenate is to be
used as an accelerator, it should be added to the reaction mixture
toward the end.

Characterization

Soxhlet extraction with a mixture of benzene and 2-butanone
showed that the organotin group was attached to the polymer network.
Tin assay revealed that very little Sn was lost in the sol fraction.

The cured polyesters, however, were found to break down on prolonged treatment with the solvent mixture. Cured polyurethanes, on the other hand, had swollen under the attack of solvents; even though they had reverted to their original dimensions on drying, the samples had cracked seriously. Epoxy- and aziridine-cured plastics underwent no apparent changes on solvent extraction for two weeks. The epoxy samples did not show any cracks even under scanning electron microscope. The change in structural integrity was in no way related to the percentage of extractables.

REFERENCES

1. R.V. Subramanian and M. Anand, in: "Chemistry and Properties of Crosslinked Polymers," S.S. Labana, Ed., Academic Press, New York (1977). p. 1.

2. R.V. Subramanian, B.K. Garg, J.J. Jakubowski, J. Corredor, J.A. Montemarano, and E.C. Fischer, Am. Chem. Soc., Fiv., Org. Coat. Plast. Chem., Pap. 36(2):660 (1976).

3. R.V. Subramanian and B.K. Garg, in: "Proceedings of the 1977 International Controlled Release Pesticide Symposium," R.L. Goulding, ed., Oregon State University, Corvallis (1977). p. IV-154.

4. R.V. Subramanian, R.S. Williams, and K.N. Somasekharan, Am. Chem. Soc., Div. Org. Coat. Plast. Chem., Pap. 41:38 (1979).

5. R.V. Subramanian, B.K. Garg, and J. Corredor, in: "Organometallic Polymers," C.E. Carraher, Jr., J.E. Sheats, and C.U. Pittman, Jr., eds., Academic Press, New York (1978). p. 181.

6. R.V. Subramanian, B.K. Garg, and K.N. Somasekharan, Am. Chem. Soc., Div. Org. Coat. Plast. Chem., Pap. 39:572 (1978).

7. K.N. Somasekharan and R.V. Subramanian, in: "Modification of Polymers," C.E. Carraher and M. Tsuda, eds., American Chemical Society, Washington (1980). p. 165.

8. V.J. Castelli and W.L. Yeager, in: "Controlled Release Polymeric Formulations," D.R. Paul and F.W. Harris, eds., American Chemical Society, Washington (1976). p. 239.

9. K.N. Somasekharan and R.V. Subramanian, in: "Controlled Release of Bioactive Materials," R.W. Baker, ed., Academic Press, New York (1980). p. 415.

10. K.N. Somasekharan and R.V. Subramanian, Am. Chem. Soc., Div. Org. Coat. Plast. Chem., Pap. 40:167 (1979).

11. H.W. Godbee and D.S. Joy, Assessment of the Loss of Radioactive Isotopes from Waste Solids to the Environment. Part 1; Background and Theory, ORNL-TM-4333 Oak Ridge National Laboratory, Oak Ridge, Tennessee (1974).

12. R.S. Williams, Ph.D. Thesis, Washington State University, Pullman, Washington (1980).

13. R.F. Bennett and R.J. Zedler, J. Oil Colour. Chem. Ass. 49:928 (1966).

14. V. Stannett, <u>in</u>: "Diffusion in Polymers," J. Crank and G.S. Park, eds., Academic Press, New York (1968). Chapter 2.

SYNTHESIS AND PROPERTIES OF NEW COPOLYMERS AND

TERPOLYMERS WITH PENDENT ORGANOTIN MOIETIES

N.A. Ghanem, N.N. Messiha, N.E. Ikladious,
and A.F. Shaaban

Laboratory of Polymers and Pigments
National Research Centre
Dokki, Cairo, Egypt

INTRODUCTION

The growing interest in using acrylic polymers containing pendent hydrolyzable toxic groups as fungicides, pesticides, wood preservatives, and antifouling coatings stimulated basic research aiming at understanding and controlling the parameters which affect the content and distribution of the effective component in the macromolecules, the size of the macromolecule useful as film former, the quality of the film upon application, and the stability of the copolymer solution during storage.[1-4]

The interest stemmed from the much higher effectiveness of the organotin compounds over cuprous oxide, say, in antifouling formulations; organotin polymers present the additional feature of hydrolysis and may be esterasis prior to release, thus providing a molecular layer-by-layer consumption of the film instead of leaching from inner voids.

On one hand, homopolymers of tri-n-butyltin methacrylate and tri-n-butyltin acrylate are unsuitable as film formers; on the other hand, their copolymerization and terpolymerization with other monomers reduce the polymer's general effectiveness and in view of vast differences in monomer reactivities in these processes it is really rare to ensure structure uniformity based on their molar portions in the feed. The problem is further complicated by that even when this is ensured the film properties might not be acceptable.

Guidelines defining the type of copolymerization behavior and
distribution of the active monomer in the chain may be provided
by a knowledge of the so-called monomer reactivity ratios which
can be determined at the early stages of building up the macromolecules.

EXPERIMENTAL

Tri-n-butyltin acrylate (BTA) and tri-n-butyltin methacrylate
(BMTA) were prepared according to the method of Cummins and Dunn,[5]
by the reaction of tri-n-butyltin oxide with acrylic or methacrylic
acids, respectively. All other monomers used in the copolymerization reactions (acrylic acid esters, methacrylic acid esters, acrylonitrile, and styrene) were obtained from E. Merck, Germany, and
were freed from inhibitors by distillation under reduced pressure
and the center cuts retained for use. Azobisisobutyronitrile (AIBN)
was crystallized from alcohol, m.p. 102°C.

Organotin copolymers were obtained by solution polymerization
in toluene so that the total monomer concentration was about 3 mol/l.
The polymerization was commenced by adding AIBN in a concentration
of 1 mol/100 mol monomers, and the solutions were heated at 70°C
for 15-60 min depending on the comonomer pair and composition.

For determinations of monomer reactivity ratios, conversions
were limited within 7-10%, evaluated as weight of copolymer with
respect to the total weight of comonomers. The copolymers were
purified by reprecipitation from 90% methanol, washed several times,
dried, and weighed. Certain azeotropic copolymers and selected
terpolymer compositions were similarly prepared over a wide range
of conversion. Tin contents of the organotin monomers and copolymers were determined by the method of Gilman and Rosenberg,[6] and
nitrogen was determined by a modified Kjeldahl method. The results
of the analyses were used to calculate copolymer and terpolymer
compositions.

RESULTS AND DISCUSSION

In the present investigation the copolymerization parameters
for the copolymerization reactions of tri-n-butyltin acrylate (BTA)
or methacrylate (BTMA) with methyl methacrylate (MMA), n-propyl
methacrylate (PMA), n-butyl methacrylate (BMA), allyl methacrylate
(AMA), methyl acrylate (MA), ethyl acrylate (EA), n-butyl acrylate
(BA), acrylonitrile (AN), and styrene (St) were determined. The
monomer reactivity ratios (r_1 and r_2) for each system were deduced
from the analytical data by both the Fineman-Ross[7] and Kelen-Tudos[8]
methods, and the standard deviations of the results were calculated
by regression analysis as illustrated in Table I. Figures 1 and

TABLE I. MONOMER REACTIVITY RATIOS FOR COPOLYMERIZATION REACTIONS OF BTMA AND BTA WITH METHACRYLIC ACID ESTERS, ACRYLIC ACID ESTERS, ACRYLONITRILE AND STYRENE.

M_1-M_2	Fineman-Ross Method			Kelen-Tudos Method			Azeotropic Composition (Mole %)
	r_1	r_2	$r_1 r_2$	r_1	r_2	$r_1 r_2$	
BTMA-MMA	0.789±0.012	1.004±0.034	0.792	0.790±0.010	1.023±0.009	0.808	no azeotrope
BTMA-PMA	0.580±0.012	0.900±0.046	0.522	0.571±0.014	0.893±0.024	0.510	19.23 : 80.77
BTMA-BMA	0.623±0.016	0.646±0.048	0.402	0.642±0.022	0.678±0.028	0.435	48.43 : 51.57
BTMA-AMA	2.306±0.100	1.013±0.104	2.336	2.380±0.145	1.058±0.078	2.518	no azeotrope
BTMA-MA	1.747±0.028	0.644±0.004	1.160	1.730±0.025	0.649±0.024	1.120	no azeotrope
BTMA-EA	1.259±0.016	0.606±0.032	0.763	1.262±0.014	0.613±0.024	0.773	no azeotrope
BTMA-BA	0.846±0.005	0.572±0.015	0.484	0.855±0.008	0.578±0.008	0.494	73.00 : 27.00
BTA-MMA	0.401±0.012	2.199±0.060	0.881	0.395±0.013	2.180±0.058	0.861	no azeotrope
BTA-PMA	0.323±0.010	1.713±0.048	0.553	0.314±0.017	1.684±0.033	0.528	no azeotrope
BTA-BMA	0.196±0.005	1.650±0.032	0.323	0.197±0.012	1.668±0.028	0.328	no azeotrope
BTA-AMA	0.195±0.005	2.257±0.054	0.440	0.201±0.009	2.619±0.040	0.526	no azeotrope
BTMA-AN	0.465±0.006	0.467±0.009	0.217	0.471±0.026	0.474±0.008	0.223	50.00 : 50.00
BTMA-St	0.256±0.003	1.104±0.039	0.282	0.259±0.029	1.108±0.009	0.287	no azeotrope
BTA-AN	0.243±0.001	1.008±0.011	0.244	0.240±0.004	0.997±0.007	0.239	no azeotrope
BTA-St	0.213±0.010	1.910±0.049	0.406	0.219±0.048	1.939±0.038	0.424	no azeotrope

2 show the Fineman Ross and Kelen Tudos plots, respectively, for the copolymerization reactions of BTMA with methacrylic acid esters, as an example of the systems studied.

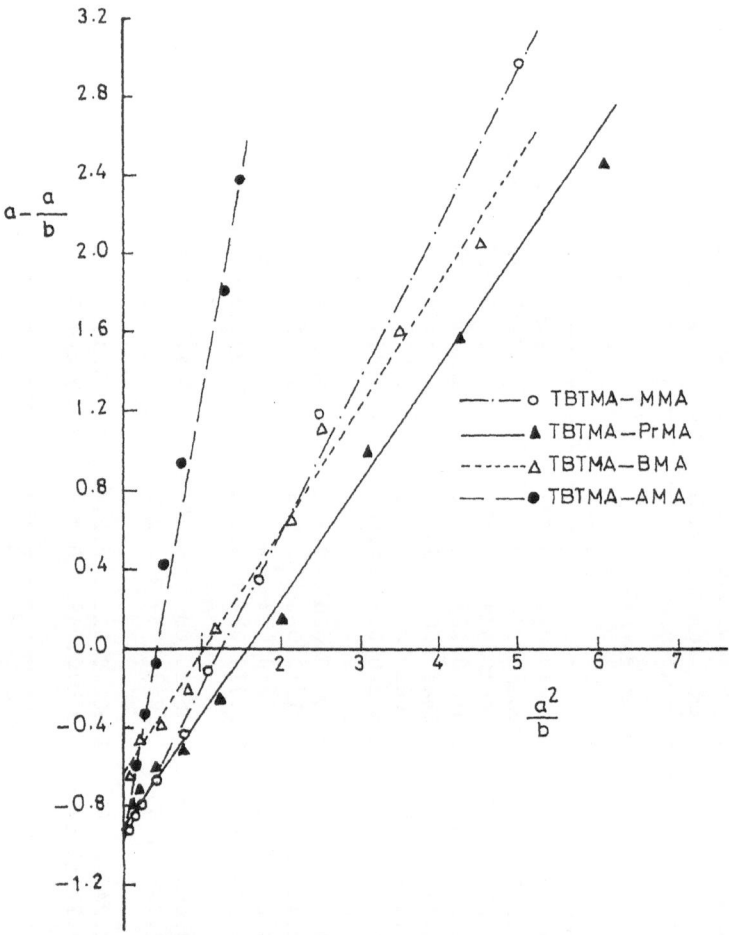

Figure 1.   Fineman-Ross plots for copolymerization reactions of BTMA with methacrylic acid esters. (a and b are comonomer feed and copolymer compositions in molar ratios, respectively).

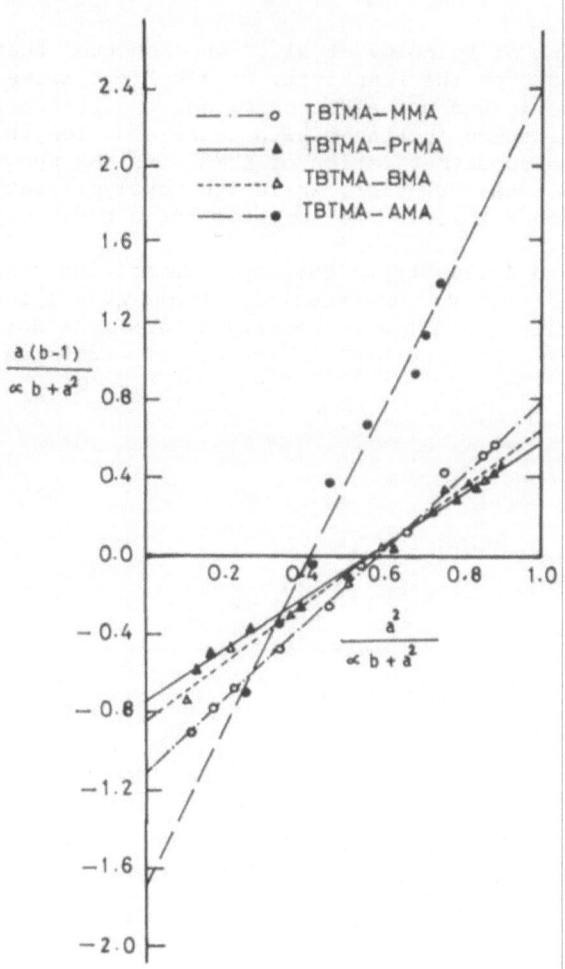

Figure 2.   Kelen-Tudos plots for copolymerization reactions of
            BTMA with methacrylic acid esters. (a and b are
            comonomer feed and copolymer compositions, respectively,
            and
$$\propto \ = \ \frac{a_{min.} \ a_{max}}{\sqrt{b_{min.} \ b_{max}}}$$

     The $r_1 r_2$ values illustrated in Table I indicate that most of
the studied copolymer systems should have random distribution of
the monomer units in the copolymer chain and the tendency towards
alternation increases with increasing the alkyl chain length of
methacrylic or acrylic acid esters used. This behavior is in agree-

ment with the work of Eginbaev et al.,[9] who reported that the predominant influences on the reactivity of alkyl acrylates or methacrylates were steric and not electronic, and the steric hinderance in the copolymerization increased with increasing length of the alkyl chain. The copolymerization of BTMA with MMA shows greater tendency towards ideal behavior, while its copolymerization with AMA shows a tendency towards the formation of a block copolymer.

Figures 3 and 4 illustrate the copolymerization composition curves for the fifteen systems studied. From Table I and Figures 3 and 4, it is clear that the reactivity ratios r_1 and r_2 for BTMA-PMA, BTMA-BMA, BTMA-BA, and BTMA-AN systems are both less than

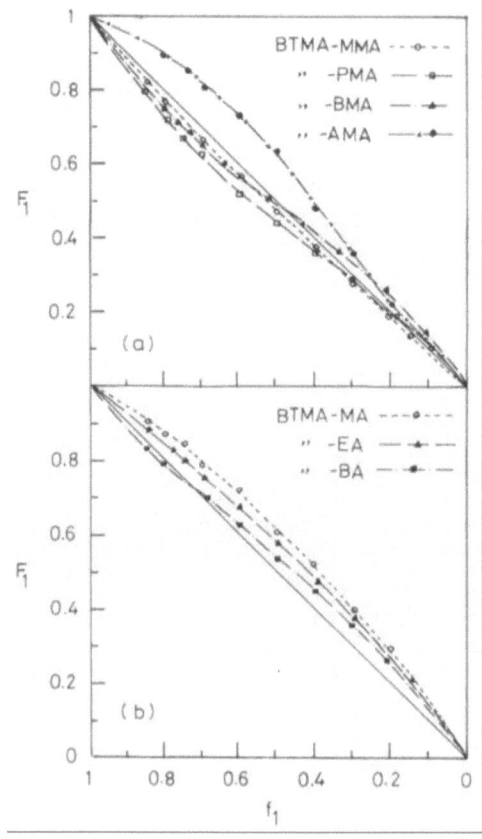

Figure 3.   Composition curves for copolymerization reactions of: (a) BTMA with methacrylic acid esters, and (b) BTMA with acrylic acid esters. (f_1 and F_1 represent mole fraction of organotin monomer in comonomer feed and in copolymer, respectively).

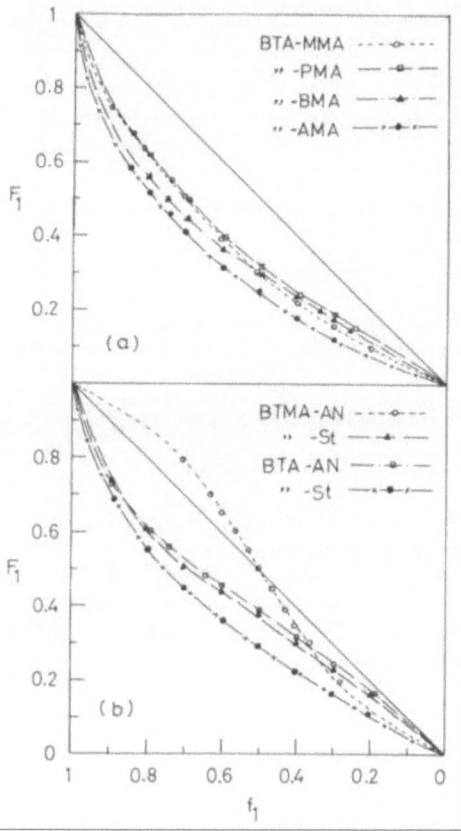

Figure 4. Composition curves for copolymerization reactions of:
(a) BTA with methacrylic acid esters, and (b) BTA and
BTMA with acrylonitrile and styrene. (f_1 and F_1 represent mole fraction of organotin monomer in comonomer
feed and in copolymer, respectively).

unity, and the copolymerization reactions of these systems should
have azeotropic compositions as illustrated in Table I; the copolymerization reactions studied for BTA did not show any azeotropic
compositions. Thus, the four azeotropic compositions were polymerized to different levels of conversion covering a wide range,
and each sample was analyzed for its tin content. Figure 5 shows
F_1 (mole fraction of BTMA in copolymer) as a function of conversion,
which indicates that the experimental points, calculated from the
tin content of each sample, are in good agreement with the lines
representing the mole fractions of BTMA in the four azeotropic
copolymer compositions.

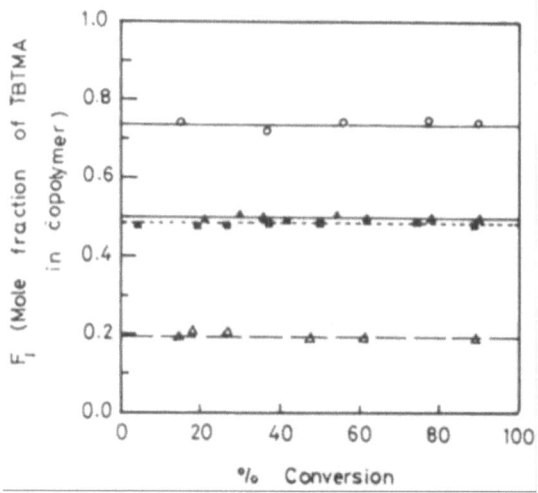

Figure 5.   Mole fraction of BTMA as a function of conversion for
azeotropic copolymerizations of:
BTMA-PMA ———— △ ————, BTMA-BMA ---- ■ -----,
BTMA-BA ————O———— and BTMA-AN ———▲———
(lines represent theoretical values and points from
experimental results).

The terpolymerization reactions of EA-BTMA-AN, BA-BTMA-AN,
MMA-BTA-AN, and BMA-BTA-AN systems were studied to check the cor-
rectness of the reactivity ratios determined by us (Table I) and
the literature values for the binary copolymerizations of EA-AN,[10]
BA-AN,[11] MMA-AN,[12] and BMA-AN[13] systems. The selected feed compositions for the four systems studied (Table II) were polymerized
to low conversions (less than 10%), and the terpolymers produced
were analyzed for their tin and nitrogen contents from which the
terpolymer composition of each sample could be calculated. The
initially formed terpolymer composition of each system was calculated by using the terpolymer composition equation in the form proposed by Khan and Horowitz.[14] Table II shows the results of the
analysis of the four terpolymer compositions, which are in good
agreement with the calculated values.

It is well known that molecular heterogeneity has a direct
effect on the physical properties of polymers. The four terpolymer
systems illustrated in Table II were polymerized to different
extents of conversion, and the terpolymer composition of each sample

TABLE II. TERPOLYMER COMPOSITIONS FROM TIN AND NITROGEN
ANALYSES

System	Feed Composition Mole %	Sn%	N%	Terpolymer Composition Mole % Found	Calcd
EA	29.96			22.80	21.21
BTMA	19.97	21.65	4.48	27.98	27.87
AN	50.07			49.28	50.92
BA	40.02			34.14	32.95
BTMA	19.95	19.70	3.16	27.86	27.37
AN	40.03			37.99	39.78
MMA	40.46			59.89	58.48
BTA	19.64	10.80	3.71	10.24	8.87
AN	39.90			29.86	32.65
BMA	29.51			5.07	51.72
BTA	29.99	13.30	3.00	16.77	15.54
AN	40.50			32.15	32.74

was determined on the basis·of tin and nitrogen analyses. Prediction of both the instantaneous and average terpolymer composition
at each level of conversion was calculated for each terpolymer
system by integration of the terpolymer composition equation according to the method of Skeist.[15] The variations of the calculated
instantaneous terpolymer composition (Mole %) and average terpolymer
composition (Wt %) as a function of conversion for the four terpolymer systems studied are illustrated in Figures 6-9. From the
conversion-composition curves for EA-BTMA-AN and BA-BTMA-AN systems,
it is clear that BTMA is completely consumed at 95% conversion in
both systems, after which copolymers of EA-AN and BA-AN are formed,
and that the AN contents of the two terpolymers remain almost constant up to 90% conversion. Also, Figures 8 and 9 for MMA-BTA-AN
and BMA-BTA-AN systems show that MMA and BMA decreased continuously
with conversion and disappeared at 85% and 77% conversions respectively. BTA content for both systems increased continuously with
conversion up to 100% conversion. Figures 6-9 also show that the
experimental points obtained from tin and nitrogen analyses of the
four terpolymer systems studied at different levels of conversions
are in good agreement with the predicted lines.

The prepared copolymers and terpolymers were soluble, colorless,
transparent, and suitable for film formation. A set of co- and
terpolymer compositions was selected with the aim to prepare co-
and terpolymers at high conversions (about 90%) having suitable

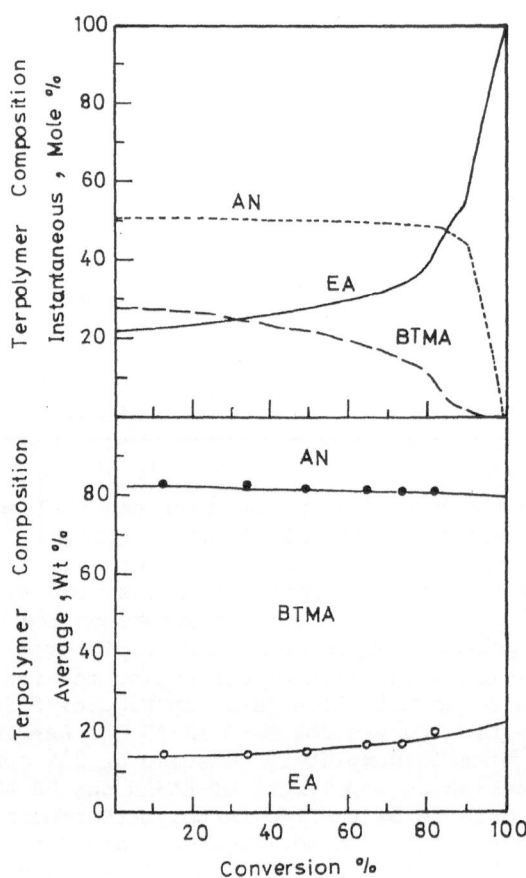

Figure 6. Variation of instantaneous and average terpolymer
compositions with conversion for EA-BTMA-AN, feed
29.96:19.97:50.07 mole % (lines represent predicted
values and points from nitrogen and tin analyses).

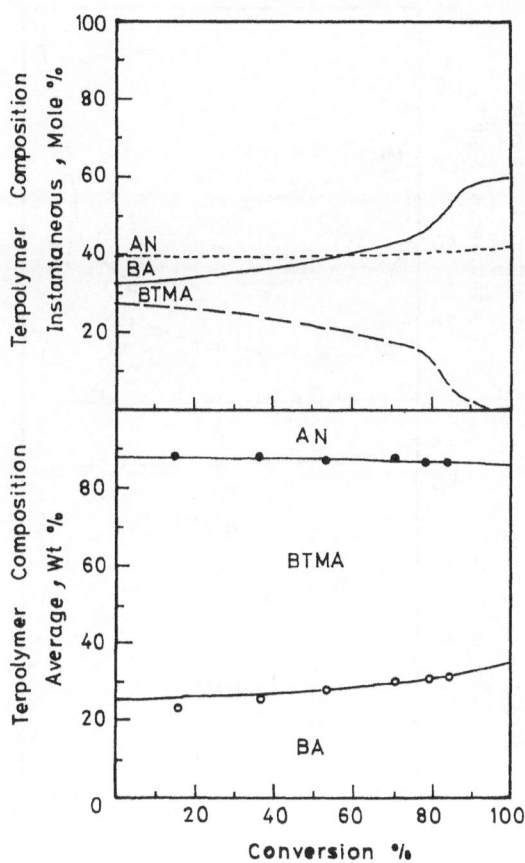

Figure 7. Variation of instantaneous and average terpolymer
           compositions with conversion for BA-BTMA-AN, feed
           40.02:19.95:40.04 mole % (lines represent predicted
           values and points from nitrogen and tin analyses).

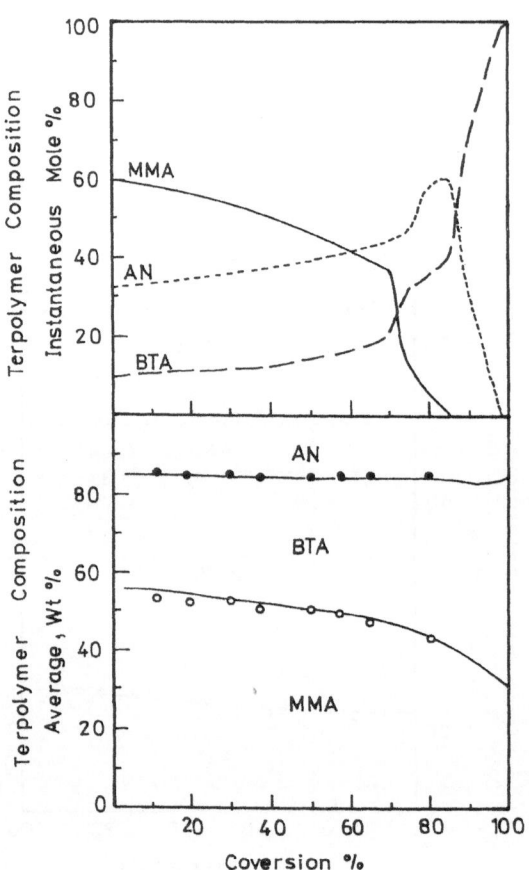

Figure 8. Variation of instantaneous and average terpolymer
compositions with conversion for MMA-BTA-AN, feed
40.46:19.65:39.90 mole % (lines represent predicted
values and points from nitrogen and tin analyses).

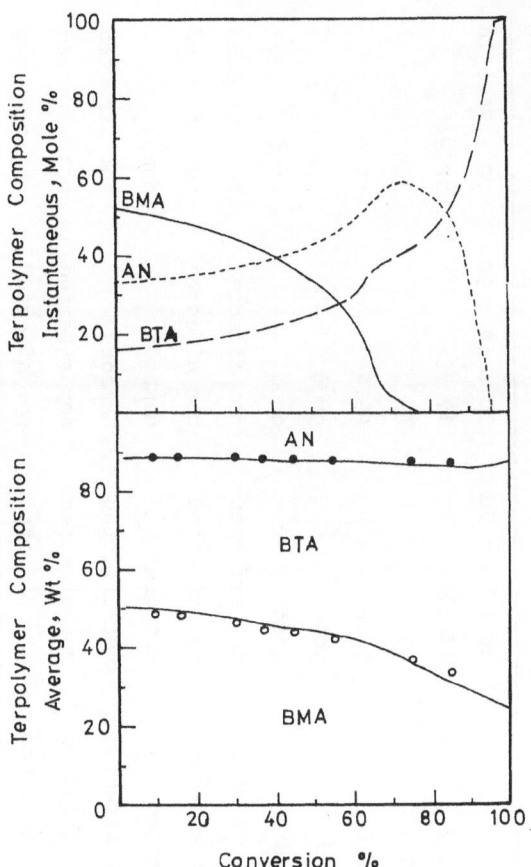

Figure 9. Variation of instantaneous and average terpolymer
           compositions with conversion for BMA–BTA–AN, feed
           29.51:29.99:49.50 mole % (lines represent predicted
           values and points from nitrogen and tin analyses).

film properties. Films were prepared from the purified organotin
polymer solutions on glass, tin, and PVC plates and left at room
temperature to complete drying for evaluation and testing[16] for
hardness (pendulum), adhesion, elasticity, resistance to cold and
hot water, and resistance to dilute alkaline and acid solutions.
The experimental conditions and testing results are summarized in
Tables III and IV.

TABLE III. FILM PROPERTIES OF SELECTED COPOLYMER AND TERPOLYMER COMPOSITIONS INVOLVING BTMA AND MMA

Test	BTMA-MMA	BTMA-MMA-BMA	BTMA-MMA-AN	BTMA-MMA-BTA
Molar Ratio	30 : 70	30 : 50 : 20	30 : 50 : 20	20 : 70 : 10
Tin Content (%)	18.72	18.59	19.98	18.94
Thickness (μm)	100	95	85	120
Hardness (seconds)	101.0	81.6	95.6	97.9
Adhesion	good	good	good	fiar
Elasticity	good	good	good	good
Cold water	not affected	not affected	not affected	not affected
Hot water	not affected	not affected	not affected	not affected
5% NaOH soln	damaged	damaged	damaged	damaged
5% Na$_2$CO$_3$ soln	not affected	not affected	damaged	not affected
5% H$_2$SO$_4$ soln	not affected	not affected	not affected	not affected
Synthetic sea water	not affected	not affected	not affected	not affected

TABLE IV.   FILM PROPERTIES OF SELECTED COPOLYMER AND TERPOLYMER COMPOSITIONS
INVOLVING BTMA AND St

Test	BTMA-St	BTMA-St-BMA	BMA-St-AN	BTMA-St-BTA
Molar Ratio	40 : 60	40 : 40 : 20	40 : 40 : 20	20 : 60 : 20
Tin Content (%)	20.85	29.54	21.70	22.38
Thickness (μm)	90	100	90	100
Hardness (seconds)	tacky	tacky	tacky	20
Adhesion	good	good	good	good
Elasticity	good	good	good	good
Cold water	not affected	not affected	not affected	not affected
Hot water	not affected	not affected	not affected	not affected
5% NaOH soln	damaged	damaged	damaged	damaged
5% Na$_2$CO$_3$ soln	not affected	not affected	not affected	not affected
5% H$_2$SO$_4$ soln	not affected	not affected	not affected	not affected
Synthetic sea water	not affected	not affected	not affected	not affected

From Tables III and IV it is clear that all films of the selected organotin compositions possess good film properties. However, compositions involving St showed slight tackiness, which may be due to its high organotin moieties (50 mole %). All films showed sensitivity towards dilute sodium hydroxide solution; they were not affected by the carbonate solution.

REFERENCES

1. N.A. Ghanem, N.N. Messiha, N.E. Ikladious and A.F. Shaaban, Europ. Polymer J. 15:823 (1979).
2. N.A. Ghanem, N.N. Messiha, N.E. Ikladious and A.F. Shaaban, Europ. Polymer J. 16:339 (1980).
3. N.A. Ghanem, N.N. Messiha, N.E. Ikladious, M.M. Abd El-Malek, and A.F. Shaaban, 26th International Symposium on Macromolecules (IUPAC), Vol. I, p. 632, Mainz, September 1979.
4. D. Atherton, J. Verborgt, and M.A.M. Winkeler, J Coatings Technol. 51(657):88 (1979).
5. R.A. Cummins and P. Dunn, Aust. J. Chem. 17:185 (1964).
6. H. Gilman and D. Rosenberg, J. Am. Chem. Soc. 75:3592 (1953).
7. M. Fineman and S.D. Ross, J. Polymer Sci. 5:259 (1950).
8. T. Kelen and F. Tudos, J. Macromolek. Sci.-Chem. 9:1 (1975).
9. Ah.E. Eginbaev, K.A. Ayapbergenov, and Z.M. Muldakhmetov, Deposited Doc. USSR, 1977, c.f. C.A. 91:124043q (1979).
10. W.M. Ritchey and L.E. Ball, J. Polymer Sci. B4:557 (1966).
11. J. Muller, Chem. Listy, 48:1593 (1954), c.f. C.A. 49:5077d (1955).
12. F.M. Lewis, F.R. Mayo, and W.F. Hulse, J. Am. Chem. Soc. 67:1701 (1945).
13. A.S. Nair and M.S. Muthana, Makrolmol. Chem. 47:138 (1961).
14. D.J. Khan and H.H. Horowitz, J. Polymer Sci. 54:363 (1961).
15. I. Skeist, J. Am. Chem. Soc. 68:1781 (1946).
16. A. Gardner and G. Sward, in: "Physical and Chemical Examinations of Paints, Varnishes, Lacquers and Colours," 12th Edition, Gardner Laboratory, Inc. Bethesda 14, MD, U.S.A. (1962).

CHARACTERIZATION OF BIOACTIVE ORGANOTIN POLYMERS:

FRACTIONATION AND DETERMINATION OF MW BY SEC-GFAA

E.J. Parks and F.E. Brinckman

Chemical and Biodegradation Processes Group
Center for Materials Science
National Bureau of Standards
Washington, D.C. 20234

INTRODUCTION

Organometallic polymers (OMP's), incorporating biocidal tri-organotin moieties, chemically bonded to carboxyl groups pendant along polymer chains, are undergoing intensive development as long-term controlled-release, marine antifouling agents.[1] Materials in this general class have been prepared by copolymerizing methyl-methacrylate and organotin-substituted methacrylates in a free radical initiated process.[2] The polymers are incorporated within a polymeric binding substrate and coated over surfaces that are to be exposed to a marine-service environment. Tin-containing fragments tailored[3] to prevent build-up of fouling micro-organisms[4] are slowly leached out of the coating.[5] The protective mechanism is not necessarily a simple chemical or physical process, and the macromolecular materials break down over a period of years.[1,2]

To devise a useful and predictable slow release OMP, it is desirable to incorporate most of the tin within a high polymer matrix,[1] to control the molecular weight (MW) and MW distribution (MWD) and, ultimately, to correlate degradation, leaching rates, and other parameters of field performance with measurable and controllable molecular size properties. Consequently, our major objectives in the present investigation were to determine the relative quantities of organotin-containing polymer in the high- and low-MW fractions of OMP formulations of current interest and to estimate the molecular weight of these fractionated polymers.

Brinckman et al.[6] introduced methods and apparatus for the speciation of trace metal- or metalloid-containing molecules by high-performance liquid chromatography (HPLC) automatically coupled with a metal-specific graphite furnace atomic absorption (GFAA)

spectrophotometric detector. Parks et al.[7] extended the HPLC-GFAA
method for fractionating metal-containing macromolecules according
to differences in MW and determining the relative amount of metal
associated with each fraction. This approach is based on size-
exclusion chromatography (SEC) similarly coupled with a concentra-
tion-sensitive differential refractive index/ultraviolet absorption
(RI/UV) dual detector in-line with element-specific GFAA.

The GFAA detector offers significant advantages over conventional RI or UV detectors in selectivity, sensitivity, and freedom
from eluent matrix effects.[5] For many macromolecules, especially
the OMP materials studied here, where neither strong chromophores
nor index of refraction changes occur during elutions, this alternative proved useful. In our previous work[7] with organotin-containing copolymers of MMA, at high column loadings, we obtained RI and
UV chromatograms that appeared to indicate well-resolved fractions
of both high- and low-MW. Nonetheless, the concurrent GFAA chromatograms showed that serious peak overlap and tailing was occurring
with the tin-containing eluates, indicating that poor resolution
of the bioactive macromolecules was obtained because of column over-
loading.

In the present investigation, we have exploited the desirable
features of the GFAA detector at the expense of obtaining no concurrent RI and limited UV information. Thus, we injected approximately five percent of the amounts of organotin polymers conventionally required for RI detection in tetrahydrofuran (THF), the
solvent/eluent of choice. Our selections of OMP materials are those
also undergoing concurrent evaluation as candidate marine antifoul-
ants in field tests.

EXPERIMENTAL*

Instrumental Methods

The HPLC-UV/RI-GFAA system is outlined schematically in
Figure 1.[7] A high-pressure pump (Altex Model 110A, Berkeley, CA),
equipped with a single sapphire piston in conjunction with precision
inlet and outlet valves, was used to deliver solvent at the controlled flow rate of one mL min^{-1} in the present work. Isocratic con-

---

* Certain commercial materials and equipment are identified in this
  paper in order to specify the experimental procedures. In no case
  does such identification imply recommendation or endorsement by the
  National Bureau of Standards nor does it imply that the material or
  equipment identified is necessarily the best available for the
  purpose.

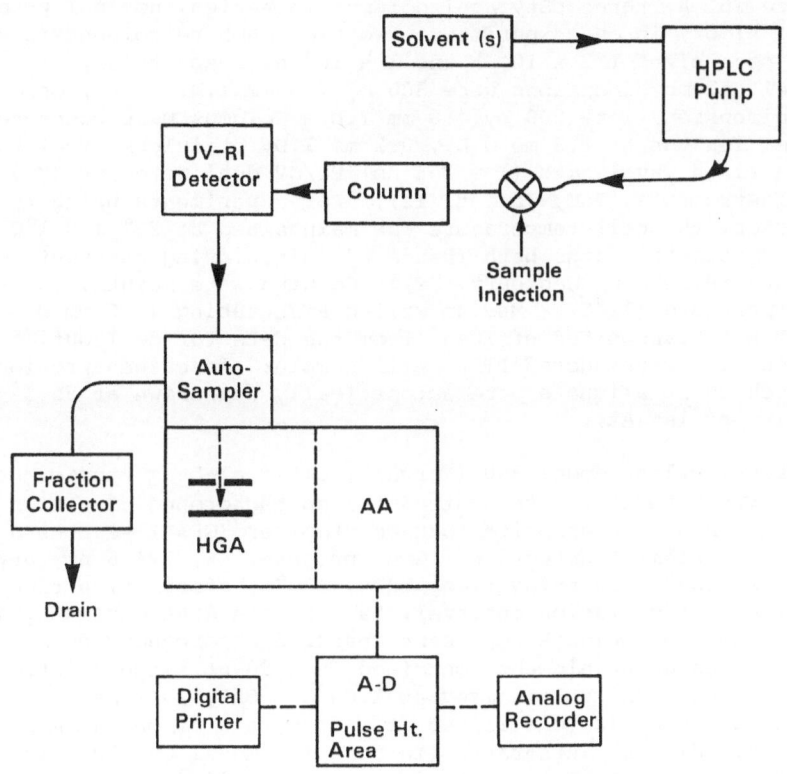

Figure 1.   Block diagram summarizing the SEC-GFAA system, including
accessory devices.[7]   In the present work, the auto
sampler continuously aliquoted 20-μL specimens into the
graphite furnace at intervals of 55.5 seconds.   With
a flow rate of one mL min^{-1}, the amount of sample consumed
in GFAA is 2.14 percent of the effluent.   Excess sample
can be collected for off-line analysis.

ditions were employed. Solutions of organometallic compounds, or
compounds of standard MW, were injected in solution (50 μL) into
the SEC system via an on-line high-pressure syringe loading sample
injector (Rheodyne Model 7120, Berkeley, CA). An in-line precolumn
filter, pore size 2 μm (No. 84560, Waters Associates, Milford, MA),
was used to protect columns employed for SEC. The columns were
packed with porous, highly crosslinked polystyrene-divinylbenzene
(PS-DVB) copolymer (μStyragel, Waters Associates), or with microspheres of silica (LiChrosphere, Merck, Darmstadt, West Germany),
each packing material having a particle size of ten μm. Columns

used for separations were: two μStyragel columns in series, nominal
pore size 10^2 Å; three μStyragel columns in series, nominal pore
size 10^3 Å; or, in one experiment, two LiChrosphere columns in series,
nominal pore size of 3×10^2 Å and 1×10^2 Å, respectively. The
μStyragel column dimensions were 300 by 7.8 mm I.D. The LiChrosphere
column dimensions were 250 by 4.6 mm I.D. Columns were connected
by 100-mm lengths of 1.5 mm O.D., 0.2 mm I.D. stainless-steel tubing,
and to a fixed wavelength (λ = 254 nm) RI/UV dual detector (Knaur,
Utopia Instruments, Inc, Joliet, IL). For experiments using the
RI detector, the cell temperature was maintained at 22° ± 0.1°C
by a thermostatted water bath (Lauda K4R circulating constant temperature bath, Brinkman, Westbury, NY). Columns were maintained at
room temperature (22°C). Medium-walled PTFE tubing (1.6 mm O.D.,
0.7 mm I.D.) transported effluent from the detector cell outlet
to a specially constructed PTFE "well sampler" described previously,[6]
from which 20-μL aliquots were automatically withdrawn at 55.5-
second intervals (Δt).

A Perkin-Elmer Model 360 (Norwalk, CT) dual-beam atomic absorption spectrophotometer with deuterium lamp background corrector
and a Model HGA 2100 graphite furnace atomizer (GFAA) were used
for specific element detection. GFAA program: λ, 224.6 nm; drying
time, 10 s, 100°C; charring time, 10 s, 200°C; atomization time,
10 s, 2700°C; atomization interval, 55.5 s. In GFAA chromatograms,
the observed peak heights represent measured absorbances due to
the quantities of an element contained in a 20-μL aliquot introduced
into the furnace and volatilized at 2700°C. Only 2.14 percent of
the total effluent is volatilized at a flow rate of one mL·min^{-1}.
An automatic digital integrator (Infotronics Model CRS-204, Infotronics Corp., Austin, TX) was used to obtain a direct record of
AA absorption intensities.

Chemical Reagents and Polymer Samples

Samples of organometallic polymers in solution were provided
by the U.S. Naval Ship Research and Development Center, Annapolis,
MD. Dyckman and Montemarano have described the preparation, structure, and empirical testing of a number of formulations of these
materials.[2] A representative terpolymer of methyl methacrylate,
tri-n-butyltin methacrylate, and tri-n-propyltin methacrylate (OMP-
1) is depicted in Figure 2.[2] Macromolecules of polystyrene and
polymethyl methacrylate serving as MW standards, obtained from
commercial sources, are listed in Table I. OMP-1 and OMP-2 were
provided in the form of solutions in Stoddard solvent (mineral
spirits) containing approximately 50 percent by weight of the
polymer. OMP-S and OMP-R were provided in the form of solutions
in benzene containing approximately 40 percent by weight of polymer.
These samples were diluted with THF and analyzed by SEC-GFAA in

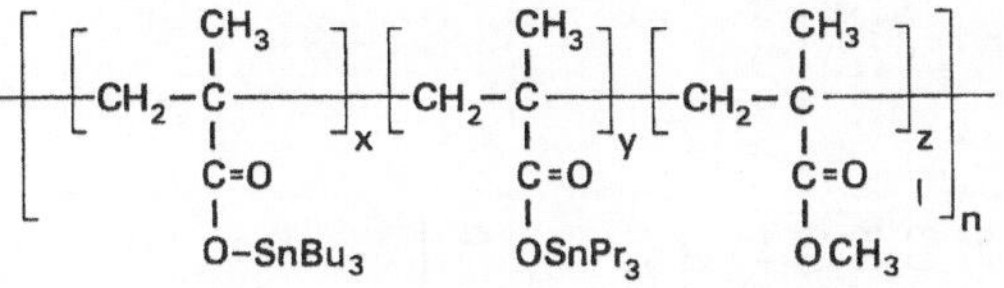

n, x, y, z = repeating monomeric units

Figure 2. Suggested formula for a representative OMP, the terpolymer of methylmethacrylate, tributyltin methacrylate,
and tripropyltin methacrylate. The subscripts x, y and
z represent numbers of monomers. Actual numerical values
may not be assigned,[2] and are not assumed to be constant.

0.1-percent solutions showing strong UV absorbance due to the benzene.
The major portion of benzene then was removed by permitting the
samples to stand overnight under ambient conditions in a vented
hood, and the samples were taken up in tetrahydrofuran (THF) prior
to fractionation by SEC. All other OMP samples were provided in
the form of solutions in the THF, containing about one percent by
weight of polymer.

THF (Eastman-Kodak, Rochester, NY) was used throughout as both
solvent and eluent. In one experiment using the LiChrosphere columns
described above, THF was modified by the addition of 0.05 percent
by weight of polyethylene glycol (Carbowax, Fisher Scientific Co.,
Silver Spring, MD) of MW 20,000. Solvent was purified by filtration
before use, by means of organic-clarification kits with filters
of 0.5-μm pore size (Millipore, Bedford, MA), and degassed daily
by magnetic stirring at ambient temperature under vacuum. Insoluble
materials were removed from sample solutions in THF by filtration
with organic sample clarification kits of 0.45-μm pore size (Millipore, Bedford, MA).

Methods of Data Reduction

Weight-average and number-average molecular weights (M_w and
M_n) were determined from chromatographic GFAA peaks corresponding
to individual polymeric fractions, by the methods described in
detail by Yau, Kirkland and Bly.[8,9] The intensities of individual
tin peaks (h_i), proportional to experimental peak heights, were
obtained from the digital integrator record. Molecular weights
(M_i) corresponding to each (h_i) value were obtained by comparing
the corrected elution volume (V_R') with a corresponding point on
the column calibration curve shown in Figure 4. The logarithm of
the molecular weight of the tin-containing species is assumed for

TABLE I. STANDARDS FOR COLUMN CALIBRATION

Compound	Source	Nominal MW Value	Analytical Data[a]		
			M_n[b]	M_w[c]	MWD[d]
Polystyrene	Arro[e]	600	600 7%	---[f]	<1.10
Polystyrene	Arro	800	811 7%	---	---
Polystyrene	Arro	2,100	2,115 7%	---	<1.10
Polystyrene	Arro	4,000[g]	3,100 5%	---	---
Polystyrene	Arro	12,000	12,000	12,200	1.10
Polystyrene	Arro	19,000	18,900	19,400	1.03
Polystyrene	Arro	50,000	50,400	52,100	1.03
Polystyrene	Arro	111,000	111,000	111,000	1.00
Polystyrene	Arro	233,000	217,000 ± 6%	257,000 ± 6%	1.17
Polystyrene	Arro	390,000	383,000	392,000	1.02
Polystyrene	Arro	630,000	632,000	694,000	1.10
Polystyrene	Arro	1,500,000	---	1,500,000	<1.10
Polymethyl-methacrylate	Polysciences[h]	75,000	---	---	<1.10

[a] All data provided by manufacturer.

[b] Number average molecular weight.

[c] Weight average molecular weight.

[d] Molecular weight dispersion (Mw/Mn).

[e] Arro Labs, Joliet, IL.

[f] A blank line indicates data not provided.

[g] In preparing the calibration curve, our best estimate value of 3100 was substituted for the manufacturer's nominal MW of 4000.

[h] Polysciences, Inc., Warrington, PA.

present purposes to be that of the Polystyrene standard sample that elutes with a corresponding elution volume. From the (h_i) and $M_i)$ values, M_w, M_n and molecular weight dispersions (MWD) are calculated according to the following relationships:[9]

$$M_w = \frac{\sum_{i=1}^{n} (h_i M_i)}{\sum_{i=1}^{n} h_i}$$

$$M_n = \frac{\sum_{i=1}^{n} h_i}{\sum_{i=1}^{n} (h_i/M_i)}$$

$$MWD = \frac{M_w}{M_n}$$

The area of each polymeric peak was calculated by summation of the individual tin peaks.[6,10] GFAA chromatograms usually were separated into fractions at a V_R' of 30 ml, corresponding to a species having a molecular weight of about 500. Occasionally, there appeared to be peak overlap involving not more than one individual tin signal of relatively low intensity, shared by two polymeric fractions. In these instances, 50 percent of the tin signal was attributed to each fraction in summing up total areas.

The percent of tin in each fraction was obtained by summing up the total of GFAA tin signals, dividing that quantity into the sum of tin associated with the polymer fraction, then multiplying by 100.

RESULTS AND DISCUSSION

Dyckmann and Montemarano[2] prepared various OMP's, typically from monomers of organotin acrylate esters and methyl methacrylate

(MMA), in the presence of a free-radical initiator at the reflux
temperature of benzene (80°C). Under similar reaction conditions,
MMA alone forms homopolymers of polymethyl methacrylate (PMMA)
having a predominantly syndiotactic configuration.[11] The free
radical reaction of this homopolymer terminates by disproportiona-
tion above 60°, producing an end group in which a carbon-to-carbon
double bond is conjugated with a carbonyl group,[12] viz.

$$H_2C = C\!\!\begin{array}{c} H \\ | \\ C \\ | \\ C=O \\ | \\ O\text{-Me} \end{array}\!\!\!\!-(C\!\!\begin{array}{c} CH_3 \\ | \\ C \\ | \\ C=O \\ | \\ O\text{-Me} \end{array}\!\!)_n$$

The mechanism of copolymerization of organotin methacrylate esters
with methyl methacrylate has not been studied in as much detail
as the free-radical homopolymerization. Ghanem et al.[13] demonstrated
that tri-n-butyltin methacrylate (TBTM) and MMA in the molar ratio
of 50:50 in the presence of a free-radical initiator at 60°C react
in a closed system to form an azeotropic polymer, i.e., a polymer
that maintains a constant composition ratio of TBTM and MMA at all
degrees of conversion.

Side reactions reasonably expected during the copolymerization
of TBTM and MMA include competitive homopolymerization of TBTM and
of MMA to polymethyl methacrylate (PMMA). Complications may ensue
if oxygen is not excluded from the reaction process, since reaction
of PMMA and MMA with oxygen[14] results in low MW polymeric peroxides,
formaldehyde and methyl pyruvate.

Initially, it was necessary to develop a method for determining
the molecular weight of OMP's. The calibration of a system comprised of three μStyragel column in series, each having an average
pore size of 10^3 Å, is illustrated in Figures 3 and 4. A composite
of individual UV chromatograms (Figure 3) of a series of polystyrene
(PS) standards of known MW and narrow molecular weight distribution
(MWD) was assembled and eluted under the same experimental conditions employed in fractionating OMP's. The retention volume (V_R')
of each PS standard is determined[15] as the intersection point of
tangents extrapolated from the straight-line portions of each absorption chromatogram. Between the extremes of total exclusion
and total permeation, molecules are eluted in linear SEC in direct
proportion to the log of molecular weight.[16]

In Figure 4 are plotted average V_R's obtained from duplicate
chromatograms of toluene and a series of PS standards of increasing
MW. The expected[16,17] direct relationship of V_R' and log MW yields
a linear regression slope of -0.1498 with an intercept at +7.166

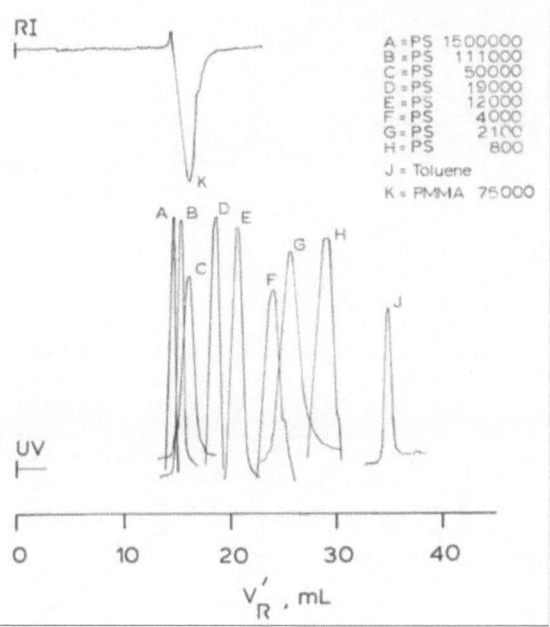

Figure 3. Size-exclusion chromatography (SEC) of polystyrene (PS)
standard samples of known molecular weight (MW), polymethyl methacrylate of MW 75,000 and toluene. Solvent
THF. Columns: Waters Styragel columns (three) in
series, average pore size 10^3Å. Mobile phase THF. Flow
rate one mL $\min^{-1}$ Detector: Knauer UV/RI Dual Detektor.
UV detector operating at 254 nm; UV sensitivity 0.003
absorption unit per full scale deflection (AUFS). RI
sensitivity: (6×10^{-8}) ΔRI per full scale deflection
(DRIFS). Injected volume: 50 µL. Injected concentrations: PS standards 25 µg/50 µL; toluene 16 µg/50 µL;
PMMA, 1250 µg/50 µL. This figure represents a composite
of individual sample injections.

and a linear correlation coefficient of 0.997, for PS standards
having MW between toluene and PS 111,000. The standard deviation
from the mean of each value is represented by bars in Figure 4,
or else is exceeded by the dimensions of the plotted symbols.

The molecular weights of tin-bearing species responsible for
individual signals in the GFAA chromatograms are estimated from
the column calibration data by the following working formula:

$$\log_{10}MW = 0.1498 \ \Delta V_R' + 1.923$$

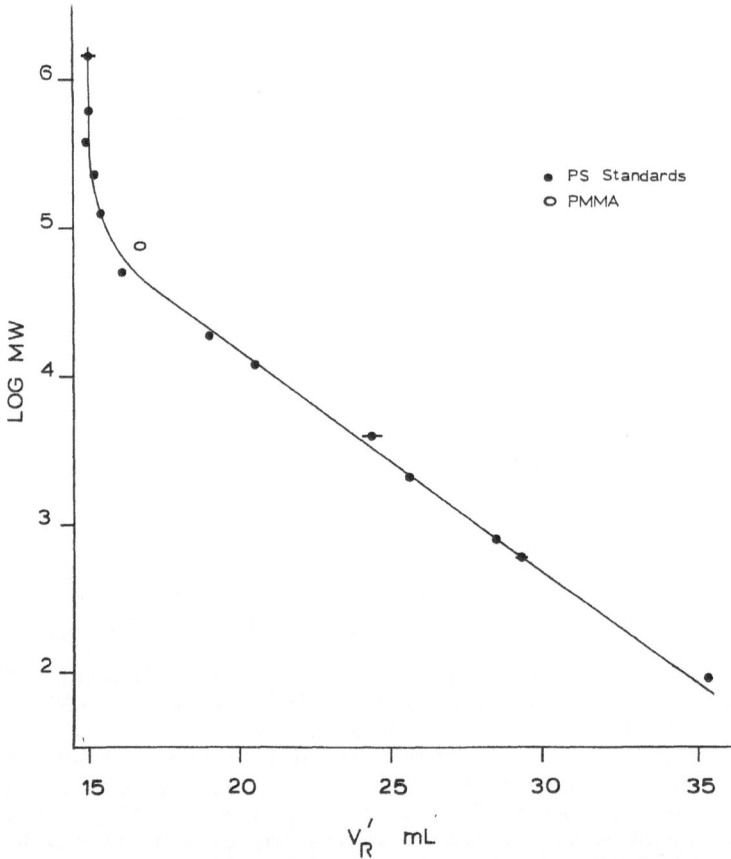

Figure 4.   Column calibration based on elution volumes of PS and
            toluene. Each point represents the intersection of
            tangent extrapolated from straight line portions of the
            respective chromatographic absorption spectra in
            Figure 2. V_R' represents retention volume corrected
            for 0.1 mL of dead volume between the column and the
            UV/RI detector. The point for PMMA (open oval) was
            omitted in calculating slope and correlation coefficient
            (0.997) of the plot of log MW vs V_R'.

In this relationship, $\Delta V'$ is taken to be $(V_R' - 35)$ mL, where V_R'
is the elution volume of the unknown species, 35 mL is an arbitrarily
selected point on the linear portion of the calibration curve, and
1.923 is the logarithm of the MW predicted for the PS standard that
would exhibit an elution volume of 35 mL.

Where Δt is the distance between observed composite tin signals in the GFAA chromatogram, in relating pulsed GFAA signals to continuous UV chromatograms, there exists an uncertainty factor of $\pm$ 1/2 Δt.[6] With an experimental Δt of 55.5 sec, the maximum error is $\pm$ 27.5 sec, and the maximum uncertainty in determining the logarithm of the MW is 27.75/60 x 0.1498, or 0.0693. Thus, for a molecule having an apparent MW of 111,000, the log of the actual MW is 5.045 $\pm$ 0.0693, and the MW lies between 94,559 and 130,107 for an error of $\pm$ 14.8 percent. For a molecule having an apparent MW of 300, log MW = 2.477, and the actual MW lies between 256 and 352 for a potential error of $\pm$ 17.2 percent. The M_w and M_n assignments listed in Table II similarly are subject to maximum errors in the range of 15 percent. The MWD values, being ratios of M_w and M_n, are not subject to this source of error.

The SEC mechanism can be complicated by the presence of other retention modes, depending on stereoelectronic interactions between stationary phase materials and solvents and solutes.[18] Figure 5 shows the culmination of a series of unsuccessful experiments in which fractionation of an OMP on a series of LiChrosphere columns was attempted. The THF used as sample solvent and mobile phase was modified by adding 0.05 percent of polyethylene glycol in order to set up competitive surface adsorption and allow the SEC mechanism to take place.[19] It is seen in Figure 5 that none of the tin-bearing polymer species is eluted prior to PS 600, even though OMP-2 was demonstrated to include a fraction of MW about 111,000.[7] This is consistent with the predominance of an adsorption mechanism, and it is not possible to determine whether the SEC mechanism exerts any influence on the retention of this OMP on this substrate.

μStyragel does not evince the strongly adsorptive retention of OMP-2 shown in Figure 5.[7] However, PS-DVB is not entirely free of surface adsorptivity toward polar molecules.[20-23] For this reason, an attempt was made to acquire a series of polymethyl methacrylate (PMMA) samples of standard MW for comparison of their retention volumes with those of OMP fractions. We were able to obtain only a single commercial PMMA standard sample of MW 75,000. As shown in Figure 4, the data point (open oval) falls somewhat to the right of the point to be expected for a PS standard of equal MW, indicating slower elution of PMMA. The need for better calibration standards than PS in this field is evident. However, a comparison of Figure 3 with Figure 5 shows the effect of adsorption of μStyragel is much smaller than that of adsorption on LiChrosphere. Pending availability of additional PMMA standards, or methods for absolute determination of MW,[24] the $V_R{'}$ values of OMP fractions eluted from columns packed with μStyragel are satisfactorily comparable with those of PS standards, at least for the purposes of the present research.

TABLE II. SEC CHARACTERIZATION OF FRACTIONATED ORGANOTIN
MOIETIES IN ORGANOMETALLIC POLYMERS

Sample[a]	Peak A				Peak B			
	M_n	M_w	MWD[b]	Sn (%)	M_n	M_w	MWD	Sn (%)
OMP-1	14030	39330	2.80	87.4	181	206	1.14	9.5
OMP-2	9130	32110	3.52	67.0	146	238	1.63	16.2
OMP-B-2	6940	20380	2.94	85.55	161	229	1.42	11.7
OMP-B-3	5260	15880	3.02	84.3	171	221	1.29	15.7
OMP-B-4	6870	20890	3.04	89.8	168	252	1.50	10.2
OMP-B-6	9690	21490	2.22	67.4	191	398	2.08	20.8
OMP-B-9	8220	21600	2.63	72.2	97	116	1.19	14.8
OMP-B-11	5790	17750	3.07	94.4	195	318	1.63	5.6
OMP-B-12	4320	11490	2.66	70.5	117	150	1.28	19.4
OMP-B-13	5810	15130	2.60	85.3	133	159	1.20	14.7
OMP-B-14	7510	19770	2.63	86.9	156	265	1.70	13.1
OMP-B-15	4855	19720	4.06	80.7	150	218	1.46	17.0
OMP-B-16	6690	17680	2.64	81.4	155	212	1.37	11.3
OMP-B-17	5310	24680	4.65	85.8	116	222	1.91	12.3
OMP-B-18	8270	21040	2.54	85.6	144	162	1.13	14.4
OMP-B-20	8960	20170	2.25	74.5	146	203	1.80	17.2
OMP-B-23	7390	21540	2.91	82.5	163	253	1.55	11.6
OMP-R	17860	38370	2.15	85.6	171	198	1.16	11.5
OMP-S	24330	49150	2.02	81.5	212	377	1.78	11.7

[a] Sample designation provided by USNRDC personnel.

[b] MWD = M_w/M_n.

Figure 6 depicts the RI and UV chromatograms of PMMA of MW
75,000, eluted from two columns in series packed with µStyragel
of average pore size 10^2 Å. Figure 7 represents chromatograms of
OMP-S and three PS standard samples on these same columns. Because
of the lower pore size, these columns exhibit a lower exclusion
limit than that observed with the 10^3-Å columns discussed above.
The V_R' of PS 111,000 and PS 50,000 on these 10^2-Å columns is that
of total exclusion, since it is equal to the V_R' of PS 19,000 in
another chromatogram (not shown).

Figure 6 shows that the PMMA sample contains at least two fractions of very different MW. As shown in the RI chromatogram, most
of the compound exhibiting a refractive index different from the
mobile phase (DRI), is totally excluded; i.e., the V_R' is that of
excluded PS standards. A second fraction exhibits much lower DRI,
presumably because it is present in much lower concentration. This
fraction is assigned a MW of less than 600 by comparison with the

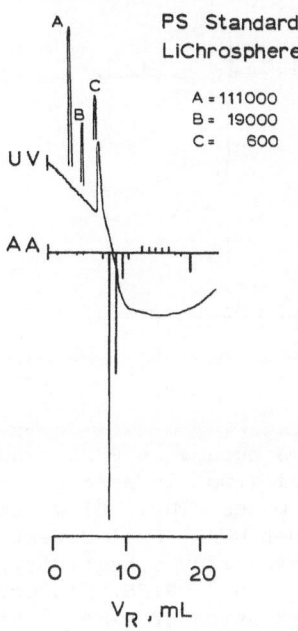

Figure 5.   SEC-UV-GFAA chromatogram of OPM-2.   Solvent, THF.
            Columns: LiChorsphere columns (two) with average pore
            size 3×10^2 Å and 1×10^2 Å, in series. Mobile phase,
            THF containing 0.05 percent polyethylene glycol of MW
            20,000. Flow rate 1.0 mL min^{-1}. GFAA detector Perkin-
            Elmer 460. UV detector, Altex Model 153, operating at
            254 nm. UV sensitivity 0.002 AUFS. Injected volume:
            50 µL. Injected concentrations: PS standards, 5 µg/50
            µL; OMP-2, 5 µg/50 µL.

UV chromatograms of PS standards shown in Figure 7. This low MW
fraction, however, strongly absorbs UV light at a wavelength of
254 nm. As expected, the intensities of the UV absorption peaks
are a quantitative measure of chromophoric group concentrations,
rather than the relative concentrations of high and low MW polymeric
fractions in the PMMA sample.

     Similarly, in the chromatograms of Sample OMP-S, (Figure 7)
a fraction having a comparatively low MW absorbs UV light much more
strongly than the fraction of high MW. The amounts of tin detected
by GFAA, however, indicate a much greater quantity of organotin
incorporated in the high MW than the low MW fraction (Table II).
These data suggest, by analogy with the PMMA chromatograms, that

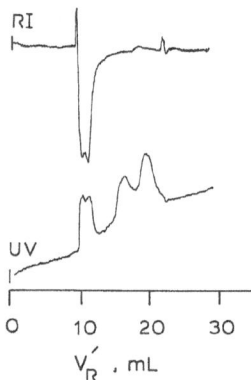

Figure 6.   SEC-UV/RI chromatograms of PMMA. Solvent THF. Columns:
            Waters μStyragel (two) in series, average pore size
            10^2 Å. Mobile phase, THF. Flow rate 1.0 mL min^{-1}.
            Detector: Knauer UV/RI Dual Detektor. UV detector
            operating at 254 nm; UV sensitivity, 0.003 AUFS. RI
            sensitivity, 6 x 10^{-8} DRIFS. Injected volume: 50 μL.
            Injected concentration of PMMA: 1650 μg/50 μL.

the GFAA chromatographic peak sizes are much more nearly proportional than UV signals to the relative concentration of the polymeric fractions.

     Figure 8 shows UV and GFAA chromatograms of OMP-S eluted from
the 10^3-Å μStyragel columns (three in series) whose calibration
is depicted in Figures 2 and 3. The salient features of Figure
7 again are evident. A weakly absorbing, early peak in the UV
chromatogram coincides with a very strong peak in the GFAA chromatogram, and relatively weak AA peaks. By comparison with Figure
2, the initial UV/AA peak is not that of a totally excluded polymer.
Calculations from the GFAA data show fraction A of OMP-S (Table
II) to have a M_w of 49,150, a M_n of 24,330, and a MWD of 2.02.
The MWD is somewhat broad but in line with dispersities reported
in the literature for PMMA.[25,26] The M_w, M_n, and MWD of fraction
B are 377, 212, and 1.78. Although the formula weight of TBTM also
is 377, the agreement with the calculated M_w is probably fortuitious,
since a range of M_w species is involved in the calculation of M_w.
The high MW fraction contains 81.5 percent of the detected tin,
the low MW fraction 11.7 percent. Tailing accounts for 6.8 percent
of the detected tin. The observed tailing may result from either
partial absorption of a polar, tin-bearing species, or total permeation and slow continuous elution of low MW tin-bearing moieties.[18]

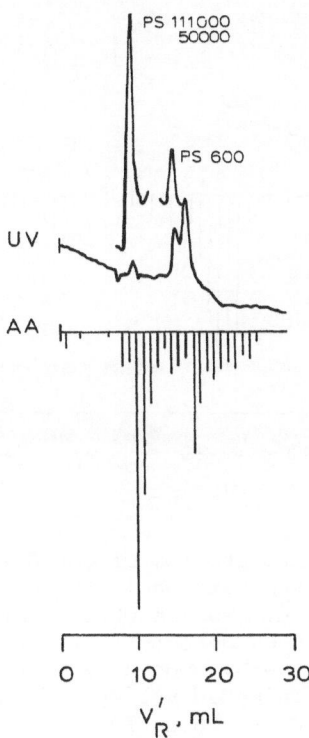

Figure 7.   SEC-UV-GFAA chromatograms of OMP-S and PS standards.
            Solvent, columns, mobile phase and flow rate the same
            as for Figure 6. Knauer UV/RI detector operating in the
            UV mode at 254 nm. Sensitivity 0.003 AUFS. Injected
            volume: 50 µL. Injected concentration of OMP-S:
            50 µg/50 µL. Injected concentration of PS standards
            25 µg/50 µL.

      Figure 9 depicts chromatograms of OMP-23 similarly obtained.
Comparison of Figure 8 with Figure 9 further demonstrates the power
of the experimental technique using tandem means of detection for
differentiating between OMP's prepared from the same types of
monomer by different polymerization methods, as mentioned earlier.
The methods of synthesis differ only in the relatively high charge
of MMA used in synthesizing OMP-23 (Figure 9). On the basis of
UV chromatograms alone, it would seem that OMP-23 contained a significantly greater proportion of high MW polymer than OMP-S, but the
GFAA chromatograms show conclusively that this possibility is not
true of the relative amounts of tin-bearing high polymer species

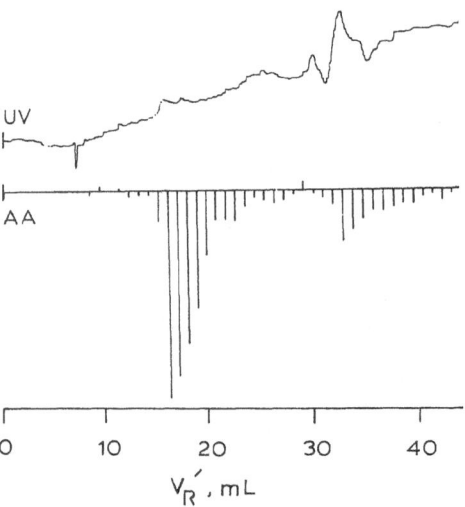

Figure 8.   SEC-UV-GFAA chromatogram of OMP-S.   Solvent THF.
            Columns: Waters μStyragel (three) in series, average
            pore size 10^3 Å. Mobile phase, THF.   Flow rate
            1.0 mL min^{-1}.   UV detector: Knauer UV/RI Dual Detektor
            operating in the UV mode at 254 nm.   UV sensitivity:
            0.003 AUFS.   Injected volume: 50 μL.   Injected concen-
            tration of OMP-S: 25 μg/50 μL.

in the respective OMP's. The relative amount of tin in fractions
A and B of the respective OMP's is nearly the same.

      The elution volume of the initial UV chromatographic peak of
OMP-23 is approximately two mL less than that of the initial GFAA
chromatographic peak of the same polymer, strongly indicating the
presence of two high MW species in this formulation. The first
probably is PMMA of MW 111,000 or greater, having a narrow MWD and
essentially free of tin; and the second is a copolymer of MMA and
TBTM having M_w of 21,540 and MWD of 2.9. The tandem chromatograms
of OMP-S do not indicate the presence of a low-tin, high polymer
species like that responsible for UV absorption in OMP-23.   These
data may be explained by the simple hypothesis that a copolymer
of MMA and TBTM is formed initially during the synthesis of OMP-23,
and that PMMA then continues to be synthesized from excess MMA.
In contrast, MMA and TBTM appear to copolymerize over the entire
course of the conversion resulting in OMP-S.

      The tin-containing low MW fractions of OMP-23 and OMP-S have
molecular weights ranging from 500 to less than 100, suggesting
the presence of unreacted TBTM and unidentified low MW tin species

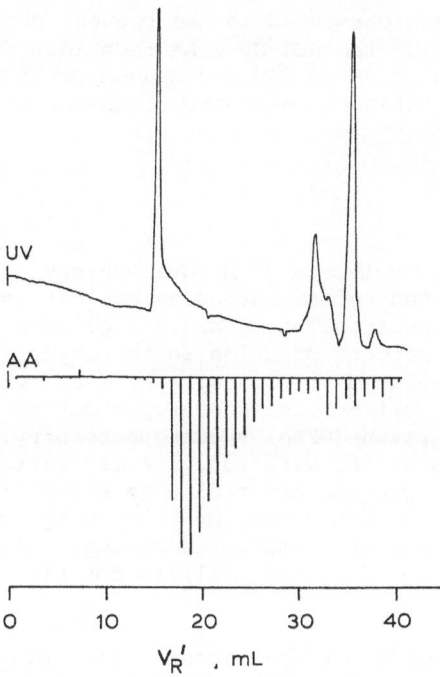

Figure 9. SEC–UV–GFAA chromatogram of OMP-23. All conditions the
           same as for Figure 8. Injected concentration on OMP-23:
           50 µg/50 µL.

in the OMP. Their presence would result in the relatively rapid,
early leaching of tin-containing species into an aqueous environment
that has been observed by Jewett et al.,[5] which is followed by the
slower zero-order leaching that others have observed[2] over much
longer periods of time. Table II shows the relative amounts of
tin associated with the two major MW fractions of each of a variety
of OMP's undergoing current study. All of these contain from 5.6
to 20.8 percent of the total amount of detected tin within species
of low MW, and from 67.0 to 94.4 percent of their total tin within
species having comparatively high MW. Work currently in progress
is directed to the kinetic optimization of the polymerization procedure, using SEC–UV–GFAA criteria to realize two major objectives:
to concentrate tin within a narrow, high polymer fraction; and cor-
respondingly to diminish the relative amount of low polymer, tin-
containing species.

     Off-line analytical techniques, such as ^{119}Sn and ^{13}C FT–NMR,
infrared and Mossbauer spectroscopy, will be required to fully

characterize OMP fractions typed in the present chromatograms.
The unique advantage of the SEC-UV-GFAA technique lies in its
capacity to differentiate rapidly and conveniently between polymer
formulations on the basis of chromophoric and metal-bearing species
of different MW.

CONCLUSION

Organometallic copolymers of methylmethacrylate and organotin
acrylate esters are undergoing extensive evaluation as candidate
slow-release marine antifouling agents. Organotin polymer (OMP)
formulations in 0.1 percent solution in tetrahydrofuran (THF) were
subjected to size-exclusion chromatography (SEC) with continuous
eluent monitoring by ultraviolet spectrophotometry (UV) and graphite
furnace atomic absorption (GFAA) spectrophotometry. High-resolution
chromatographic separations were successfully performed with THF
as mobile phase on a packing material consisting of microspheres
of styrene crosslinked with divinylbenzene (μStyragel). Microspheres
of silica gel (LiChrosphere) exhibited strong adsorption of OMP
material in THF and could not be utilized for size-dependent separations.

On μStyragel, OMP's are fractionated into tin-bearing components
whose relative concentrations were determined by the intensity of
tin-specific GFAA signals, and whose molecular weights were estimated
from elution volumes compared with the elution volumes of polystyrene
samples of known molecular weight. The weight-average- and number-
average-molecular weights (M_w and M_n) of polymer fractions were
calculated from the observed concentrations and MW's of the tin
containing species composing each fraction. M_w's of 20,000 to
50,000 and 100 to 400 were obtained, with molecular-weight dispersions (MWD) of 2.0 to 5.0 and 1.1 to 2.1, respectively. The MWD's
of the high MW fraction are comparable in magnitude to MWD's for
polymethyl methacrylate (PMMA) reported in the literature.

The intensity of UV chromatographic peaks obtained concurrently
with GFAA chromatograms is not directly proportional to the concentration of tin-bearing species, but in at least one formulation
demonstrates the presence of a high MW species with which little
or no tin is associated. Tentatively, this is attributed to a homopolymer of PMMA, an undesired side product. Although differential
refractive index (DRI) detectors are mass sensitive, the threshold
of detection of OMP's in THF by DRI is orders of magnitude less
sensitive than that of tin specific GFAA, and it is of little value
at the concentration levels necessary and employed here to optimize
SEC column efficiencies.

Tandem UV and GFAA detection is shown to provide a more powerful tool for the chromatographic evaluation of the extent of conversion of monomer to polymer and for comparing OMP's prepared by different polymerization processes. Off-line techniques (FT-NMR, IR) will be required for determining differences in polymer structure that influence interaction of the tin-containing moieties and their service environment. Such methods will be effective with preparative SEC-GFAA monitoring, because less than five percent of the material is consumed in the GFAA analysis. Thus more than 95 percent of eluent peaks can be recovered.

ACKNOWLEDGEMENTS

The authors thank Dr. K.L. Jewett for assistance and helpful discussions of HPLC separation techniques. Financial support of this research, provided by the Office of Naval Research and the Naval Ship Research and Development Center, Annapolis, MD, is gratefully acknowledged.

REFERENCES

1. W.L. Yeager and Y.J. Castelli, in: "Organometallic Polymers," C.E. Carraher, Jr., J.E. Sheats and C.J. Pittman, eds., Academic Press, New York (1978). pp. 175-180.
2. E.J. Dyckman and J.A. Montemarano, Antifouling Organometallic Polymers: Environmentally Compatible Materials, Report No. 4186, Naval Ship Research and Development Center, Bethesda, MD (1974).
3. P.J. Smith and L.Smith, Chem. Britan 11:208-212 (1975).
4. W.A. Corpe, in: "Proc. 3rd International Congress Marine Corrosion and Fouling," Northwestern University Press, Gaithersburg, MD (1973). pp. 593-608.
5. K.L. Jewett, W.R. Blair, and F.E. Brinckman, in: "Proceedings 6th International Symposium on Controlled Release of Bioactive Materials," R.W. Baker, ed., New Orleans (1979).
6. F.E. Brinckman, W.R. Blair, K.L. Jewett, and W.P. Iverson, J. Chromatogr. Sci. 15:493 (1977).
7. E.J. Parks, F.E. Brinckman, and W.R. Blair, J. Chromatogr. 185:563 (1979).
8. W.W. Yau, J.J. Kirkland, and D.D. Bly, "Modern Size-Exclusion Liquid Chromatography, Practice of Gel Permeation and Gel Filtration Chromatography," Wiley-Interscience, New York (1979). pp. 4-8.
9. Ibid, pp. 318-322.
10. F.E. Brinckman, K.L. Jewett, W.P. Iverson, K.J. Irgolic, K.C. Erhardt, and R.A. Stockton, J. Chromatogr. 191:31 (1980).
11. F.W. Billmeyer, Jr., in: "Textbook of Polymer Science," Wiley-Interscience, New York (1971). p. 143.

12. J.C. Berington, N.W. Melville and R.P. Taylor, J. Polymer Sci. 12:449 (1954).

13. N.A. Ghanem, N.N. Messiha, N.E. Ikaldisus, and A.F. Shaaban, European Polymer J. 15:823 (1979).

14. A. Ravve, in: "Organic Chemistry of Macromolecules," Marcel Dekker, New York (1967). p. 216.

15. Reference 8, pp. 57-59.

16. Reference 8, pp. 309-312.

17. R.V. Vivilecchia, B.G. Lightbody, M.Z. Thimot and H.M. Quinn, J. Chromatogr. Sci. 15:424 (1977).

18. J.V. Dawkins, J. Liquid Chromatogr. 1:279 (1978).

19. L.R. Snyder and J.J. Kirkland, in: "Introduction to Modern Liquid Chromatography," 2nd Ed., Wiley-Interscience, New York 503 (1979).

20. H.J. Mencer and Z. Grubisic-Gallet, J. Liquid Chromatogr. 2:649 (1979).

21. Augustin Campos and J.E. Figuerelo, Makromol. Chem. 178:3249 (1977).

22. M. Minarik, Z. Sir, and J. Coupek, Die Angewandte Makromole- kulare Chemie 64:147 (1977).

23. M. Popl, J. Fahnrich, and M. Stejskal, J. Chromatogr. Sci. 14:537 (1976).

24. R.C. Jordan, J. Liquid Chromatogr. 3:439 (1980).

25. J.R. Weakley, R.J.P. Williams, and J.P. Wilson, J. Chem. Soc. London 3963 (1960).

26. L. Letot, J.Lesec, and C. Quivoron, J. Liquid Chromatogr. 3:427 (1980).

CONTROLLED-RELEASE ORGANOTIN PESTICIDES BIOCHEMISTRY :

TOXICOLOGY : ENVIRONMENTAL FACTORS

Nate Cardarelli and William Evans

Environmental Management Laboratory
University of Akron

Daniel Smith

Department of Chemistry
University of Akron

INTRODUCTION

Organotin compounds have long been used as pesticidal agents in antifouling preparations, agricultural fungicides and miticides, mildewcides, and bactericides. Trialkyl organotins were incorporated in elastomers as early as 1964 and long-term (over ten years) protection against marine fouling observed in commercial applications.[1,2] Evaluation of such compounds showed considerable merit as molluscicides.[3] Small-scale field evaluations of bis tri-n-butyltin oxide, "TBTO", and tributyltin fluoride, "TBTF" slowly released from natural rubber and other elastomers demonstrated successful long-term snail controls.[1,4,5]

Release of an agent from select elastomers is based upon a diffusion-dissolution mechanism relying upon the degree of solubility of the organotin within the polymer and various matrix factors.[6] It was later discovered that non-matrix soluble molluscicides could be incorporated in elastomers if they were highly water soluble and the loading was sufficiently high. Copper sulfate, for instance, was successfully released for a six-month period from ethylene-propylene-diene elastomers provided the agent loading was in excess of 40% and a secondary releasant was used to adjust interfacial pH.[7] More importantly, in the far less expensive thermoplastics, the incorporation of a water-soluble porosity enhancing agent (porosigen) proved useful. As the porosigen leached slowly from the system, water penetration of the developing pores allowed contact, solvation, and egress of the organotin agent.[8] Organotins, per se, are not effective aquatic insect larvicides due to their affinity for organic matter and soil when used in the conventional mode. Emission of TBTO and/or TBTF at ultralow levels retards metamorphic changes in larva leading to eventual mortality.[9]

DISPENSING SYSTEMS

     Unlike conventional pesticide formulations, controlled-release elastomers and plastics can be formed in a wide variety of geometries--granules, pellets, flakes, chips, tapes, strands, tubes, etc; with densities conducive to floating, hovering, or sinking in a given water course. Anchored systems encompassing a floating tape, strand, or chip successfully overcame dispenser loss in flowing water and deactivation by silting over as observed with conventional or controlled-release pellets.[10,11] Molluscicidal and larvicidal materials are now commercially available that will provide from three to five years continuous agent emission.

ENVIRONMENTAL EFFECTS

     The organotin of choice as a snail, mosquito, and black fly control agent is TBTF. In an aquatic system TBTF is non-persistent hydrolyzing to TBTO through a hydroxide intermediate described elsewhere.[12] Presently, in-house data apparently indicate that TBTF has a relatively low toxicity and the actual control agent is TBTO whether the dispenser in question contains TBTF or TBTO. Reportedly TBTO, in turn, degrades via hydrolytic cleavage and when exposed, photolytic cleavage to dibutyltin oxide, butylstannoic acid and finally the non-toxic ubiquitous stannic oxide.[4] Intermediate hydroxide and halogen compounds (especially the chloride) can be postulated. Plant, fish, mammal, and bird toxicities are known and occur at concentrations 100X to 1000X higher than that necessary to destroy the stated targets.[1,4,5] The aquatic life of the principles and mildly toxic degradant (dibutyltin oxide) probably does not exceed 60 days.

     Both TBTO and TBTF are rapidly purged from the water course through absorption on cellulosic and other organics, with the major loss being into bottom soil. High Freundlich isotherms preclude desorption.[5] Emission patterns and organotin movement through the aqueous medium and soil have been described.[5,13] Snail intoxication arises through ingestion of organotin containing soil and organic matter via browsing activities. The unique physiology involved in snail digestive processes releases the organotin absorbants, physiological accumulation occurs, and the target succumbs. The

actual kill mechanism is possibly proteolytic arising from dena-
turing of proteins and gross interference in histidine transamination.[14] TBTO and TBTF are non-mutagenic, non-teratogenic, and
probably non-carcinogenic.[5] In fact alkyl organotin complexes are
used as anti-tumor drugs.[15]

ORGANOTIN BIOCHEMISTRY

Mouse Tissue

C^{14}-labelled TBTO was provided to mice in their drinking water.
Periodic sacrifice, dissection of select organs, and analysis by
liquid-scintillation techniques indicated that 92 to 96% of the
ingested label passed unaltered in the feces.[16] One to two percent
was found in the urine, indicating metabolism, and the remainder
accumulated mainly in liver, lung, kidney, and fat tissue. Once
the C^{14}-source was removed, tissue clearance was rapid and essentially complete within 15 days (see the Figure).

The possibility of transmission to the fetus by the parent
ingesting TBTO was investigated. In this study, female mice were
fed C^{14}-TBTO water for two weeks prior to impregnation and during
the gestation period. Analysis of the selected tissues of the
parent and offspring was performed immediately after birth. The
tissues were processed as previously described and counted by LSC.

Initial results indicate a low level of transmission to the
fetus with the major sites of accumulation being the liver and
kidney. The results from the parent mice indicate a lower amount
of accumulation of the C^{14} label than was observed in previous
studies[16] although the relative levels among the sample tissues
remained approximately the same. One anomoly was the kidney tissue
which exhibited a higher relative accumulation than was noted in
adult mouse tissue. These differences in the parent are believed
to be due to the metabolic changes which occur during pregnancy
and possibly modify the mechanisms by which the TBTO is accumulated
and excreted.

The modified phenylfluorone analytical technique was used in
the analysis of adult and neonate mice for organotin and inorganic
tin content.[17] Inorganic tin is present, as expected, in all organs
examined. Surprisingly, hexane extractable organotin was found,
though at very low levels in non-exposed mouse tissue. Neonates
similarly contained extractable organotin, as did the lactates of
the mother found in the neonate stomach.

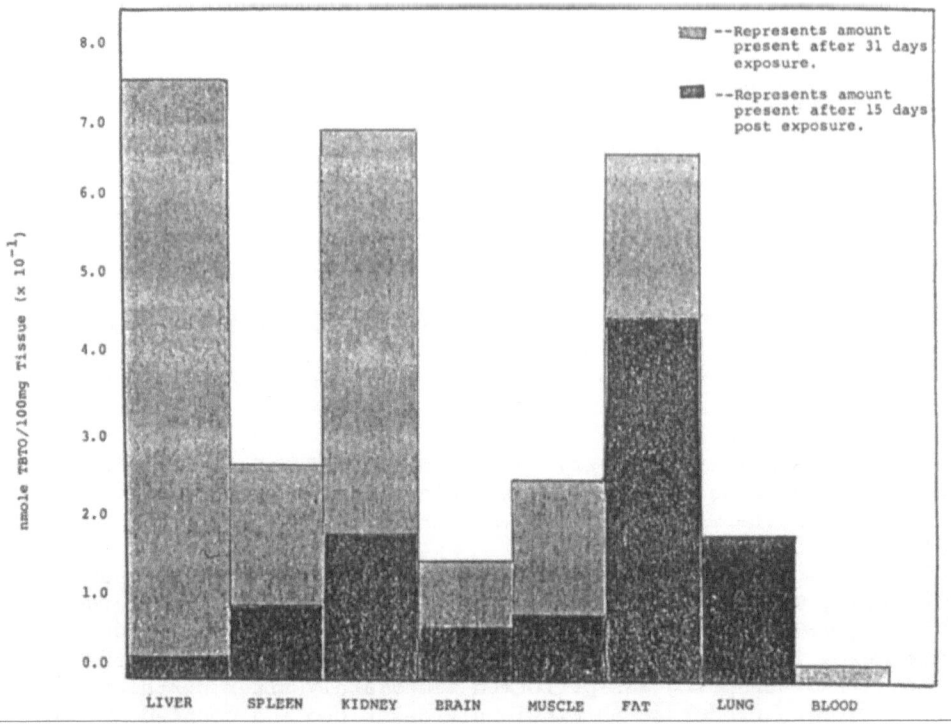

Clearance of [^{14}C-TBTO] from tissues. Light shading
represents accumulated TBTO after 31 d of exposure.
Dark shading represents the amount remaining after
15 d postexposure.

Human Tissue

It has been well recognized for over a century that the human
body contains appreciable tin, measured as inorganic, in most of
the organ systems.[18,19] Schwartz and his colleagues, in elaborate
isolation systems, have demonstrated that tin is an essential trace
nutrient for the rat.[20] They have also shown that this necessary
element can be supplied as inorganic or organic tin as a dietary
supplement. Since humans and rats have similar physiologies, and
all known trace elements essential to the rat have been found essential to humans, it is hypothesized that tin will be found to be
necessary in human nutrition. It is likely that the tin biochemi-
cal(s) so needed are in organic form. Recently trimethyltin has
been discovered in human urine although industrial pollution may
be causative.[21]

Analysis of human organs from select cadavers for hexane extractable organotin has qualitatively indicated their presence in the liver and other organs. Quantification has not yet been achieved with any degree of accuracy as the levels are too low for good reproducibility by the phenylfluorone method (>10 ng/g). Speciation has yet to be attempted. Data will be published when present studies are complete. All data to date are supportive of our basic hypothesis that TBTO and/or TBTF ingested by humans, at the expected levels arising from ingestion of treated water, can be utilized as a source of a nutritional need.

Snail Tissue

The accumulation sites of TBTO in <u>Biomphalaria glabrata</u> were probed by use of C^{14}-TBTO. A time versus concentration profile was determined for various tissues by placing the snails in C^{14}-TBTO laden water. The results indicate a non-linear accumulation pattern for most of the tissues samples. The most significant accumulation is observed in the head-foot region, which parallels the onset of snail morbidity. The accumulation in this region is generally quite rapid with levels peaking at 72 hrs for the 10 ppm test and 120 hrs for the 0.05 ppm test.

Gradual movement into the body cavity is seen in the order, renal tissue > reproductive tissue >> digestive tissue. This increase is coupled with a concommitant decrease in the head-foot region. Peak levels for the renal tissue being reached at 96 hrs (10 ppm) and 168 hrs (0.05 ppm).

The digestive tissue exhibited the least accumulation with no label detectable in 10- and 1-ppm test time periods and peak levels for the other test occurring at 120 to 168 hrs. In all cases examined, the levels in the digestive tissue were significantly below those for the other organs.

These results indicate the primary mode of adsorption is due to cutaneous adsorption along the head-foot and mantle cavity, both of which are highly vasculated and in direct contact with the C^{14}-TBTO/water solution. Transport to the body interior is most likely via the hemolymph with a large portion being extracted by the renal tissue. The C^{14}-TBTO concentration of the hemolymph tends to support this scheme since TBTO hemolymph concentrations rise rapidly during the first 24 hours after exposure and reach a maximal value in 48-72 hours. It is interesting that the snails actively accumulate TBTO, in opposition to a concentration gradient with levels in the tissue reaching 20-40 times the original water concentration, indicating a high affinity.

REFERENCES

1. N.F. Cardarelli, in: "Controlled Release Pesticide Formulations,"
    CRC Press, Cleveland (1976).
2. G.A. Janes and R.L. Senderling, in: "Proceedings Controlled
    Release of Bioactive Materials Symp.," R.W. Baker, ed., New
    Orleans (1979). p. II.3.
3. N.F. Cardarelli and H.F. Neff, U.S. Patent 3639583 (1972).
4. N.F. Cardarelli, in: "Controlled Release Molluscides," mono-
    graph, Pub. Univ. Akron (1977). 136 pp.
5. N.F. Cardarelli and W.H. Evans, in: "Proceedings Controlled
    Release of Bioactive Materials Symp.," R.W. Baker, ed., New
    Orleans (1979). p. II.23.
6. N.F. Cardarelli, and S.V. Kanakkanatt, in: "Controlled Release
    Pesticides," H.B. Scher, 60-73, ACS Symp. Ser. No. 53, Washing-
    ton (1977). pp. 60-73.
7. N.F. Cardarelli and K.E. Walker, U.S. Patent 4012221 (1977).
8. N.F. Cardarelli, U.S. Patent 4166111 (1979).
9. N.R. Cardarelli, Mosquite News 38:328 (1978).
10. T.J. Quick, Controlled Release Temephos: Laboratory and Field
    Evaluations, to be published 1980.
11. R. Himel, et al., Field Evaluation of Controlled Release
    Mosquito Larvicide Dispensers, Rep. Amer. Mosq. Control Assoc.
    Mtng., Salt Lake City, Nevada (1980).
12. J.C. Jackson, J.L. Everetts, and L.R. Sherman, in: "Controlled
    Release of Bioactive Materials Symp.," D.H. Lewis, ed., Fort
    Lauderdale (1980).
13. P.J. Gingo, in: "Proceedings Controlled Release Pesticide Symp.,"
    R. Goulding, ed., Oregon State University, Corvallis (1977).
14. A.J. Allen, B.M. Quitter, and C.M. Radick, in: "Proceedings
    Controlled Release of Bioactive Materials Symp.," R.W. Baker,
    ed., New Orleans (1979). p. II-47.
15. S. Ozaki and H. Saki, Japanese Patent 76,100,089 (1976).
16. W.H. Evans, N.F. Cardarelli, and D.J. Smith, J. Toxicol. Environ,
    Hlth. 5:871 (1979).
17. L.R. Sherman and T.L. Carlson, J. Analyt. Tox. 4:31 (1980).
18. A.P. Luff and J.H. Metcalfe, Brit. Med J. 1:833 (1980).
19. C.J. Benoy, P.A. Hooper, and R. Schneider, Food Cosmet. Tox.
    9:645 (1971).
20. K. Schwarz, D.B. Milne, and E. Vinyard, Biochem. Biophys. Res.
    Comm. 40:22 (1970).
21. M. Tompkins and R.S. Braman, Rep. Amer. Chem. Soc. 4th Biannual
    Rocky Mountain Regional Meeting, Boulder (1978).

OPTIMAL FORMULATIONS WITH PHANTOLID FOR EXTENDING THE DURATION
OF EFFECTIVENESS OF TRIMEDLURE AND METHYL (E)-6-NONENOATE AS
ATTRACTANTS TO MALE MEDITERRANEAN FRUIT FLIES[a]

Irving Keiser

Tropical Fruit and Vegetable Research Laboratory
Agric. Res., Science and Education Administration
U.S. Department of Agriculture
Honolulu, Hawaii 96804

Martin Jacobson

Biologically Active Natural Products Laboratory
Agricultural Environmental Quality Institute
Agric. Res., Science and Education Administration
U.S. Department of Agriculture
Beltsville, Maryland 20705

James A. Silva

Hawaii Agricultural Experiment Station
College of Tropical Agriculture and Human Resources
University of Hawaii
Honolulu, Hawaii 96822

In 1976 we reported[1] that certain perfume fixatives controlled
the release of trimedlure,[2] an attractant of male Mediterranean
fruit flies, Ceratitis capitata (Wiedemann), and thereby enhanced
the duration of effectiveness of this lure. The perfume fixatives
were evaluated in an olfactometer stocked with laboratory mass-
reared flies, and included tonalid, musk R-1, ambrettozone, galaxo-
lide, astrotone, hibiscolide, phantolid, and musk BRB.

All of the perfume fixatives were found to be similar in effectiveness for prolonging the duration of trimedlure attractiveness
under laboratory conditions. Therefore, phantolid (a standardized
mixture of structural isomers of 1-(2,3-dihydro-1,1,2,3,3,6-hexa-
methyl-1H-inden-5-yl)ethanone was selected for extensive field trials
on the island of Maui in Hawaii under natural conditions with wild
Mediterranean fruit flies, since it was the least expensive of those

---

[a] Mention of a proprietary product in this paper does not constitute
an endorsement of this product by the USDA.

tested. The results, reported in 1978,[3] showed that the duration
of effectiveness of formulations with as little as 50% of trimedlure,
plus phantolid added either as a 25% solution in ethyl alcohol or
as 100% phantolid incorporated directly into the trimedlure, was
increased at least 25% over that of trimedlure at 100% concentration
(no added fixative) when applied as a single treatment to wicks
in traps emplaced in the field.

The present studies were conducted to determine an optimal
trimedlure-phantolid formulation, since we found earlier that this
perfume fixative is operative under field conditions against wild
populations of Mediterranean fruit flies. The tests were conducted
in the Kula area on the island of Maui in Hawaii, and traps for
nine treatments were positioned at each of seven different locations
a mile or more apart. The plastic traps[4] were fitted with 2.4-cm
wicks suspended by a wire, and each trap received a single application of 2 ml of formulation pipetted onto the wick. A complete set
of treatments was installed at each test location; therefore, each
treatment was replicated seven times. The traps with the different
treatments were positioned at least 15.24 m apart at each test site
and were serviced at biweekly intervals, at which times the flies
were removed and the traps rotated to other positions within the
test site. For example, the trap with treatment 1 would be moved
to the tree that held the trap of treatment 2; the trap with treatment 2 would be moved to the tree that held the trap of treatment
3, etc., until finally the trap with treatment 9 would be positioned
in the tree that held the trap of treatment 1.

The formulations tested contained trimedlure at 100, 75, and
50% concentrations. The 75 and 50% trimedlure formulations included
25 and 50%, respectively, of phantolid either dissolved directly
into the trimedlure, or 25 and 50%, respectively, of a 25% solution
of phantolid in ethyl alcohol or diethyl phthalate. Capilure®,
a proprietary product containing trimedlure and a fixative, was
included in these studies for purposes of comparison. It was marketed after our disclosure in 1976 that perfume fixatives enhanced
the duration of trimedlure effectiveness. The results are shown
in Table I.

We averaged the total number of flies from all seven replicates
of each treatment collected on the indicated number of days after
trap emplacement. An analysis of variance was conducted on these
data after they were first normalized with the transformation
$\sqrt{x + 1}$. Differences between means were tested with the Bayes least-
significant-difference test for multiple comparisons.[5]

As noted in Table I, variability in the data was high. Coefficients of variance ranged from 25 to 80%, but this is not uncommon
in trapping data of natural populations under field conditions.
Therefore, although demonstration of statistically significant

TABLE I. COMPARATIVE EFFECTIVENESS OF TRIMEDLURE (TML) ALONE AND IN COMBINATION WITH PHANTOLID IN VARIOUS PROPORTIONS AND FORMULATIONS. KULA, MAUI, HAWAII, 1979

Treatment (% ingredients)	Male Mediterranean fruit flies (mean of total of 7 replicates) caught on indicated no. of days after treatment of wicks and emplacement of traps in the field[a]/										
	6	20	27	34	48	57	69	83	97	111	124
TML 100	7.29 bc cd	12.84 ab bc	4.60 a a	5.62 a a	7.86 a a	6.53 a a	3.68 a a	3.21 b b	1.95 bc c	2.33 ab bc	2.45 a a
TML 75+ phantolid 25[b]/	7.51 bc cd	9.10 b d	5.01 a a	7.06 a a	8.29 a a	5.92 a a	6.09 a a	6.40 ab ab	5.41 ab ab	5.53 a a	2.55 a a
TML 50+ phantolid 50[b]/	7.67 bc cd	10.10 b cd	5.95 a a	6.94 a a	7.14 a a	6.06 a a	4.98 a a	8.46 a a	5.62 ab ab	4.09 ab abc	2.08 a a
TML 75+ solution A[c]/ 25	5.51 c d	12.40 ab bc	5.35 a a	4.85 a a	7.14 a a	5.53 a a	4.35 a a	6.00 ab ab	2.41 abc bc	1.96 ab bc	1.10 a a
TML 50+ solution A[c]/ 50	8.92 ab bc	12.41 ab bc	4.49 a a	6.98 a a	6.64 a a	4.20 a a	5.00 a a	5.66 ab ab	1.59 c c	1.41 b c	1.21 a a
TML 75+ solution B[d]/ 25	10.83 a ab	11.51 b bcd	6.38 a a	7.41 a a	7.28 a a	6.19 a a	7.40 a a	9.33 a a	4.09 abc abc	4.05 ab abc	1.74 a a
TML 50+ solution B[d]/ 50	10.16 a abc	14.95 a a	6.01 a a	5.85 a a	6.15 a a	7.13 a a	6.64 a a	7.50 ab ab	6.14 a a	4.95 ab ab	2.95 a a
TML 50+diethyl phthal. 50[e]/	10.42 ab ab	10.46 b bcd	5.97 a a	5.19 a a	6.23 a a	4.98 a a	5.07 a a	5.62 ab ab	3.86 abc abc	2.07 ab bc	1.85 a a
Capilure® 100	11.30 a a	13.26 ab a	5.54 a a	5.71 a a	7.23 a a	5.80 a a	4.80 a a	7.61 ab ab	4.71 abc abc	4.45 ab ab	2.89 a a

a/ Values are averages of 7 replicates after normalization with the transformation $\sqrt{x + I}$. Means in the same column followed by the same letter are not significantly different at the 5% level (upper letters) or at the 10% level (lower letters) according to Bayes least significant difference test for multiple comparisons.

b/ Phantolid dissolved directly into trimedlure.

c/ Solution A: phantolid 25%; ethyl alcohol 75%. Ethyl alcohol denatured with 1% dimethyl phthalate, as supplied to the perfume industry.

d/ Solution B: phantolid 25%; diethyl phthalate 75%.

e/ Control.

(P = 0.05) differences was not uniform, the consistent trends in
trap catches were highly indicative of the relative effectiveness
of the various treatments. Delineation was greater at the 10% level
of probability, and the differences were more distinct.

The data are also presented in graphs as total numbers of flies
trapped rather than as normalized means and are therefore without
statistical significance. Nevertheless, they show the patterns
of differential attraction among the various formulations. Phantolid dissolved in diethyl phthalate (solution B) gave consistently
better results than when dissolved in ethyl alcohol (solution A),
both in the trimedlure 75:phantolid solution 25 (Figure 1) and in
the trimedlure 50:phantolid solution 50 (Figure 2) proportions.
When phantolid was dissolved directly into trimedlure, trimedlure
75:phantolid 25 and trimedlure 50:phantolid 50, formulations were
essentially similar in effectiveness (Figure 3.). However, trimedlure 75:solution B 25 was superior to trimedlure 75:phantolid 25
(Figure 4); and trimedlure 50:solution B 50 was superior to trimedlure 50:phantolid 50 (Figure 5). Therefore, not only were the
trimedlure:phantolid solution (in diethyl phthalate) formulations
superior to those of trimedlure:solid phantolid, but much less
phantolid is present in the solutions which contain only 25% phantolid, the actual amount of phantolid being only 6.25% at the 75:25
and only 12.5% at the 50:50 proportions.

Of all formulations tested, the trimedlure 50:solution B 50
proportion was found to be the optimal trimedlure-phantolid formulation. It was better than the trimedlure 75:solution B 25 proportion
in most instances (Figure 6) and was also superior to Capilure in
8 of the 11 collutions (Figure 7).

In a second study,[6] methyl (E)-6-nonenoate (MEN), which was
found recently to be attractive to male Mediterranean fruit flies,
was evaluated in the field alone and in combination with phantolid
as a 25% solution in diethyl phthalate (solution B of the earlier
studies) at MEN 75:phantolid solution 25 and MEN 50:phantolid solution 50 proportions. The optimal trimedlure-phantolid formulation
as noted in the study just reported was included in these tests
as a standard of comparison. The study was conducted also on the
island of Maui, and traps were positioned at five different locations. The test methods--plastic traps, single treatments, rotation
on each collection data, etc.--were identical to those of the first
study. Table II lists the total trap catches of the five replicates
and also the analysis of variance conducted on the means after
normalization with the transformation $\sqrt{x + 1}$. The results indicate
that phantolid extends the duration of effectiveness of MEN and
that the 50% MEN + 50% of 25% solution of phantolid in diethyl
phthalate formulation is as good as the optimal trimedlure formulation of like proportions.

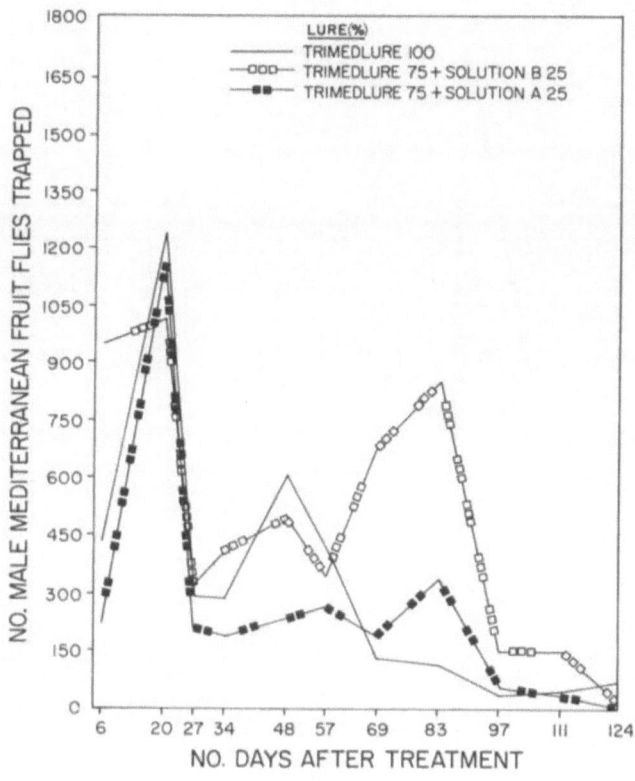

Figure 1.   Relative effectiveness of phantolid as 25% solution in
            ethyl alcohol (A) and in diethyl phthalate (B) at trimed-
            lure 75:solution 25 proportions.

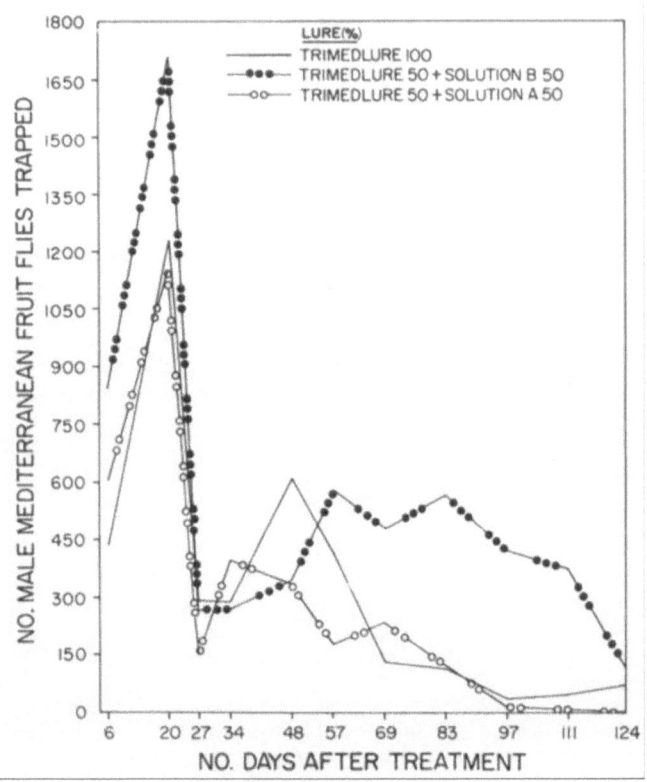

Figure 2.   Relative effectiveness of phantolid as 25% solution in
            ethyl alcohol (A) and in diethyl phthalate (B) at
            trimedlure 25:solution 25 proportions.

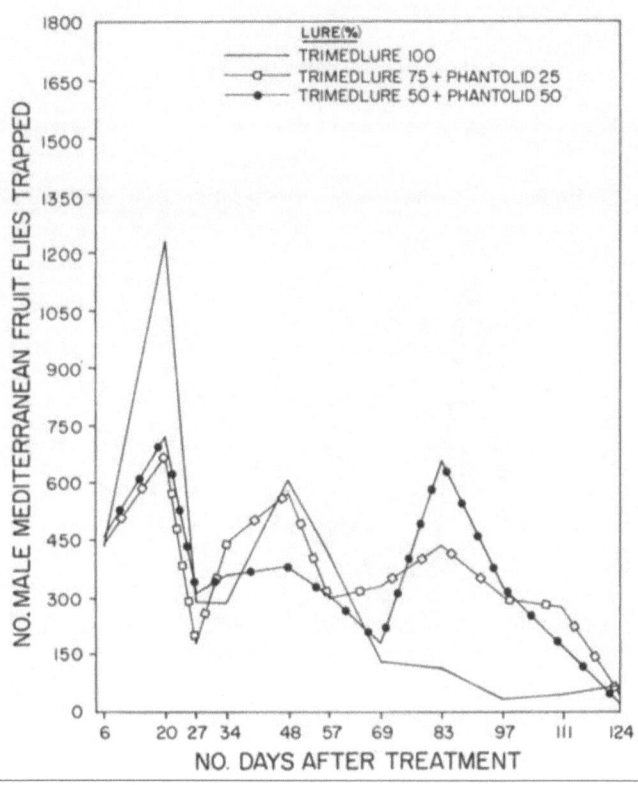

Figure 3.   Relative effectiveness of phantolid dissolved into
            trimedlure at 75:25 and 50:50 proportions.

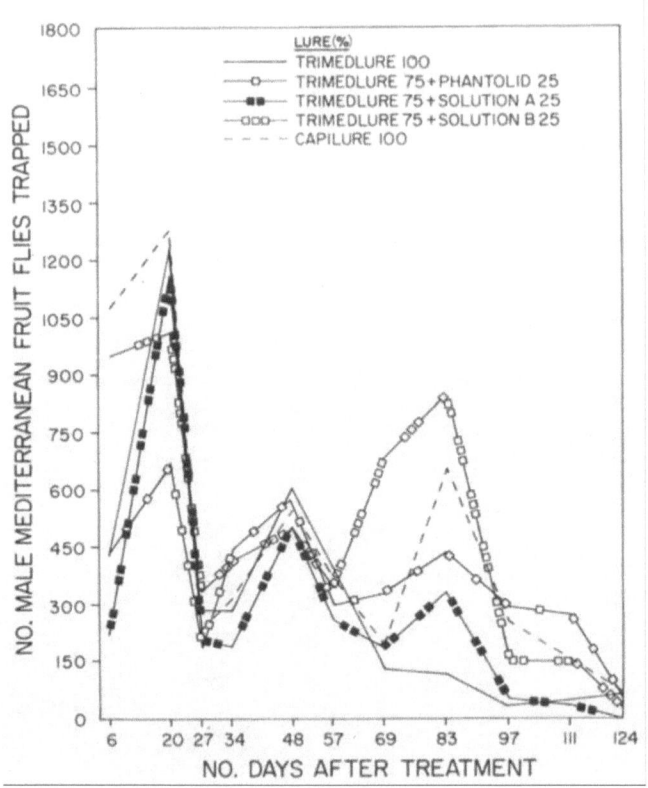

Figure 4.   Relative effectiveness of phantolid dissolved directly
into trimedlure at 75:25 proportions.

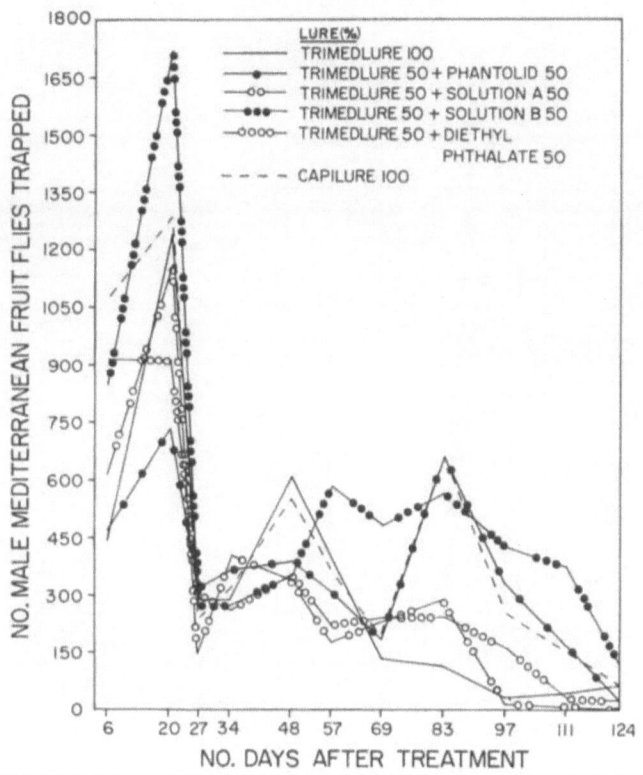

Figure 5.   Relative effectiveness of phantolid dissolved directly
             into trimedlure at 50:50 proportions.

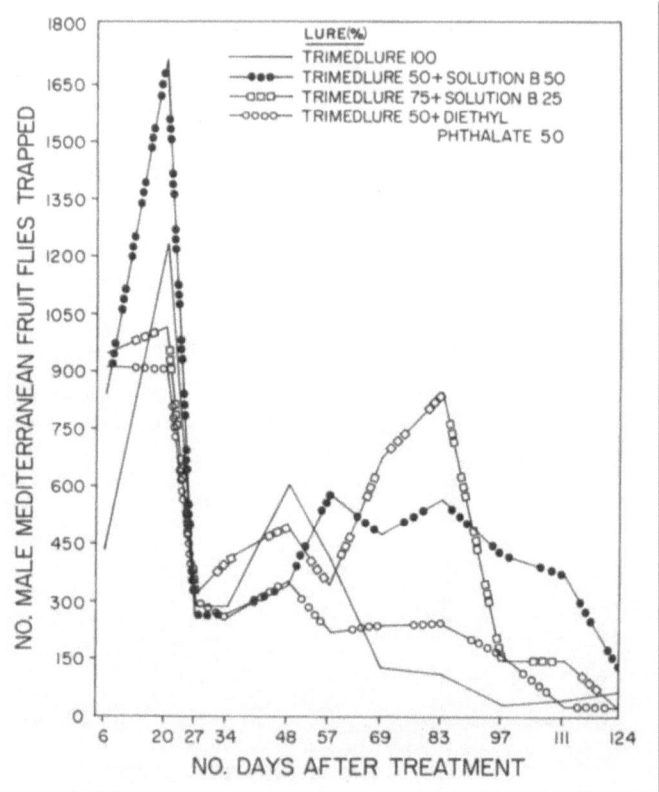

Figure 6.   Relative effectiveness of phantolid as 25% solution
            in diethyl phthalate when combined with trimedlure at
            75:25 and 50:50 trimedlure:solution proportions.

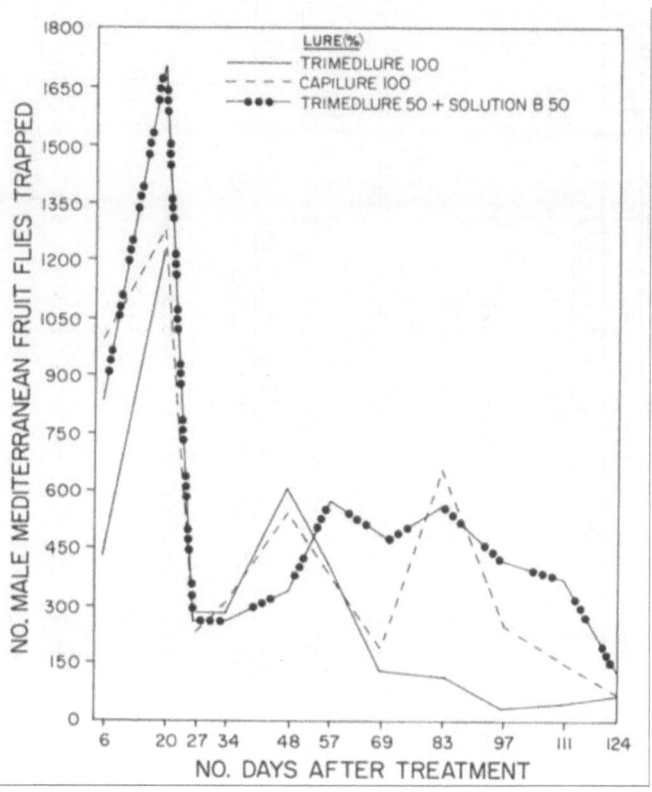

Figure 7.   Relative effectiveness of the optimal trimedlure-
phantolid formulation and Capilure®.

TABLE II. COMPARATIVE EFFECTIVENESS OF TRIMEDLURE (TML) AND METHYL (E)-6-NONENOATE (MEN) ALONE AND WITH THE INCLUSION OF PHANTOLID. KULA, MAUI, HAWAII, 1979

Treatment (% ingredients)	Male Mediterranean fruit flies caught on indicated no. of days after treatment of wicks and emplacement of traps in the field									
	14	28	42	69	83	104	118	139	153	174
	Number (total of 5 replicates)									
TML 100	712	583	1732	1163	119	8	0	0	1	1
TML 50+phantolid solution[a]/50	562	612	1724	1512	220	435	15	99	69	130
MEN 100	707	784	1489	372	131	16	1	0	0	1
MEN 75+phantolid solution[a]/25	858	461	1101	815	226	238	15	43	4	1
MEN 50+phantolid solution[a]/25	610	828	684	984	183	227	260	154	90	1
	Means of totals normalized with the transformation $\sqrt{x+1}$[b]/									
TML 100	11.75	10.55	17.50a	14.38ab	2.99b	1.49b	1.08b	1.00b	1.00a	1.08b
TML 50+phantolid solution[a]/50	9.99	10.73	16.21a	17.15a	6.03a	7.72a	5.06a	4.20a	3.46a	3.71a
MEN 100	11.50	11.46	16.23a	7.93c	3.17b	1.89b	1.08b	1.00b	1.00a	1.08b
MEN 75+phantolid solution[a]/25	13.01	9.29	13.22ab	12.52b	6.03a	6.00a	1.90b	2.78a	1.33a	1.08b
MEN+phantolid solution[a]/50	10.81	11.99	11.31b	12.65ab	5.49ab	5.99a	6.40a	3.92a	2.95a	1.08b

a/ 25% solution of phantolid in diethyl phthalate.

b/ Numbers in the same column followed by the same letter are not significantly different at the 5% level according to Bayes least significant difference test for multiple comparisons.

ACKNOWLEDGEMENT

We acknowledge the assistance of Raymond Y. Miyabara, Biological Technician, in the conduct of the field trials.

REFERENCES

1.   I. Keiser, R.M. Kobayashi, and E.J. Harris, _in_: "Proceedings 1976 Controlled Release Pesticide Symp.," N.F. Cardarelli, ed., The University of Akron, Akron (1976).
2.   M. Beroza, N. Green, S.I. Gertler, L.F. Steiner, and D.H. Miyashita, _J. Agric. Food Chem_. 9:361 (1961).
3.   I. Keiser, R. Miyabara, J. Silva, and E. Harris, _in_: 5th Int. Symp. on Controlled Release of Bioactive Materials," E. Brinkman and J. Montemavano, eds., Gaithersburg (1978).
4.   L.F. Steiner, _J. Econ. Entomol_. 50:508 (1957).
5.   D.B. Duncan, _Technometrics_ 7:171 (1965).
6.   K. Ohinata, M. Jacobson, S. Nakagawa, T. Urago, M. Fujimoto, and H. Higa, _J. Econ. Entomol_. 72:648 (1979).

CONTROLLED-RELEASE FORMULATIONS AND THEIR USE

IN INSECT CROP PROTECTION

Norman L. Gauthier

Agway Inc.
Syracuse, New York 13221

The use of chemical and biorational pesticides formulated into
various powdered, solid, or liquid products represents the basis
of our present crop protection programs. The use of any pesticide
under field conditions is subject to many factors which regulate
efficacy and residuality. Biological compounds may have high selectivity but show low persistence or half-life under field conditions
and may be relatively unstable to sunlight or oxidants.[1] With application of insecticides to the soil, additional loss and poor persistence may be caused by hydrolysis, volatilization, leaching, differential photo decomposition, or other deactivation of the toxicant.
Detailed tests by Read[2] demonstrated that most pesticide materials
placed on the soil surface were initially highly toxic but showed
a continuous and relatively rapid loss of toxicity. In soil insect
control for corn, potatoes, and other crops, granular formulations
are widely used as banded or broadcast applications. Type and
method of application of a pesticide also affects toxicity. With
a given insect such as cabbage root maggot, banded treatments of
insecticide granules were shown to be more effective than broadcast
treatments.[3] However, granular insecticide formulations are not
just limited to soil applications. Lynch, et al.[4] obtained excellent control of European corn borer with granular Bacillus thuringi-
ensis Berliner formulations. In these tests, granules were significantly more effective than sprays in providing borer control.
Method of application, insecticide selectivity, placement of toxicant, type of application, and formulation used: all influence
degree of control obtained.

During the past few years, a growing interest in encapsulating
the insecticide toxicant through controlled-release polymeric formulation systems has emerged. These systems offer great promise for

enhancing the efficacy of some existing insecticides as well as
reducing breakdown and deactivation of the active ingredient. Most
of the organic chemicals used as insecticides represent short-lived
compounds of high mammalian or acute toxicity. Controlled-release
technology can be used to increase biological and residual activity
as well as providing added protection and safety in the handling
of organic pesticides.

There has been great effort in the pharmaceutical and veterinary field in the controlled-release area, but this effort has not
extended into pesticide use. Although microencapsulation of pesticides has been investigated and at least two commercially available
encapsulated insecticide formulations are now produced by Pennwalt,[5,6] additional pesticide research is needed.

Pest-control strategies for the future demand that novel formulations be examined. In this interest, preliminary field insect-
control studies with macroencapsulated polyvinyl and polymeric
laminates and resin systems were conducted from 1975 to 1977.
Results of these studies were reported at previous symposia in 1977
and 1978.[7,9] Based on this work additional laboratory formulation
studies were made to improve formulation techniques and select
candidate compounds for extensive small-plot field programs.
Several systems of encapsulation were evaluated over a three-year
period during 1977 to 1979 at the Agway Farm Research Center, Fabius,
NY. The formulations of controlled-release insecticides tested
included granules, flowables, polyvinyl laminated strips, tapes,
and other forms. Candidate insecticides used in controlled-release
systems included primarily diazinon, chloropyrifos, and acephate.
Several crops, including field and sweet corn, cabbage, alfalfa,
potatoes, onions, and beans, received treatment.

Objectives of these continuing annual programs are threefold.
Certain crops receive many prophylactic chemical applications for
insect control. A single application of controlled-release insecticide has been shown effective for seasonal insect control on corn
and cabbage.[8] This aspect of investigation and application was
expanded to evaluate both foliar and soil treatments on many crops
in order to confirm earlier studies. Also, determination of the
factors of improved efficacy and residuality were attempted. A
final objective was to evaluate new encapsulation systems for insecticides and their performance in the field on crop insect
control. In the 18 studies conducted over this three-year period,
the performances were compared to standard commercial insecticide
formulations and treatments. Where possible, data are analyzed
for the total test period.

MATERIALS AND METHODS

The encapsulated controlled-release granular formulations used in these studies were based on four different systems. Insecticides formulated into these controlled-release systems were O,O-Diethyl O-2(2-isopropyl-4-methyl-6-pyrimidinyl) phosphorothiote (diazinon), O,O-Diethyl O-(3,5,6-trichloro-2-pyridyl)-phosphorothioate (chlorpyrifos), and O,S-Dimethyl acetylphosphoramidothioate (acephate). Efficacy comparisons were made between encapsulated and non-encapsulated standard commercial insecticide products. The standard commercial formulations used, considered to be short-residual, quick-release types, were chemical impregnations on inert carriers such as corn cob or clay granules.

The Herculite formulations of chlorpyrifos and diazinon utilized consisted of laminated polymeric membrane systems with release through the permeation process.[10,11] The use of these insecticidal strips for cockroach control was reported by Quisumbing, et al.[12] Use of the diazinon insecticide strips for cluster fly control were also reported at the symposium in 1978.[9] Granular formulations used in the above process were obtained by grinding impregnated laminated polymeric sheets containing the active ingredient into particles ranging in size from 100-500μ (microns).

Starch-encapsulated pesticide systems were also utilized for diazinon. These systems for encapsulating pesticides involve introducing sulfur bonds in soluble starch by xanthating it, then crosslinking the starch xanthate to encapsulate the pesticide as described by Doane and Shasha.[13,14]

Acephate controlled-release formulations used, all produced by Ortho, consist of resin-plasticized, quick- and slow-release systems. Other formulations of diazinon and chlorpyrifos were produced at Agway based on macroencapsulation by imbibing polyvinyl beads and forming flowable slurries or dry-coated granular products. In 1978 and 1979, Agway formulations of starch xanthate diazinon were also investigated and formulated.

All field studies utilized the randomized complete-block design for small plots with three replications. Specific insect control data and damage injury ratings were obtained on specified post-treatment samplings or at normal crop harvest time. Specific insect control ratings were made on the following pests:

Pieris rapae L., imported cabbageworm
Plutella xylostella L., diamondback moth
Phyllotreta cruciferae (Goeze), cabbage flea beetle
Hylemya brassicae (Bouche), cabbage root maggot
Melanotus sp., wireworms
Agromyza frontella (Rondani), alfalfa blotch leafminer

Emposasca fabae (Harris), potato leafhopper
Diabrotica longicornis (Say), Northern corn rootworm
Ostrinia nubilalis (Hubner), European corn borer
Spodoptera frugiperda (J.E. Smith), fall armyworm
Heliothis zea (Bodie), corn earworm
Hylemya platura (Meigen), seed corn maggot
Hylemya antiqua (Meigen), onion maggot

Field plots for vegetables and other crops were established at the
Agway Farm Research Center located in Fabius, NY. Soil types in
this area range from a Genesee alluvial fan to a Halsey gravel loam.
Soil analyses indicate a range in pH of 6.4 to 6.6 with organic
matter content of 5.0 to 6.0%. All treatments were applied with
small-plot hand equipment. Granular formulations were banded to
the soil or broadcast over tops of plants with a hand-held shaker
can or small screw-cap glass jars (2 oz.). Flowable or liquid formulations were drenched or sprayed on using a small-plot CO_2 bottle
sprayer attached to a six-foot aluminum boom to deliver 30 GPA
(gallons per acre). Plot sizes varied from 200 to 450 square feet.
All tests involved a single application of candidate formulations
prior to the actual pest infestation applied at planting or for
sweet corn and cabbage, applied post emergence to the growing crop.

Insect sampling surveys were made post treatment at specified
days by counting live insects or assessing their damage with a crop
injury indexing system. This injury index system varies by crop
or pest and is specified in each table.

RESULTS AND DISCUSSION

Cabbage Granular Whorl Application Studies

All chemical treatments resulted in reduced foliar injury to
cabbage applied as a single directed post emergence application
to heading white cabbage. As indicated in Table I, these treatments
replaced several weekly protective foliar sprays used to protect
plants from feeding by larvae of the imported cabbageworm and
diamond-back moth. Starch xanthate formulation of diazinon improved
its efficacy compared to other encapsulation systems and the standard
formulation. However, this improvement is the result of only one year
of testing. Acephate formulations indicate that both types of quick
and slow encapsulated systems were equal in performance at one pound
over three years of tests. This finding supports preliminary
results reported earlier in 1978,[8] but in one test the quick-release
formulation CC-2271 was not as effective as the slow-release CC-
7135 formulation at one pound ai/acre. Combined, these tests do
indicate an important new method of insecticide application that

TABLE I. COMPARISON OF SINGLE POST EMERGENCE WHORL APPLICATIONS OF INSECTICIDES ON CABBAGE FOR WORM AND FLEA BEETLE CONTROL AT AFRC, FABIUS, NY FROM 1977 TO 1979

Material and Rate AI/Acre	Compound Type*	Avg. Foliage Injury Rating**			Avg. % FB Damage 1979***
		1977	1978	1979	
Carbofuran 10G, 1 lb	ST	1.06	1.20	1.00	3.8
Carbofuran 10G, 2 lbs	ST	----	----	0.26	6.7
Diazinon 14G, 1 lb	ST	1.00	1.00	0.60	37.0
Herculite Diazinon 10G, 1 lb	SR	1.26	1.06	1.00	27.0
Agway Diazinon 2E, 1 lb	SR	----	----	0.66	45.3
Agway Diazinon 17.3G SXE, 1 lb	SR	----	----	0.60	47.6
Acephate CC-7135 10G, 1 lb	SR	1.00	1.03	0.46	20.3
Acephate CC-7135 10G, 2 lb	SR	0.76	1.00	0.73	29.8
Acephate CC-2271 10G, 1 lb	QR	1.46	1.06	1.06	22.7
Acephate CC-2271 10G, 2 lb	QR	0.66	1.00	0.66	37.6
Untreated Check	--	2.73	2.56	3.26	70.0

* Compound Type: ST=Standard commercial formulation; SR=Slow release, encapsulated; QR=Quick release, encapsulated.

** Foliar feeding injury index ratings on head leaves: 1=Only slight damage or a trace of chewing; 2=Less than 10% chewing on leaves; 3=Moderate feeding on 25% of leaves; 4=Severe feeding on 50% of leaves; 5=100% severely injured.

*** Average % flea beetle damage on head leaves rated only in 1979.

may replace or reduce the number of foliar spray treatments now
required for worm control on cabbage.

Direct Seeded Cabbage Root Maggot Studies

Data presented in Table II provide average percent reduction
in root maggot tunneling in cabbage roots based on the untreated
check values. These ratings taken at harvest by digging up whole
roots and plants indicate that over a three-year period, this insect
can cause extensive root damage to a given planting, but a crop
is still obtained. The greatest response to crop protection with
chemical applications was observed in 1978. It is interesting to
note that the variation observed in Herculite diazinon controlled-
release formulations can be attributed to the use of three different
formulations. Percent maggot reduction can be directly converted
to percent control. In the tests, a level of 60% would be deemed
commercially acceptable, as these treatments would have experienced
two complete generations of maggot.

Wireworm Control Studies on Potato

Wireworm problems in potato are observed as tuber damage at
harvest. With the use of systemic compounds at planting, little
insecticide is left at maturation of the crop to prevent tuber
damage. As evidenced in Table III, a 10% damage level is economic.
Encapsulated formulations of diazinon and chlorpyrifos look very
promising in this type of control.

New Seeding Alfalfa Study

A new practice to protect new pure seedings of alfalfa is to
incorporate a systemic insecticide such as carbofuran at planting
with the seed. This application of chemical then gives residual
insect crop protection over the critical crop establishment period.
As documented in Table IV, both carbofuran and acephate granules
applied in this manner protected the alfalfa from blotch leafminer
infestation and increased average stand over the untreated check.
Only carbofuran, however, had any effect on suppressing potato leafhopper which was assessed by measuring the amount of terminal yellows
resulting from leafhopper feeding.

Northern Corn Rootworm Control Studies

As shown in Table V, all chemical treatments reduced larval
rootworm damage to corn roots when compared to the untreated check.

TABLE II. COMPARISON OF CABBAGE ROOT MAGGOT DAMAGE ON DIRECT SEEDED CABBAGE TREATED WITH CONTROLLED-RELEASE INSECTICIDE FORMULATIONS AT AFRC, FABIUS, NY, 1977 TO 1979

Material and Rate AI/Acre	Compound Type*	Avg. % Reduction in Maggot Root Tunneling at Harvest		
		(69 Days) 1977	(62 Days) 1978	(65 Days) 1979
Diazinon 14G, 1 lb	ST	23.0	90.4	37.1
Chlorpyrifos 15G, 1 lb	ST	73.0	86.3	40.0
Herculite Diazinon 10G, 1 lb**	SR	20.7	86.3	42.9
Herculite Chlorpyrifos 10G HL90-3B, 1 lb	SR	60.0	92.5	----
Carbofuran 10G, 1 lb	ST	34.6	84.3	61.6
Acephate CC-7135 10G, 1 lb	SR	42.3	----	----
Acephate CC-2271 10G, 1 lb	QR	51.5	----	----
Agway Diazinon AG500, 1 lb	ST	47.7	85.9	62.8
Diazinon AG500 + Soil Penetrant 1 lb + 3%	ST + SP	----	----	70.5
Diazinon 16G, SXE, 1 lb	SR + SXE	----	89.8	15.1
Agway Chlorpyrifos, 2E, 1 lb	SR + PVB	----	----	50.0
Agway Diazinon 2#, PVB, 1 lb	SR + PVB	----	----	61.6
Pennwalt Knox Out 2FM, 1 lb	SR	----	----	33.6
Diazinon 10% Insectape Strip	SR	----	----	41.6
Untreated Check		130 Tunnels / 30 Roots	441 Tunnels / 30 Roots	396 Tunnels / 30 Roots

* Compound Type: ST=Standard commercial formulation; SR=Slow release, encapsulated; QR=Quick release, encapsulated; SP=Soil penetrant adjuvant; SXE=Starch xanthate, encapsulated; PVB=Polyvinyl bead encapsulated.

** 3 Different Formulations Tested Successively Each Year: HL90-3A-10G; HSM-1087-10G; and EOP-1 10G, respectively.

TABLE III. COMPARISON OF WIREWORM CONTROL IN POTATOES WITH CONTROLLED-RELEASE SOIL APPLICATIONS OF INSECTICIDE AT AFRC, FABIUS, NY, FROM 1977 TO 1979

Material and Rate AI/Acre	Compound Type*	Avg. % Wireworm Control on Tubers at Harvest		
		1977	1978	1979
Diazinon 14G, 3 lbs	ST	90.9	80.0	70.0
Herculite Diazinon 10G, 3 lbs	SR	100.0	100.0	100.0
Aldicarb 15G, 3 lbs	ST	90.9	90.0	----
Chlorpyrifos 15G, 2 lbs	ST	----	90.0	----
Herculite Chlorpyrifos 15G, 2 lbs	SR	----	90.0	----
Diazinon 10% Insectape	--	----	100.0	----
Diazinon 17.3G SXE, 3 lbs	SR	----	100.0	90.0
Acephate CC-7135 10G, 3 lbs	SR	----	----	90.0
Untreated Check**	--	----	----	----

* Compound Type: ST=Standard commercial formulation
                  SR=Slow release, encapsulated.

** Check had 33.3%, 10% and 16.6% tuber wireworm damage at harvest for each respective year.

TABLE IV. INSECT DAMAGE RATINGS AND STAND COUNTS ON NEW PURE SEEDING OF 'SARANAC' ALFALFA WITH GRANULAR INCORPORATED INSECTICIDES AT AFRC, FABIUS, NY, 1978

Material and Rate AI/Acre	Compound Type*	A** Avg. Stand	B Avg. Ablm Mines	C Avg. Ablm Mines	D Avg. PL Nymphs	E Avg. % Yellows
Carbofuran 10G, 1½ lbs	ST	63.6	18.2	7.6	0.8	20.0
Carbofuran 10G, 2 lbs	ST	41.0	15.7	4.3	1.1	56.6
Carbofuran 10G, 3 lbs	ST	42.6	10.5	3.5	0.3	33.3
Acephate CC-7135 10G, 2 lbs	SR	60.6	15.4	4.0	1.5	73.3
Untreated Check	--	38.6	22.6	18.4	1.1	53.3

* Compound Type: ST=Standard commercial formulation; SR=Slow release, encapsulated.

** Key to Ratings: A = Rated June 28, 1978 - Avg. counts/sq. ft. @ 20 lbs/acre
B = Rated July 20, 1978 - Avg. No. blotch leaf miner mines per terminal
C = Rated Aug. 29, 1978 - Avg. ablm mines/terminal at 100 days post
D = Rated July 20, 1978 - Avg. No. potato leafhopper nymphs/terminal
E = Rated June 10, 1978 - Avg. % pl yellowing on terminals
stand planted and treated May 19, 1978.

TABLE V. COMPARISON OF NORTHERN CORN ROOTWORM LARVAL CONTROL ON FIELD CORN AT AFRC, FABIUS, NY, 1977 TO 1978

Material and Rate AI/Acre	Compound Type	Avg. Root Damage Injury Ratings*		
		NO-TILL 8/16/77	LAY-BY 9/2/77	NO-TILL 8/22/78
Carbofuran 10G, 1 lb	ST	2.43	3.33	3.46
Terbufos 15G, 1 lb	ST	2.73	3.26	2.93
Chlorpyrifos 15G, 1 lb	ST	2.63	3.26	----
Herculite Diazinon 10G, HL90-3A, 1 lb	SR	2.56	3.00	----
Diazinon 14G, 1 lb	ST	2.33	3.33	3.20
Herculite Chlorpyrifos 10G, HL-903B, 1 lb	SR	----	3.20	----
Herculite Diazinon 10G, HSM-1087, 1 lb	SR	----	2.80	3.13
Agway Diazinon 2G, PVB, 1 lb	SR	----	3.13	----
Agway Chlorpyrifos 2G, PVB, 1 lb	SR	----	2.86	----
Diazinon 16G, SXE, 1 lb	SR	----	----	3.26
Untreated Check	--	4.06	4.13	3.66

* Root Rating Injury Index: (Iowa System)
1=No noticeable feeding; 2=Feeding scars by NCR larvae present; 3=At least 3 roots pruned to 1½" of base of root node; 4=One full node (whorl) of roots pruned; 5=Two full nodes (whorls) of roots pruned; 6=Three or more nodes of roots pruned - system completely destroyed.

Encapsulated formulations of diazinon and chlorpyrifos did not appear to greatly enhance efficacy as observed in the 1977 study with diazinon.[7] However, the polyvinyl bead encapsulated formulation of chlorpyrifos in 1977 was more efficacious than all other chemicals in that year of study, but was not included in the 1978 study. Other research reported by Kydonieus, et al.[15] indicated that a study with Hercon encapsulated phorate for Southern corn rootworm control lasted for 164 days; the standard 15G formulation was completely ineffective after 73 days.

Sweet Corn Insect Control Studies

Table VI presents the results of encapsulated formulations compared to fonofos and carbofuran standard formulation treatment in controlling corn earworm, fall armyworm, and European corn borer in sweet corn. Broadcast post emergence directed applications were made to the whorls of corn plants at the early green tassel stage. Percent worm ear damage was made approximately 30 days post treatment by sampling 100 ears combined from three replicates. All chemical treatments, with the exception of diazinon 14G, reduced ear insect damage. In 1979, results from timing post emergence applications at early green tassel and at tasseling were compared. The later at tasseling treatment was not as effective as early treatment in reducing ear damage. Encapsulation of diazinon enhanced insect control with polymeric laminate and starch xanthate formulations.

Seed Corn Maggot Control in Vegetables

Seed treatment is a prophylactic insurance program to prevent seed corn maggot damage to large seeded crops. In Table VII, results show the seed furrow encapsulated diazinon tape and the polyvinyl bead flowable diazinon formulation to be as effective as their counterpart commercial hopperbox seed treatment all applied at planting. An important note is that both encapsulated diazinon formulations were applied over or next to the planted seeds and did not completely cover the seed coats as did the hopperbox treatment. Because of the large size of lima bean seed, it is not surprising to have observed reduced stand, since this tape was placed next to or over the seed. Some separation away from the seed could have occurred when seed furrows were closed. However, it would be possible to combine seed and tape into a single unit.

Onion Maggot Control Study

Onion maggot damage to seedlings is exhibited in reduced stand. As indicated in Table VIII, all chemicals greatly improved stand

TABLE VI. SWEET CORN INSECT CONTROL STUDIES WITH INSECTICIDE WHORL TREATMENTS AT AFRC, FABIUS, NY FROM 1977 TO 1979

Material and Rate AI/Acre***	Compound Type*	Average % Ear Damage by Worms**			
		(ECB & CEW) 1977	(ECB & CEW) 1978	(DEW & FAW) 1979	(Tasseling)
Carbofuran 10G, 1 lb	ST	3.3	3.3	25.0	31.7
Fonofos 20G, 1 lb	ST	6.6	----	25.0	28.3
Herculite Diazinon 10G, HL90-3A, 1 lb	SR	16.5	----	----	----
Diazinon 14G, 1 lb	ST	16.5	----	35.0	46.7
Diazinon 10G, EOP-1, 1 lb	SR	----	----	27.5	26.7
Fonofos 20G, DEG, 1 lb	SR	----	3.3	27.5	28.3
Diazinon 17.3G, SXE, 1 lb	SR-SXE	----	----	27.5	36.7
Diazinon 2E, PVB, 1 lb	SR-PVB	----	26.6	42.5	28.3
Untreated Check	----	26.5	40.0	45.0	40.0

* Compound Type: ST=Standard commercial formulation; SR=Slow release, encapsulated; SXE=Starch xanthate, encapsulated; PVB=Polyvinyl bead, encapsulated.

** ECB=European corn borer; CEW=Corn earworm; FAW=Fall armyworm.

*** Materials applied as directed whorl applications at EGT except where rated at tasseling.

TABLE VII. INSECTICIDES AS SEED TREATMENTS FOR THE CONTROL OF SEED MAGGOTS ON VEGETABLES AT AFRC, FABIUS, NY, 1979

Treatment and Rate*	Sweet Corn Avg. Stand/ 30 Seeds	Snap Beans			Lima Beans		
		Avg. Stand/ 30 Seeds	% Germ.	% SCM Stand Damage	Avg. Stand/ 30 Seeds	% Germ.	% SCM Stand Damage
Protector II (HB**), 2 oz	27.3	23.0	76.7	36.2	13.3	44.4	62.5
Protector II, 4 oz	29.0	24.3	81.1	45.3	14.7	48.9	59.1
Diazinon 10% SFT****	27.3	21.0	70.0	36.5	9.0	30.0	59.2
Diazinon 25% PVB S***, 4 oz	25.7	22.3	74.4	35.9	16.3	54.4	53.1
Untreated Check	26.0	19.6	65.5	93.2	14.3	47.7	93.1

* Expressed in oz of product/60/lb Bu. of seed or lbs/AI/furrow.

** HB=Hopper box treatment; S=Slurried seed treatment; protector II=25% diazinon + 37.5% captan

*** Polyvinyl bead encapsulated flowable slurry containing 2 lb. AI/gal. diazinon.

**** In-furrow seed treatment with SR granular 10% formulation of diazinon on a 1/4" wide tape.

TABLE VIII. ONION MAGGOT CONTROL STUDY ON MUCK SOILS AT CANASTOTA, NY, 1978

Material and Rate AI/Acre	Compound Type*	Average Onion Stand Counts/10' Row			
		6/30	7/10	7/26	Averaged Stand
Chlorpyrifos 15G, 1 lb	ST	56.0	55.0	56.0	55.6
Herculite Chlorpyrifos 10G, HL90-3B, 1 lb	SR	54.0	62.3	62.0	59.4
Diazinon 14G, 1 lb	ST	63.3	71.3	71.3	68.6
Herculite Diazinon 10G	SR	59.3	65.6	64.7	63.2
Diazinon 10G, SXE, 1 lb	SR-SXE	49.0	61.7	58.3	56.3
USDA Diazinon 16G, SXE, 1 lb	SR-SXE	50.6	54.3	53.0	52.6
Fensulfothion + Thiram 5+7, 5G, 1 lb	ST	64.3	63.0	55.0	60.8
Untreated Check	--	40.3	48.7	60.3	49.7

* Compound Type: St=Standard commercial formulation; SR=Slow release, encapsulated; SXE=Starch xanthate, encapsulated.

over the untreated check. Encapsulation of diazinon formulations used in this test did not enhance activity, whereas the polymeric laminated chlorpyrifos formulation did.

CONCLUSIONS

Differences in insecticide release rates between standard and encapsulated insecticides are shown in the degree of insect control observed. This varies with the insecticide formulation used and the control of the insect pest compared. Specific formulations consistently indicated higher degrees of pest control than their standard commercial counterparts at equal active ingredient rates. Coppedge, et al.[16] demonstrated that slow-release formulations of disulfoton were less effective against cotton aphids than the standard granular formulation, whereas the reverse was true of aldicarb slow-release formulations compared to the fast-release standard. Thus, controlled-release formulations designed to enhance efficacy are compound specific. With certain types of applications such as cabbage, single properly timed applications of controlled-release acephate formulations tested for the last four years provided effective and residual season-long insect control. Continued research conducted since 1977 also indicated that controlled-release formulations of diazinon, acephate, and chlorpyrifos provided effective wireworm control in potato and sweet-corn insect control whereas standard chemical treatment was much less effective. The potential use of controlled-release technology for insect crop protection offers a new research area. Future research in controlled-release insecticide formulations should provide opportunities for new product development.

REFERENCES

1. B.A. Bierl and D. DeVelbiss, in: "Proceedings International Controlled Release Pesticide Symposium," F.W. Harris, ed., College of Science and Engineering, Wright State University, Dayton (1975).
2. D.C. Read, J. Econ. Entomol. 69(4):429-437 (1976).
3. R.K. Chapman and E.J. Eckenrode, J. Econ. Entomol. 66(5):1153-1158 (1973).
4. R.E. Lynch, L.C. Lewis, E.C. Berry, and J.F. Robinson, J. Econ. Entomol. 70(3):389-391 (1977).
5. Agrichemical Age, Pennwalt Sees Bright Future for Microencapsulation May (5)76 (1976).
6. R.C. Koestler, in: "Proceedings 6th International Symposium on Controlled Release of Bioactive Materials," R.W. Baker, ed., New Orleans (1979).
7. N.L. Gauthier, in: "Proceeding of 1977 Controlled Release Pesticide Symposium," R. Goulding, ed., Orgon State University, Corvallis (1977).

8. N.L. Gauthier, in: "Proceedings of 5th International Symposium on Controlled Release of Bioactive Materials," E. Brinkman and J. Montemareno, eds., National Bureau of Standards, Gaithersburg (1978).

9. A.R. Quisumbing, A.F. Kydonius, and N.L. Gauthier, in: "Proceedings of 5th International Symposium on Controlled Release of Bioactive Materials," E. Brinkman and J. Montemareno, eds., National Bureau of Standards, Gaithersburg (1978).

10. A.F. Kydonieus, in: "Proceedings of American Chemical Society Controlled Release Pesticides Symposium," New Orleans (1977).

11. Anonymous, Controlled Release Pesticides Attract Interest, Chem & Engin. News 52(30):20-22 (1974).

12. A.R. Quisumbing, D.J. Lawatsch, and A.F. Kydonieus, in: "Proceedings International Controlled Release Pesticide Symposium," F.W. Harris, ed., College of Science and Engineering, Wright State University, Dayton (1975).

13. W.M. Doane, Starchy Protecter Agricultural Research 25(5):6-7 (1976).

14. B.S. Shasha, W.M. Doane, and C.R. Russell, J. Polym. Sci. 14:417-420 (1976).

15. A.F. Kydonieus and S. Baldwin, in: "Proceedings 1976 Controlled Release Pesticides Symposium," N.F. Cardarelli, ed., University of Akron, 4.23-4.35 (1976).

16. J.R. Coppedge, R.A. Stokes, R.L. Ridgeway, and D.L. Bull, J. Econ. Entomol 68(4):508-510 (1975).

CONTROLLED RELEASE TEMEPHOS: LABORATORY AND

FIELD EVALUATIONS

Thomas J. Quick and Nathan F. Cardarelli

Environmental Management Laboratory
The University of Akron
Akron, Ohio

Ruben J. Ellin and Larry R. Sherman

Department of Chemistry
The University of Akron
Akron, Ohio

INTRODUCTION

The development of controlled-release pesticides based upon
the monolithic dispersion of a chemical agent in a polymer has been
described in detail elsewhere.[1] Temephos, 0,0,0',0'-tetramethyl-
0,0-thiodi-p-phenylene phosphorothioate (C.A. Registry #3383-96-8),
was incorporated in elastomeric matrices and a diffusion-dissolution type release mechanism was established.[2] Although a continuous
release of the agent occurred for over three years, commercialization was not undertaken. Later it was discovered that long-term
toxicant release from a plastic matrix could be achieved through
a leaching process keyed to the use of a water-soluble additive
whose emission led to the development of the necessary porosity
in the matrix.[3] The processing costs for such materials are relatively inexpensive, and consequently a number of controlled-release
temephos materials are now commercially available. Unlike conventional formulations which are limited to solutions, emulsions,
granules, and wettable powders, controlled-release plastic dispensers
can be manufactured in any geometry conducive to the particular
environment to be treated.

Technical grade temephos is a light brown semi-viscous liquid
which may crystallize below 15°C. Its specific gravity is 1.3 at

275

$25°C$. Temephos has a solubility in water of 25 ppb at $25°C$ and
is stable indefinitely at room temperature. However, there may
be hydrolysis at high pH for prolonged periods of time. The LC_{50}
for Culex p. quinquefasciatus is ≈ 0.0016 ppm and LC_{90} is ≈ 0.0019
ppm. Residual efficacy of temephos depends on the degree of dilution
and the type of water that is to be treated.

MATERIALS AND METHODS

    The commercial temephos formulations examined consisted of
ECOPRO-1707 FPW, a 1 3/8" x 1 1/4" x 1/16" floating chip anchored
by a metal washer and a nylon line, designed for use in tropical
rain barrels and other potable water devices; ECOPRO-1707F, three
14" x 1/2" x 1/32" floating ribbons attached to a sigmoid metal
anchor for use in a catch basin environment; and ECOPRO-1700 sinking
granules. The ECOPRO formulations are products of Environmental
Chemicals Inc., Barrington, IL. Figure 1 depicts dispenser geometries.

    The basic formulation consists of 7.2% temephos monolithically
dispersed in a plastic matrix containing a porosity-inducing material
(porosigen). Agent release rate is constant, once steady-state
is achieved in several days.

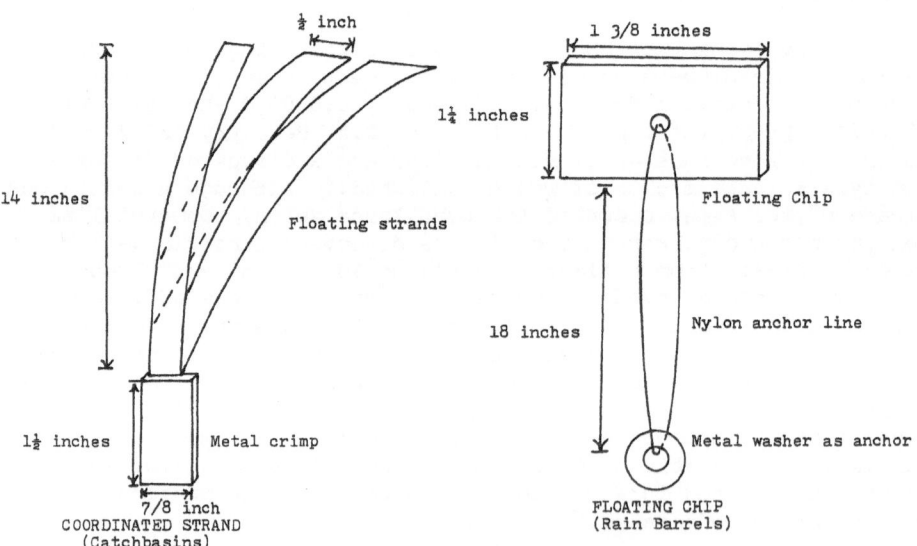

Figure 1.   Controlled-release temephos dispensers.

Laboratory evaluations are performed according to the periodic challenge bioassay method described in an earlier report.[4] First and second instars Culex pipiens quinquefasciatus are used. Dispensers are soaked continuously in demineralized water with periodic water change.

In one field trial, eight 55-gallon-capacity steel drums were used for simulated catch basins or rain barrels or both. The location was within a shady grove of beech and ash trees within 50 feet of a septic outcrop and bog. A ditch carrying septic effluents from about 20 homesteads flowed within 200 feet of this area. The general area breeds mosquitoes, mainly Culex pipiens pipiens in large numbers.

Each drum was lined with plastic and filled to the 50-gallon mark with well water or a combination of well water and high organic content sewage from the aforementioned septic ditch. ECOPRO 1707F coordinated strand dispensers were placed as whole or half units in each drum. Table I depicts the scheme used.

Sections of coordinated strand units were immersed in water and aliquots analyzed periodically for temephos in order to determine the emission-rate and steady-state concentration.

TABLE I.

Drum No.	Gallon Water	Gallon Sewage[a]	EC 1707F Dispenser (Lot 1)
1	50	0	1 unit
2	49	1	1 unit
3	48	2	1 unit
4	45	5	1 unit
5	50	0	½ unit
6	50	0	none
7	48	2	½ unit
8	45	5	½ unit

[a] Sewage is jet black, of a soupy-globular consistency containing considerable decaying vegetation, and highly acidic (pH 3.2-3.5). Organic content was determined as 2.3%.

In emission-rate studies a 1.00-gram sample of ECOPRO 1707 strand was submerged in 1000 ml of distilled deionized water for three days. All water was removed with the flask inverted and drained for 20 minutes. The test specimens were reimmersed in 1000 ml of water. The temephos-containing water was divided into two equal portions, and each was extracted with three 10-ml aliquots of hexane. Fractions were then recombined in a 100-ml Kjeldahl flask and digested with 3 ml of concentrated sulfuric acid until the hexane was evaporated, at which time 1 ml of concentrated nitric acid is added and the mixture is digested until clear. Temephos was determined by a method similar to the classic heteropoly blue method for organic phosphorus (Treatise on Analytical Chemistry, part 2, Vol. 11, 534-544, John Wiley & Sons, Inc., 1965). It is described below:

The digested samples were transferred to 100-ml test tubes, the pH was adjusted to 1.4 with NaOH, 5.00 ml of reagent 1 (100 ml of H_2O, 150 ml of conc. H_2SO_4, and 100 ml of 10% ammonium molybdate solution) and 5.00 ml of reagent 2 (0.2 g of Elon (p-methyl aminophenol sulfate, Eastman Kodak, Rochester, NY), 40.0 g of potassium metabisulfite, and 1.0 g of sodium sulfate diluted to 300 ml) were added. The test tubes were heated for 13 minutes in a boiling water bath, diluted to 50 ml, and the absorption peak measured on a Cary 17 spectrophotometer near 830 nm by scanning over 850-770 nm range.

The calibration curve had a least-square slope of 104 ± 3 µg/A units. The temephos (13.28% phosphorus) detection limit is 2.9 µg determined as phosphate.

In the steady-state determination a 2.00-gram strand sample was submerged in 2000 ml of distilled deionized water. A 200-ml sample was volumetrically removed, extracted with three 10-ml aliquots of hexane, and the temephos determined as described above. The sample was rediluted to 2000 ml, mixed, and allowed to equilibrate until the next sample was removed.

RESULTS

Laboratory Bioassay

Table II is a compendium of repeat-challenge bioassay results from EC-1700 pellets over a 1108-day period. The LT_{100} (lethal time for 100% larva mortality) was used as the indicia. Conventional measures such as the 24-hr LD_{50} and LD_{90} are valueless, since temephos water concentrations increase with exposure time. First and second instars C. p. quinquefasciatus were used at 15 per 1000-ml

TABLE II.   LABORATORY EVALUATION OF ECOPRO 1700 PELLETS
AGAINST MOSQUITO LARVA

Water Imersion Time	LT_{100} (days) – Lethal Time to 100% Population Mortality					
	3.6ppm[a]	2.2ppm[a]	1.5ppm[a]	0.84ppm[a]	0.54ppm[a]	0.23ppm[a]
30 days	2 days	2 days	3 days	3 days	2 days	2 days
70	2	3	3	3	3	4
110	2	3	4	3	8	7
160	2	2	1	6	6	4
225	2	2	3	5	4	4
310	3	3	6	5	5	6
416	2	1	5	5	5	8
532	2	2	3	2	5	10
710	3	3	3	3	5	–
820	2	1	5	5	5	–
950	2	2	3	3	2	–
1108	1	1	5	8	7	–

[a] Temephos Concentration (Day 0) in Pellet per 1000 ml Water

test aquaria, five aquaria per test. The temephos dosage provided is that amount in the given test pellet at Day 0, and not the water concentration.

Mortality, pupation, and emergence were noted at 24-hour intervals during testing. Results indicate that temphos is not a pupacide but does prevent larva from pupating when in sufficient quantity. During tests few larva develop to the fourth instar; however, it is not uncommon to have viable first and second instars for as long as five days. Lower pellet concentrations (in 1000 ml) failed over the course of the experiment; 0.14 ppm, 0.06 ppm, and 0.035 ppm at the 310-day check point. Also some pupation was noted at 310 days at 0.23 ppm, 0.46 ppm, and 0.54 ppm formulations.[4]

Field Evaluation - 55-Gallon Drums

Drums containing well water with and without sewage content, as described in Table I, were examined periodically for the presence of mosquito larva. Numbers of a given instar below 50 were counted, over 50 estimated. Results are shown in Table III. The water was not changed, although the drums overflowed during rainstorms in the spring and summer months. Tests were initiated in Copley Township, Ohio, June 2, 1979, and were terminated 172 days later at the end of the local mosquito "season".

TABLE III.   LARVICIDAL ACTIVITY OF ECOPRO 1707F STRANDS
IN 55-GALLON OPEN TOP DRUMS

Immersion Day (check point)	No. Larva and/or Pupa							
	Drum #1	2	3	4	5	6 (control)	7	8
21	0	0	0	0	0	200	0	300
24	0	0	0	0	0	500+	20	315
27	0	0	0	0	0	500+	60	500+
32	0	0	0	0	0	500+	200	320
36	0	0	0	0	0	500+	400	25
39	0	0	0	0	0	500+	500+	30
44	0	0	0	0	10	500+	500+	500+
48	0	0	0	0	20	500+	400	60
57	0	0	0	0	0	500+	30	20
70	0	0	0	0	0	500+	0	0
76	0	0	0	0	25	500+	0	0
89	0	0	0	0	0	500+	0	0
97	0	0	0	0	0	500+	0	0
105	0	0	0	0	0	500+	0	0
117	0	0	0	0	0	500+	0	0
130	0	0	0	0	0	500+	0	0
139	0	0	0	0	0	500+	0	0
147	0	0	0	0	0	400	0	0
159	0	0	0	0	0	400	0	0
172	0	0	0	0	0	300	0	0

Full- and half-coordinated strand units provided long-term
control in clear water. Where organic matter was present, full
units provided quick control; however, half units require considerable time to bring the temephos concentration up to the lethal
dosage. Egg masses were present in all drums at all times. No
evidence of adult repellency was noted. Hatching, as evidenced
by the presence of pupa cases, was considerable in the control drum
and present in drums 7 and 8 from Day 27 to Day 57.

Snails, nematode, and water-beetle populations were profuse
in all drums containing septic material with no observed mortality.
Dead moths and flies were found at various times in all drums.

While it is recognized that this initial experiment is not
statistically sound, it is reasonable to conclude that, under the
stated conditions, one can achieve a full-season mosquito control
in static water of low-to-moderate organic content.

Collaborators Reports

Pellets and chip dispensers were furnished to a number of agencies for evaluation, and reports submitted to Environmental Chemicals, Inc. were forthcoming. These were released to the Environmental Management Lab for this report and are summarized in Tables IV and V.

TABLE IV.   COOPERATORS FIELD TEST RESULTS: TEMEPHOS CHIP
DISPENSERS (ECOPRO 1707FPW)

Location	Environment	No. of Units	Results
Salem, OR[5]	Catch Basins	100	Control
Sun River, OR[6]	Pond	1	Control
Rangoon, Burma	Drums (Rain Barrels)	100	Partial Control, 60% showed 100% control
Portsmouth, OH[7]	Catch Basins	10	Control
Elkhart, IN[8]	Catch Basins	101	Control, save in a few basins with heavy debris
Lyndhurst, OH[9]	Catch Basins	10	No control
Edison, NJ[10]	Pools	23	No control
Hinckley, UT[11]	Lake Margin	1000	Control
Hastings, NB[12]	Catch Basins	52	Control, save in 16 basins where units washed out
North Riverside, IL[13]	Catch Basins	145	No control
Gloucester City, NJ[14]	Catch Basins	200	Control, save in basins where units washed away
Rosell, IL[14]	Trenches	11	Control
St. Joseph City, IN[14]	Catch Basins	66	Control, save in units with heavy debris
Chincoteague, VI[14]	Catch Basins	200	Control
Sunbury, PA[14]	Catch Basins	25	Control
Bowling Green, OH[14]	Catch Basins	25	No control, units washed away
Columbus, OH[15]	Catch Basins	88	Partial control
Virginia Beach, VI[14]	Catch Basins	2000	Control, save in basins where units washed away

TABLE V.   COOPERATORS FIELD TEST RESULTS: TEMEPHOS
GRANULES (ECOPRO 1700)

Location	Environment	Concentration	Results
Sun River, OR[6]	Ditch	Unknown	Control
Trad, Thailand[16]	Gem Pits(50)	0.1ppm-ta to 0.3ppm-ta	Partial Control
Naperville, IL[17]	Concrete Basins(4)	4#/acre rate	No control
DuPage County, IL[18]	Swamps(4)	1.5#/acre rate	Control
Midvale, UT[19]	Irrigated Pastures	80 oz/acre	No control
Anahuac, TX[20]	Salt Marsh	48 oz/acre	Control
Williamsport, PA[21]	Pools	25 ox/acre	No control (silt over effect)
Barberton, OH[22]	Pools(4)	0.68ppm-ta	Control

Analysis of collaborators' results indicated that the anchored
chip provided control when in place, but tended to wash away when
exposed to rapid water movement. The coordinated strand dispenser
was developed in order to overcome this problem, and also to increase the agent emission rate. The anchored chip appears to be
most appropriately used in potable water reservoirs such as rain
barrels. ECOPRO 1700 sinking granules lose effectiveness upon
silting over.

Laboratory Kinetics of Coordinated Strand Dispensers

The emision-rate studies indicate that 1.00 gram of ECOPRO 1707
strand (7.2% temephos) emits 24 ± 21 µg per day into one liter of
water over a period of greater than 150 days. The results, given
in Table VI, have been normalized to 24 hours regardless of the
time interval between sampling. The large deviation was likely
due to inconsistent mixing and lack of temperature control.

Since the ECOPRO 1707F contains approximately 72 mg of temephos,
the emission study indicates that the tape has a life of more than
2400 days when 100% of water is exchanged every 24 hours. In
quiescent water a longer life would be expected.

The steady-state studies indicate that ECOPRO 1707F reaches
a steady-state concentration of 192 ± 65 ppb in about ten days when
10% of water is exchanged between sampling (Figure 2). The concentration decreases slightly after 120 days. The large deviation
is probably due to the same reasons listed above.

TABLE VI. ECOPRO 1707F COORDINATED
STRAND EMISSION RATE

Day	Temephos Concentration μg/g-l/day
1	12.70
2	62.30
3	43.70
9	30.90
21	2.59
25	7.92
48	4.53
50	6.04
52	23.10
58	46.50
97	24.10
150	23.90
	$\bar{x} = 24.0 \quad \sigma = 21.0$

Temephos has a half-life of approximately two weeks and degrades
to non-toxic compounds. Its toxic concentration is approximately
25% of the steady-state concentration. The 230-ppb bioassay sample
(Table II) probably never reached a steady-state concentration and
after 550 days was incapable of maintaining a toxic level in the
test drums.

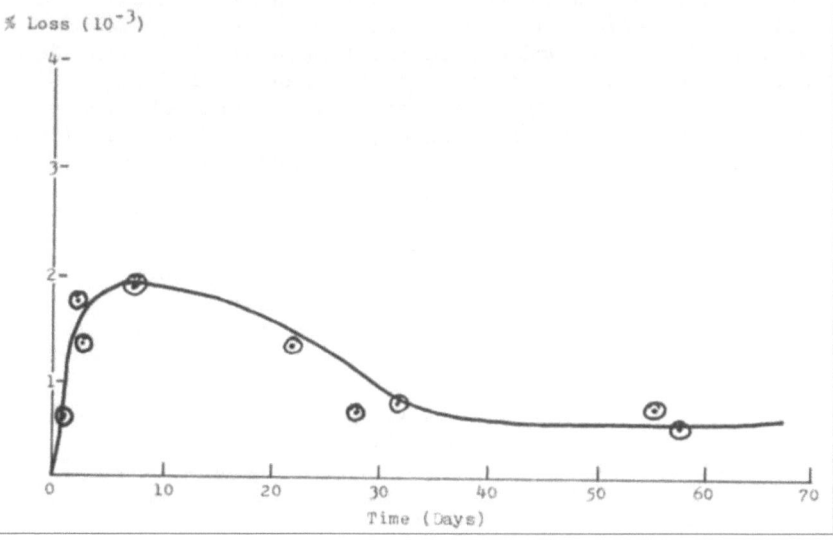

Figure 2.   Temephos loss from ECOPRO 1707F strands.

CONCLUSION

The bioassay and chemical studies of temephos controlled-release formulations indicate that they are effective larvicides, that the lethal dosage is in the range of 20–50 ppb, and that they have an active life of approximately seven years when used at one gram per liter of water in ideal circumstances.

ACKNOWLEDGEMENTS

The authors wish to acknowledge the assistance of Robert D. Boon for the chemical analysis and Linda Boswell for the bioassay work.

Financial assistance for the work was provided by Environmental Chemicals, Inc., Barrington, IL 60010.

REFERENCES

1. N.F. Cardarelli, in: "Controlled Release Pesticide Formulations," CRC Press, (1976). p. 210.
2. N.F. Cardarelli, U.S. Patent 3590119 (1971)
3. N.F. Cardarelli, U.S. Patent 4116111 (1979).
4. N.R. Cardarelli, Mosquito News 38:328–333 (1978).
5. T.L. Park, Correspondence to Environmental Chemicals, Inc., Marion County Health Department, Salem, OR, Jan 12 (1979).
6. J. Bowerman, Correspondence to Environmental Chemicals Inc., Sunriver Properties Inc., Sunriver, OR, July 13 (1978).
7. J.W. Oliver, Correspondence to Environmental Chemicals, Inc. Department of Health, Portsmount, OH, Jan 17 (1979).
8. K.M. Mackowiak, Correspondence to Environmental Chemicals, Inc., Elkhart County Health Dept., Elkhart, IN, Oct 23 (1978).
9. J.B. Jackson, A Field Evaluation of ECOPRO 1707F Larvicide in Catch Basins, Lyndhurst, OH, August–September, Unpublished Report, Cuyahoga County Board of Health, OH, p. 2 (1978).
10. R.F. Schmidt, Preliminary Report on the Effectiveness of ECOPRO 1707F, Unpublished Report, Middlesex County Mosquito Extermination Commission, Edison, NJ, Jan 6, p. 4 (1979).
11. E. Murray, Correspondence to Environmental Chemicals, Inc., West Millard County Mosquito Abatement Committee, Sept. 23 (1978).
12. L. Strommer, Correspondence to Environmental Chemicals, Inc., Department of Health, Hastings, NB, Aug. 28 (1978).
13. Anon, Field Test of ECOPRO 1707F, A Sustained Controlled-Release Chemical, Unpublished Report, Des Plaines Valley Mosquito Abatement District, Lyons, IL, p. 1 (1978).

14. R. Himel, Field Test Results of ECOPRO 1707F Mosquito Larvicide,
     Unpublished Report, Environmental Chemicals Inc., Barrington,
     IL, p. 7 (1979).
15. D.P. Ritchey, ECOPRO 1707F Evaluation, Unpublished Report,
     Dept. Health, Columbus, OH, Jan 31, p. 1 (1979).
16. Anon, Preliminary Results of a Trial with Controlled and Slow-
     Release Larvicide Formulations Against A. B. balapacensis in
     the Gem-Mining Pits in South-East Thailand, Unpub. Rep., WHO
     Regional Seminar on Anti-Malaria Operations, THA MPD 001, Trad,
     Thailand, p. 18 (1977).
17. C. Kopitke, An Evaluation of the Effectiveness of a Slow
     Release Larvicide in Controlling Mosquito Populations and a
     Survey of Macro-Invertibrates Inhabiting the Test Pools, Un-
     published Report to Environmental Chemicals Inc., p. 19 (1978).
18. C. Dancy, Unpublished Report, Microchem Inc., West Chicago,
     IL, p. 2 (1978).
19. K.H. Wagsfaff, Correspondence to Environmental Chemicals, Inc.,
     Salt Lake City Mosquito Abatement District, Midvale, UT, July
     11 (1978).
20. L.G. Terracina, Unpublished Report, Chambers County Mosquito
     Control, TX, July 3, p. 2 (1978).
21. K.C. Schuyler, Correspondence to Environmental Chemicals, Inc.,
     Pennsylvania Dept. of Environmental Resources, Williamsport,
     PA, July 10 (1978).
22. G.A. Janes and S.B. Holliday, Evaluation of Environmental Chemi-
     cals Inc., ECOPRO 1700 Controlled Release Larvicide, Unpublished
     Report Creative Biology Laboratory, Barberton, OH, p. 3 (1978).

TRI-n-BUTYLTIN FLUORIDE AS A CONTROLLED-RELEASE

MOSQUITO LARVICIDE

L.R. Sherman and J.C. Jackson

Department of Chemistry
The University of Akron
Akron, Ohio 44325

INTRODUCTION

Trialkyltin compounds have long been recognized as antifouling agents and molluscicides,[1] and more recently have demonstrated potential as mosquito larvicides.[2] Bis-n-tributyltin oxide (TBTO) and tributyltin fluoride (TBTF) are the most commonly used compounds and have been monolithically incorporated in a series of controlled-release formulations.[3][4] Both organotin compounds are non-persistent in the biosphere, degrading through a series of daughter compounds to non-toxic stannic oxide. TBTF has a half life of 6.7 days[5] and TBTO has a half life of 15.4 days in water.[6] They are probably noncarcinogenic and nonmutagenic, both effects being absent in short-term studies.[7] Teratogenicity is not evident in four successive mouse generations.[8] Field studies of formulations containing TBTO and TBTF in elastomers have demonstrated long-term snail control under environmentally adverse conditions.[9][10] Both materials are fairly specific toxicants for fresh-water snails, mosquito larvae, and certain fly larvae.

Slugs, salt-water molluscae, fish, vasular plants in general, and mammals are not affected at recommended snail control dosages. At higher concentrations fish are non-tolerant. Phytoplankton is not seriously affected until dosages are over 100x the LD_{90} for snails. The kill mechanism may arise from a blockage of transamination involving histidine and possibly other amino acids. Disturbances in blood chemistry are noted, and ^{14}C-labelled TBTO accumulated in the nuclear material of snails.[11] Yet, tin is probably an essential trace nutrient in mammals and organotin compounds may serve as a source of this essential micronutrient.[12]

287

Since the degradation of TBTO and TBTF varies with water quality,[6] it is felt that a knowledge of the rate of release and degradation scheme for TBTF in ECOPRO 1320 (20% tributyltin fluoride in a natural rubber base, Environmental Chemical Inc., Barrington, IL) is essential to determine its usefulness as a biocide. To complement this work a bioassay was performed on the Aedes aegypti larvae.

MATERIALS AND METHOD

Bioassay

One-liter aqueous solutions containing 0, 20, 100, and 200 ppb TBTF and 25 ml of the juice from rotting apples were prepared. The pH was adjusted to 6.5-7.0 with sodium bicarbonate. Fifty, third instar Aedes aegypit larvae were added to each solution. A 25-ml sample of the solution was removed each day and assayed for hexane soluble tin.

ECOPRO 1320 Leach Rate

Fifty ECOPRO 1320 pellets (assayed at 19.5% TBTF) were placed in each of three reservoirs and water was allowed to flow through them at approximately 5 ml/minute (See Figure 1). One to three pellets were removed from the reservoirs each week. The pellets were dried, cut in half, and weighed. One portion of the pellet was placed in a soxhlet extractor and extracted with reagent grade hexane for 50 hours. One ml of concentrated sulfuric acid was added to the extract. When the sulfuric acid began to reflux, 30% hydrogen peroxide was added dropwise to destroy the residual organic material, and the tin was determined as previously reported.[13]

The second half of each pellet was digested with concentrated sulfuric acid and hydrogen peroxide in a 100-ml Kjeldahl flask and the total tin determined spectrophotometrically.[13]

RESULTS

Bioassay

The bioassay of the TBTF solution is shown in Figure 2. In 20- and 100-ppb solutions, the LC_{50} for the larvae occurred within two days, whereas in 200-ppb solution the LC_{50} occurred in 7 days. This reverse phenomena has been observed with snails.[7] It is believed to occur because the organism is able to detect chronic

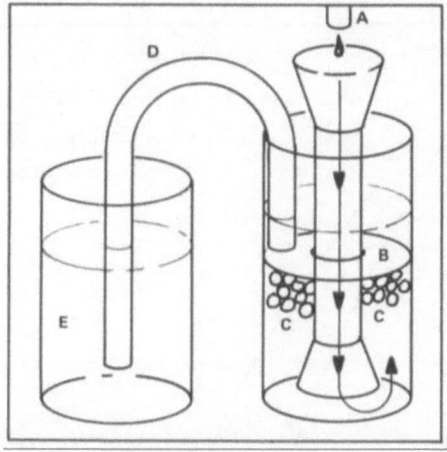

A. WATER SOURCE
B. PLASTIC TO WEIGHT PELLETS
C. ECOPRO 1320 PELLETS
D. SIPHON
E. BEAKER TO COLLECT WATER

Figure 1.

intoxication at the higher concentration and sets up a defense
mechanism. At the lower concentration the organism is unable to
detect intoxication and does not initiate a defense mechanism until
it is too late.

At $\emptyset$ ppb (the control) 50% of the larvae pupated and became
adults within nine days. Only 12% of the larvae pupated and became
adults in the 20-ppb solution. This occurred at 14 days which
indicates that larvae development was hindered by a sub-lethal dose
of TBTF. None of the larvae matured when exposed to 100- or 200-
ppb TBTF.

A repeat of the bioassay using second instar larvae at the
same TBTF concentrations resulted in an LC_{50} occurring after 24
hours. None of the larvae developed into the next instar and all
succumbed within five days. This study shows that the lethal dose
varies with size of the larvae. Since the growth of the larvae
is greatly inhibited in TBTF solutions, this work reinforces the
previous postulate that trialkyltin compounds interfere with the
protein synthesis of the target vectors.[11] Total tin concentration
remained constant during the study.

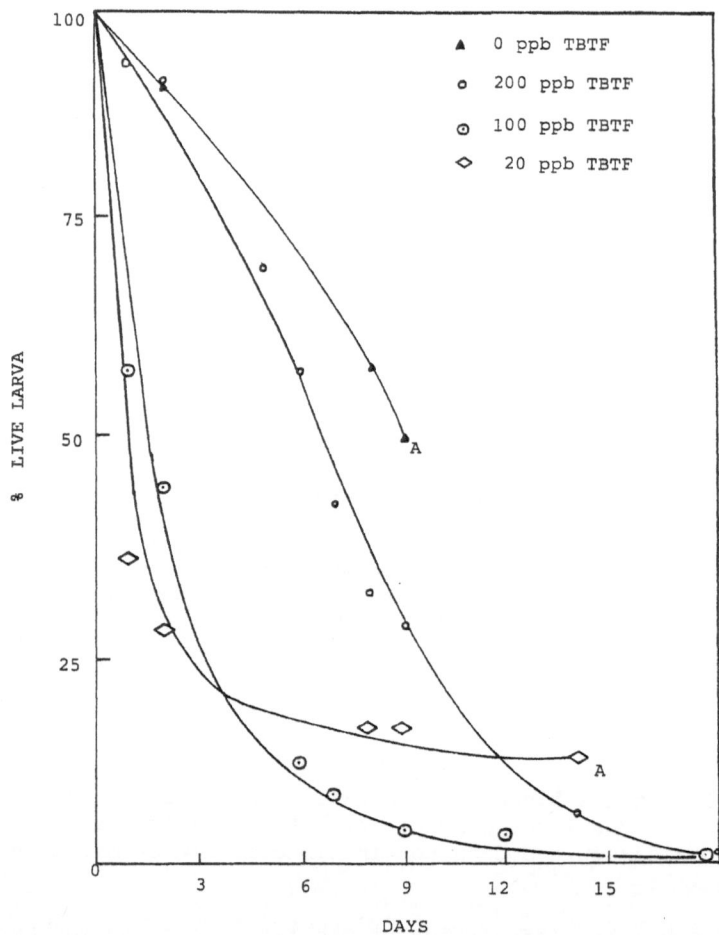

Figure 2.   Bioassay of Aedes Aegypti in TBTF
            A = all remaining larva become adults.

ECOPRO 1320 Leach Rate

     The results of the leaching study are shown in Figure 3. The
hexane-soluble materials, expressed as % TBTF on the ordinate,
rapidly decreased to a fairly constant level (approximately 2% of
the pellet) and remained at this level for about 130 days before
it increased to the 15% level. However, the total tin level decreased slowly to about 16.5% over the entire study. This laboratory study is consistent with the field testing of ECOPRO 1320

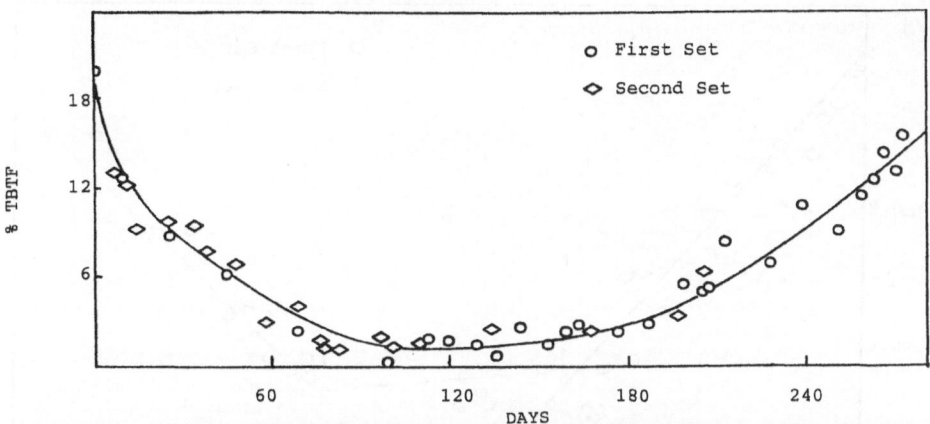

Figure 3.   Leach rate of ECOPRO 1320 hexane-soluble tin as TBTF.

pellets in Somaliland. (See Table I.) In the field test, total
tin was significantly higher than the hexane-soluble tins.

Mazaev et al.[6] reported that TBTO degradation is first order
and their work was verified by this author. Assuming the same type
of kinetics for TBTF, a first-order plot is presented in Figure 4.

Three straight lines can be drawn through the data points.
The first line is the hydrolysis of TBTF to TB(OH) which is insoluble
in hexane and less soluble in water than either TBTF or TBTO. The
second line is due to the loss of TBTO from the ECOPRO 1320 pellets
and approaches the same slope as that observed for the total tin
content. The third line corresponds to the steady-state dehydration
of TBT(OH) to TBTO. The kinetics can be expressed by equations 1-3.

$$TBTF + H_2O \rightarrow TBT(OH) + HF \tag{1}$$

$$2\ TBT(OH) \rightarrow TBTO + H_2O \tag{2}$$

$$TBTO + H_2O \rightarrow 2\ DBTO + 2\ C_4H_{10} \tag{3}$$

TABLE I.   ANALYSIS OF ECOPRO 1320 PELLETS FIELD
TESTED IN SOMALILAND

	Hexane Soluble Tin		Total Tin	
	Sn	TBTF	Sn	TBTF
22 month exposure	0.75%	3.14%	3.14%	8.16%
14 month exposure	3.75%	9.76%	5.30%	13.79%

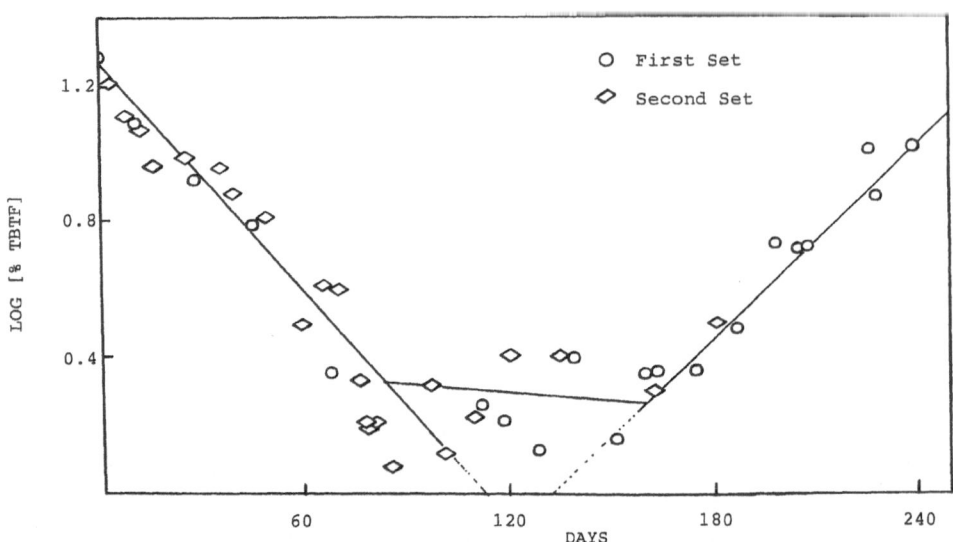

Figure 4. First-order degradation of TBTF in ECOPRO 1320.

The DBTO is hexane soluble but is probably formed in the solution after the TBTO has diffused from the pellet. The calculated half lives for the three compounds, based on these assumptions, are presented in Table II.

The half lives for TBTO and TBT(OH) were calculated assuming a static system, which is not true especially in a real environment. The chemical reactions are probably second order and dependent upon the diffusion rate of water and HF; but since the latter compounds cannot be determined in the ECOPRO 1320 pellet, the values presented in Table II are only good approximations.

TABLE II.   ECOPRO 1320 LEACH STUDY[a]

Compound	$t_{\frac{1}{2}}$	k	Ø Concentration
TBTF	26.6 days	-2.60×10^{-2}/day	194 days
TBTO	262 days	-2.65×10^{-3}/day	1250 days
TBT(OH)	30.1 days	-2.30×10^{-2}/day	N.A.

[a] Half life, first-order rate constant and time required for total leaching (99.9%) of TBTF, TBTO and TBT(OH).

The zero (Ø) concentration data correspond to the time required for 99.9% of each chemical to degrade to the next daughter compound.

The chemical kinetic study of the ECOPRO 1320 formulation shows that TBTF is rapidly hydrolyzed to TBT(OH) which dehydrates more rapidly to TBTO. It is apparent that most of the TBTF is converted to TBTO inside of the pellet and very little TBTF diffuses into the environment. If this hypothesis is true, TBTO is the primary biocide, and its long half life in the formulation accounts for the 1000-day larvicidal properties exhibited by the ECOPRO 1320 pellets.[14]

ACKNOWLEDGEMENTS

The authors wish to acknowledge the financial support from Environmental Chemical Inc., Barrington, IL 60010 and The University of Akron Faculty Research Grant #645. They also wish to acknowledge technical support from Professor N. Cardarelli and the Environmental Management Laboratory at The University of Akron.

REFERENCES

1. C.J. Shiff, in: "Molluscicides in Schistosomiasis Control," T.C. Cheng, ed., Academic Press, New York (1974). pp. 241-248.
2. N.F. Cardarelli, Mosquito News 38:328 (1978).
3. N.F. Cardarelli, U.S. Patent #3767809, Oct. 3, 1973.
4. N.F. Cardarelli and H.F. Neff, U.S. Patent #3639583, Feb. 1, 1972.
5. L.R. Sherman and H. Hoang, Anal. Proc. (Royal Society for Chemistry), (1981).
6. V.T. Mazaev, O.V. Golovanov, A.D. Igumnov, and V.H. Tsay, Gig. I. Sanit.3:17 (1976).
7. N.F. Cardarelli and W.H. Evans, in: "Proceedings Controlled Release of Bioactive Materials Symp.," R.W. Baker, ed., New Orleans (1979).
8. N.F. Cardarelli, et al., "Laboratory and Field Evaluation of Controlled Release Molluscicides and Schistolarvicides," Annual Ref. (Unpubl.) Edna McConnel Clark Found., New York, 276-0091, July 1, 1977.
9. N.F. Cardarelli, "Controlled Release Molluscicides," Monogr., Pub. Univ. Akron, Akron (1977).
10. N.F. Cardarelli, "Controlled Release Pesticide Formulations," CRC Press, Cleveland (1976). p. 210.
11. A.J. Allen, B.M. Quitter, and C.M. Radick, in: "Proceedings Cont. Release of Bioactive Materials Symp.," R.W. Baker, ed., New Orleans (1979).

12. K. Schwarz, D.B. Milne, and E. Vinyard, <u>Biochem</u>. <u>Biophysic</u>.
     <u>Res</u>. <u>Commun</u>. 40:22 (1970).
13. L.R. Sherman and T.L. Carlson, <u>J</u>. <u>Anal</u> <u>Toxicology</u> 4:31 (1980).
14. N. Cardarelli and L. Boswell, Unpublished data, Environmental
     Management Lab., The University of Akron, Akron, OH 44325.

FERMENTATION <u>PER</u> <u>SE</u> AS A BIOLOGICAL SLOW DELIVERY
MECHANISM FOR RELEASING COFACTORS OF FRUIT FLY
ATTRACTANTS[a]

Irving Keiser

U.S. Department of Agriculture
Science and Education Administration
Tropical Fruit and Vegetable Research Laboratory
Honolulu, Hawaii 96804

Nobel Wakabayashi

U.S. Department of Agriculture
Science and Education Administration
Biologically Active Natural Products Laboratory
Agricultural Environmental Quality Institute
Beltsville, Maryland 20705

Hawaii is the only place where three of the world's most
serious agricultural pests, the oriental fruit fly (<u>Dacus</u> <u>dorsalis</u>
Hendel), the melon fly (<u>Dacus</u> <u>cucurbitae</u> Coquillett), and the Mediterranean fruit fly (<u>Ceratitis</u> <u>capitata</u> [Wiedemann]), occur together.
These insects are highly destructive pests of fruits and vegetables
and of many nuts and flowers. Collectively, they attack more than
200 different hosts in Hawaii. In addition, a constant hazard
exists that one or more of these destructive fruit flies may be
introduced into the continental United States, despite constant
and rigid quarantines, because of increased tourist travel and world
trade. The melon fly is thought to have been introduced into Hawaii
about 1895, probably from Japan. The Mediterranean fruit fly was
introduced about 1910, probably from Australia, and the oriental
fruit fly about 1944, probably from Saipan. The Mediterranean fruit

---

[a] Mention of a proprietary product in this paper does not constitute
an endorsement of this product by USDA.

fly and the oriental fruit fly are major pests of citrus fruits,
mangoes, guavas, peaches, apricots, coffee, English walnuts, bread-
fruit, bananas, papayas, cantaloupes, and many other hosts, while
the melon fly is the vegetable grower's worst pest, attacking
tomatoes and cucurbits. For many years we have had an ongoing
research program to develop new and better fruit fly lures that
could be used for detection, survey, and control of these insects.

Ether extracts of peppergrass, Lepidium virginicum L., family
Brassicaceae, were found to be attractive to female Mediterranean
fruit flies, and, to a lesser extent, oriental fruit flies, and
melon flies, when evaluated in an olfactometer stocked with laboratory-reared fruit flies.[1] Subsequently, linolenic acid was isolated
as a component of this ether extract.[2] Linolenic acid worked well
in the laboratory olfactometer bioassay, catching 17X as many female
Mediterranean fruit flies as the water-only traps. However, in
field trials on the island of Maui, Hawaii, in a predominantly
Mediterranean fruit fly-infested area, linolenic acid failed to
capture male or female Mediterranean fruit flies except in one test
when a few females were attracted. We have evaluated many compounds
as fruit fly attractants over the past several years and a pattern
seems clear: male attractants discovered in the laboratory are
often active in the field, but female attractants, no matter how
active in a laboratory bioassay, have never been satisfactory in
field bioassays. The one test mentioned above constitutes the only
instance in all of our studies where a known chemical entity ever
captured female flies from a wild population in the field. Is,
then, linolenic acid an attractant for fruit flies?

Until now, only actively fermenting protein materials were
successful in capturing female fruit flies in the field.[3,4] However, no active constituents have been ever isolated from any fermenting lures. We hypothesize that, for some reason not clear to
us at the present time, male fruit flies are attracted to single-
component lures and also to multi-component lures, and that female
fruit flies are not attracted to single-component lures but require
one or more cofactors. Some speculations on the nature of the
cofactor(s) are based on the observation that only actively fermenting lures are effective for attracting females.

This means that very volatile compounds (perhaps even carbon
dioxide) may be slowly released from the fermenting mixture and,
in conjunction with some other material(s) in the mixture that are
attractive to female fruit flies, serve as effective lures.

In the present study, we tested this hypothesis by using the
fermenting lure itself as the source of slow release of the unknown
cofactors of fruit fly attractants. This approach circumvented
the difficulties of obtaining a slow-release formulation of candidate materials, which might be gases at room temperature. It also

allowed us to test our hypothesis before isolating and identifying the putative material. Studies testing this supposition in the olfactometer with laboratory-reared flies were sufficiently encouraging to warrant field evaluation. In the actual field tests described below, linolenic acid enhanced the effectiveness of fermenting lure in attracting wild populations of all 3 species of fruit flies in Hawaii as measured by the number of flies caught in the traps.

Field studies were conducted at Waimanalo on the island of Oahu and at Kula on the island of Maui, Hawaii. The former site is at sea level with moderate to high populations of oriental fruit flies and melon flies depending on the fruiting season. The latter site is at ca. 2000-m elevation with large numbers of Mediterranean fruit flies developing in peach orchards. Linolenic acid was added at 0.1% to two proteinaceous lure formulations. These consisted of (w/v) proprietary product, 9%; borax, 5%; and water, 86%. The two proprietary products were Staley's Protein Insecticide Bait No. 7® (A.E. Staley Manufacturing Co., Chicago, IL, USA) and Protein Insecticide Lure--Low Salt (Mauri Flavours Pty., Homebush, New South Wales, Australia). According to the producers the Staley product consists of total solids, 49.0%; amino acids and amino salts--31.2%; sodium chloride, 14.8%; ammonium chlordie, 3.8%. The short analysis of the Mauri Flavours product as supplied by the manufacturer is total solids, 49.3%; salt, 0.03%; total N_2, 5.7%. The Staley product with and without linolenic acid, was tested at Waimanalo and Kula, while the Mauri Flavours material was studied at Waimanalo only. Each treatment was replicated three times at Waimanalo and the entire test repeated 21 times at weekly intervals. At Kula, each treatment was replicated five times and the entire test repeated nine times for Mediterranean fruit flies, and eight times for melon flies, again at weekly intervals. A total of 300 ml of formulation was placed in 800-ml plastic traps; the flies were removed after one week, traps cleaned, and refilled with freshly prepared lure.

The results of the Waimanalo studies are shown in Tables I and II. With Protein Insecticide Base No. 7 (Table I), 4.0 and 4.6X and 2.5 and 2.0X as many male and female melon flies and oriental fruit flies, respectively, were captured when linolenic acid was included in the fermenting lure at 0.1% as were captured in the traps with fermenting lure only. With Protein-Insecticide Lure-Low Salt (Table II), 1.7 and 1.8X, 2.0 and 2.2X, and 1.4 and 1.4X male and female Mediterranean fruit flies, melon flies, and oriental fruit flies, respectively, were captured upon addition of linolenic acid to the fermenting lure at the above concentration as were captured in the traps with fermenting lure only. The results of the Kula studies are shown in Table III. When linolenic acid was included at 0.1%, 1.3 and 1.5X, and 5.3 and 4.9X male and female Mediterranean fruit flies and melon flies, respectively, were trapped as compared with fermenting lure only.

TABLE I. ATTRACTION OF PROTEIN INSECTICIDE BASE NO. 7® FERMENTING LURE ALONE AND WITH THE
ADDITION OF 0.1% LINOLENIC ACID (LA) TO FRUIT FLIES. WAIMANALO, OAHU, HAWAII

Number of Adults Caught in Traps with Indicated Formulation

| | Mediterranean Fruit Flies | | | | Melon Flies | | | | Oriental Fruit Flies | | | |
| | ♂♂ | | ♀♀ | | ♂♂ | | ♀♀ | | ♂♂ | | ♀♀ | |
Trial	Lure Only	Lure + LA	Lure Only	Lure + LA	Lure Only	Lure + LA	Lure Only	Lure + LA	Lure Only	Lure + LA	Lure Only	Lure + LA
1	1	0	2	6	3	5	0	5	17	25	288	289
2	1	1	1	8	0	1	0	1	2	27	140	247
3	0	0	6	2	1	8	0	3	12	17	134	291
4	0	0	0	0	0	1	0	0	10	29	54	156
5	0	0	1	1	0	0	0	0	28	16	104	106
6	1	1	2	1	0	0	0	0	13	52	72	111
7	0	1	0	0	2	8	0	9	30	34	90	134
8	1	1	3	5	18	12	1	4	17	18	68	89
9	0	0	0	0	0	5	0	0	4	7	17	43
10	0	0	0	7	3	13	1	7	0	15	18	122
11	0	0	7	0	20	31	14	19	7	18	94	131
12	0	1	1	2	0	32	0	10	1	10	25	81
13	0	2	2	8	0	51	1	13	4	29	22	165
14	11	2	14	9	19	23	8	17	35	40	206	30
15	1	0	3	7	4	33	0	8	3	75	60	340
16	0	0	0	2	0	6	1	4	11	27	96	253
17	0	1	0	4	1	24	1	15	10	63	71	461
18	0	0	4	5	4	4	2	3	18	7	95	48
19	2	0	0	9	0	24	0	4	8	43	49	249
20	0	1	3	2	11	17	3	8	29	55	132	338
21	0	0	2	6	5	70	3	32	14	62	80	171
Total	18	11	51	84	91	368	35	162	273	669	1915	3855

TABLE II. ATTRACTION OF PROTEIN INSECTICIDE LURE-LOW SALT FERMENTING LURE ALONE AND WITH THE ADDITION OF 0.1% LINOLENIC ACID (LA) TO FRUIT FLIES. WAIMANALO, OAHU, HAWAII

Number of Adults Caught in Traps with Indicated Formulation

| | Mediterranean Fruit Flies | | | | Melon Flies | | | | Oriental Fruit Flies | | | |
| | ♂♂ | | ♀♀ | | ♂♂ | | ♀♀ | | ♂♂ | | ♀♀ | |
Trial	Lure Only	Lure + LA	Lure Only	Lure + LA	Lure Only	Lure + LA	Lure Only	Lure + LA	Lure Only	Lure + LA	Lure Only	Lure + LA
1	1	0	2	6	0	16	1	0	32	26	474	406
2	0	0	3	0	3	4	4	3	16	2	404	404
3	0	0	0	5	2	2	0	0	15	23	276	370
4	0	0	1	0	2	0	0	0	26	26	181	280
5	0	0	2	0	0	0	0	1	11	10	56	173
6	1	0	0	0	0	4	6	0	16	9	87	87
7	0	1	2	0	2	7	1	0	14	25	73	106
8	0	0	3	2	6	13	4	3	7	13	57	82
9	0	1	3	6	8	4	3	7	5	14	82	185
10	1	0	2	2	8	24	7	0	7	5	88	95
11	0	3	1	4	14	76	23	24	7	6	90	120
12	1	1	7	12	16	34	11	50	14	19	93	141
13	2	1	4	8	30	7	3	16	36	32	130	190
14	0	0	5	1	9	9	0	8	21	28	138	248
15	1	2	1	6	7	11	1	3	36	38	157	340
16	2	3	9	9	1	6	2	2	36	84	274	625
17	3	5	0	7	5	7	4	8	43	83	309	429
18	1	2	4	4	4	23	6	3	35	30	217	239
19	0	1	1	7	5	11	7	5	27	47	225	248
20	0	1	2	5	11	14	4	3	60	43	237	177
21	0	1	2	12	6			57	47	148	194	385
Total	13	22	54	96	139	272	87	193	511	711	3842	5330

TABLE III. ATTRACTION OF PROTEIN INSECTICIDE BASE NO. 7® FERMENTING LURE ALONE AND WITH THE ADDITION OF 0.1% LINOLENIC ACID (LA) TO FRUIT FLIES. KULA, MAUI, HAWAII

Number of Adults Caught in Traps with Indicated Formulation

| | Mediterranean Fruit Flies | | | | Melon Flies | | | |
| | ♂♂ | | ♀♀ | | ♂♂ | | ♀♀ | |
Trial	Lure Only	Lure + LA	Lure Only	Lure + LA	Lure Only	Lure + LA	Lure Only	Lure + LA
1	6	43	82	164	4	23	1	30
2	21	31	58	133	0	39	5	21
3	39	26	128	182	0	8	2	11
4	36	35	135	155	9	22	5	15
5	1	0	6	23	1	3	0	0
6	9	8	2	21	0	4	0	3
7	6	17	22	52	1	14	2	21
8	19	10	141	158	16	50	15	47
9	14	20	52	71	--	--	--	--
Total	151	190	626	959	31	163	30	148

We feel that this is sufficient demonstration for the existence of one or more cofactors in the slow-release fermenting lure, and work is now underway on the identification of the cofactor(s).

REFERENCES

1.   I. Keiser, E.J. Harris, D.H. Miynshite, M. Jacobson, and R.E. Perdue, Lloydia 38:141 (1975).
2.   N. Wakabayashi, M. Jacobson, I. Keiser, D.H. Miynshite, and E.J. Harris, 177th National Meeting of the Am. Chem. Soc., Honolulu, Hawaii, April 1979.
3.   P.L. Gow, J. Econ. Entomol. 47:153 (1954).
4.   F. Lopez-D, L.F. Steiner, and F.R. Holbrook, J. Econ. Entomol. 64:1541 (1971).

IMPLANTABLE SYSTEMS FOR DELIVERY OF INSECT GROWTH

REGULATORS TO LIVESTOCK.II[a]

H. Jaffe, P.A. Giang, and D.K. Hayes

Livestock Insects Laboratory
Agricultural Research
Science and Education Administration, USDA
Beltsville, Maryland 20705

J.A. Miller

US Livestock Insects Laboratory
Agricultural Research
Science and Education Administration, USDA
Kerrville, Texas 78028

B.H. Stroud

Animal Operations Unit
Agricultural Research
Science and Education Administration, USDA
Beltsville, Maryland 20705

INTRODUCTION

During the past several years, our laboratories have been investigating the application of controlled-release technology to
the control of arthropod pests of livestock.[1] As a result we have

---

[a] This paper reports the results of research only. Mention of a
pesticide in this paper does not constitute a recommendation for
use by the USDA nor does it imply registration under FIFRA as
amended. Also, mention of a commercial or proprietary product
in this paper does not constitute an endorsement by USDA.

developed methods whereby an active ingredient can be delivered
at a controlled rate into the circulatory system of a host animal
via implanted pellets or microcapsules to affect feeding parasitic
insects or ticks. Our initial experiments involved the preparation
and bioevaluation of injectable microcapsules of the systemic
pesticide famphur (O-[p-(dimethylsulfamoyl)phenyl]O,O-dimethyl
phosphorothioate) in biodegradable polymers.[2] Subcutaneous injections of a suspension of these microcapsules into guinea pigs killed
feeding ticks over an extended period by continuously releasing
active ingredient into the host's circulatory system. However,
large injections were required because of the relatively low activity
of famphur and the volume of sesame oil used to suspend the microcapsules. Thus, this treatment was impractical for cattle. We
therefore sought to avoid these problems by developing controlled-
release implants of systemic insect growth regulators (IGR's).

    The IGR's are analogues of naturally occurring insect hormones
and are active at very low levels. They are usually specific to
a target insect parasite pest with essentially no activity or toxicity to the host or other non-target organisms.

    Our target insect pest, the common cattle grub, the larval
stage of Hypoderma lineatum (de Villers), is among the most destructive pests that attack cattle.[3] The grubs are commonly found in
cysts on the backs of cattle. Both larvae and adults are destructive. The grubs cause irritations, allow secondary bacterial infec-
tions, and create holes in the hides. Losses at slaughter include
damaged hides and reduced value of the carcasses due to trimming
of the grub-infested area. The adults, in attempting to lay their
eggs on the hairs of the cattle, cause the animals to run wildly
(gadding). As a result, cattle do not graze properly, are difficult
to handle, and occasionally injure themselves. Total losses in
the U.S. due to grubs were estimated to be about $300 million an-
nually.[4]

    Two IGR's have been utilized in our experiments, methoprene
and AI3-36206. Methoprene (isopropyl (E,E)-11-methoxy-3,7,11-trim-
ethyl-2,4-dodecadienoate) is a non-persistent insect growth regulator of minimal mammalian toxicity. The compound has been shown
to have systemic activity[5] and to be effective at very low levels
against the horn fly, Haemotobia irritans (L.), and the common
cattle grub[6] in drinking water[7-9] or in boluses permitting controlled
release. AI3-36206 (1-(8-methoxy-4,8-dimethylnonyl)-4-(1-methyl-
ethyl)benzene) is an experimental systemic[10] IGR developed at our
institute.[11] In all instances these IGR's act on the larval stage
of insects to prevent development of the adult. Thus the effect
of an IGR on cattle grubs is to limit future infestations by reduction of the adult population. Damage done by the present generation
of grubs is not prevented.

Our most promising results to date have been with methoprene formulated as implantable controlled-release pellets against cattle grubs.[12] The treatment was successful in preventing the development of adult cattle grubs, but we encountered difficulty because of the inherent liability of methoprene and its apparent incompatibility with the polymers used in formulating the pellets.

In this paper we report the subsequent preparation of (1) implantable CR pellets made of Vicryl,® a rapidly biodegradable suture material, and (2) reservoir devices made of poly(ε-caprolactone), a slowly biodegradable material. Both types of devices provided control of cattle grubs.

MATERIALS AND METHODS

Materials

The methoprene used was Altosid® technical material (91.9% AI) obtained from Zoecon Corp., Palo Alto, CA. The IGR AI3-36206 was kindly provided by Dr. M. Schwarz, Organic Chemical Synthesis Lab, AR, SEA, USDA, Beltsville, MD. Vicryl sutures (000, undyed), manufactured by Ethicon, Inc., Sommerville, N.J., were purchased locally. Poly(ε-caprolactone) tubing for reservoir devices was kindly provided by Dr. C. Pitt and Dr. A. Schindler of Research Triangle Institute, Research Triangle Park, NC 27709. Hexafluoro-isopropanol was purchased from Eastman Organic Chemicals.

Preparation of Pellets

A mixture of 12 Vicryl 000 undyed sutures (0.58 g) and methoprene (0.50 g) was completely dissolved in a minimum amount of hexafluoroisopropanol. Complete removal of the solvent on the rotary evaporator was followed by evacuation at high vacuum to form 1.17 g of a papery film. Pieces of film weighing 0.11 g were placed into the center of 10- to 15-cm lengths of 3-mm id Teflon® tubing. The center of the tubing was immersed in a water bath at 75-80° for 10 seconds to soften the film, which was then compressed by application of pressure applied by glass rods (3-mm dia) inserted into both ends of the tubing to form the pellets. The softening and compression cycle was repeated to ensure good pellet formulation. The resulting pellets (3 x 17 mm) were stored in the tubing from which they could easily be removed before use. Pellets of AI3-36206 in Vicryl were prepared similarly.

Preparation of Reservoir Devices

The poly(ε-caprolactone) reservoir devices were prepared by
the method of Pitt and Schindler.[13]   Lengths of tubing (4 cm) were
sealed at one end by pinching with warm (65-75°) Teflon-coated
forceps. The tubes were filled with IGR by use of a gas-chroma-
tography syringe to within several mm of the end. Care was exercised
so as not to wet the open end of the tube with compound. The open
end was sealed as before.

In Vitro Release Rate

The release of the IGR's from their pellets and reservoir
devices into pH 7.40 buffer at 37°C was measured in vitro by use
of a flow system previously described.[1]

In Vivo Release Rate

The release of methoprene from the reservoir devices was
measured in vivo by implanting the devices (2 x 0.3 cm) into the
ears of cattle with the Synovex Implanter®. The reservoir devices
were surgically removed periodically, washed free of tissue, air
dried, and analyzed for percent AI.

Efficacy Experiments

Experiments were designed and run to evaluate the practicality
and efficacy of our implant system against cattle grubs. Untreated
controls were also run. In the first series of experiments, four
Hereford calves (ca. 200 kg) infested with Hypoderma lineatum were
treated by implanting Vicryl pellets with the Synovex Implanter
when the grubs were visible in the back. The first animal received
three methoprene implants in each ear via two injections, a total
of six implants. The second animal received three methoprene pellets
in the right ear in one injection. The third and fourth animals
were similarly treated with Vicryl pellets of AI3-36206. In a
second series of experiments, one animal received three methoprene
reservoir devices in each ear in six injections, a total of six
devices. The second animal received two reservoir devices in the
right ear in two injections.

In both series, collection of Hypoderma lineatum was begun
at two weeks posttreatment. Larvae were collected as they emerged
from the back of the animal, allowed to pupate, and the subsequence
emergence of the adult flies was recorded. Abbott's formula was
used to calculate percent inhibition of emergence of flies from

pupae from treated animals as compared with emergence from untreated controls.

The ears of the animals treated with vicryl pellets were examined at 55 days posttreatment, at which time all grubs had emerged from the backs of the animals. Two reservoir devices were surgically removed from one animal at 139 days posttreatment and analyzed for percent methoprene remaining in the devices.

Analysis of Methoprene and AI3-36206

Pellets and reservoir devices were analyzed for percent AI by gas-chromatographic methods preceded by a chromatographic column clean-up.

RESULTS AND DISCUSSION

The types of pellets and reservoir devices are listed in Table I. In contrast to previous results, the methoprene was stable in the formulations during the time frame of the experiments.

Efficacy data are shown in Table II. As can be seen, the methoprene pellets were effective against cattle grubs. Of particular interest is the achievement of 100% control with three pellets administered by one injection. Moreover, external examination of the implant sites at 55 days posttreatment when the pellets had been almost completely absorbed showed minimum adverse tissue reaction.

TABLE I.   PELLETS AND RESERVOIR DEVICES

Type[a]	AI	Polymer	Nominal % AI[b]	Actual % AI
P	Methoprene	Vicryl	50	44.6
P	AI3-36206	Vicryl	50	34.6
R	Methoprene	poly(ϵ-caprolactone)	53.7[c]	53.7[c]

[a] P-pellet; R=reservoir device.

[b] Percent AI used to prepare formulation.

[c] Percent AI by wt. difference.

TABLE II.   CONTROLLED-RELEASE PELLETS AND RESERVOIR DEVICES
CONTAINING INSECT GROWTH REGULATORS AGAINST CATTLE GRUBS

Animal No.	Device (No. Implanted)	AI	No. Pupae Collected	% Adults Emerged	% Control
988	Vicryl pellet (6)	Methoprene	19	0.0	100
944	Vicryl pellet (3)	Methoprene	30	0.0	100
982	Vicryl pellet (6)	AI3-36206	9	67	7
961	Vicryl pellet (3)	AI3-36206	13	92	0
23	Reservoir (6)	Methoprene	45	0.0	100
27	Reservoir (2)	Methoprene	35	8.6	88
Controls[a]	No treatment	–	200	72	–

[a] Data for controls represent sum of 5 animals.

In vitro release rate studies indicate that the pellets underwent fragmentation at about one month. In vitro release rates,
however, were not reproducible, probably because of the concurrent
operation of two release rate mechanisms, diffusion and biodegradation. An additional complicating factor was the decomposition of
released methoprene in aqueous solution prior to analysis.

Reservoir devices containing methoprene were also effective
against cattle grubs. Reservoir devices with AI3-36206, however,
were not effective, possibly because the lower activity of this
active ingredient against this particular pest species or because
of its lower solubility in water. External examination of the
implant site at 139 days posttreatment indicated minimum adverse
tissue reaction. Analysis of recovered reservoir devices at 139
days posttreatment indicated that release of 43% of active ingredient had occurred.

Studies of the in vitro release rate of the methoprene reservoir devices indicated very slow release, probably because of decomposition of the methoprene in the aqueous system prior to
analysis.

In vivo release rate data are shown in Table III. The high
release during the first 20 days reflects an initial burst effect
on the type previously reported for these systems.[14,15] A release
rate of 44 μg/day/cm was observed during 20-50 days after correction
for the initial burst effect. On the basis of the measured rate
of release and our efficacy data, we conclude that the amount of
methoprene released by six 4-cm devices, or about 1 mg/day, is
required to insure 100% control of cattle grubs in a 200-kg animal.

TABLE III. IN VIVO RELEASE OF METHOPRENE FROM
            PCL RESERVOIR DEVICES

Starting AI (%)	Time (Days)	AI Released (%)	Release Rate (μg/day/cm)
53.2	20	25.6	284[a]
53.6	50	31.4	44[b]

[a] Rate during first 20 days includes burst effect.

[b] Rate during 20–50 days corrected for burst effect.

We believe that these experiments demonstrate the feasibility of using both types of systems for the control of arthropod pests of livestock throughout an entire season with one treatment. The Vicryl implants appear to meet our requirements for a short-term (1–2 months) biodegradable system; the poly(ε-caprolactone) reservoir devices are promising for use as a long-term (1 year) controlled-release system.

ACKNOWLEDGEMENTS

The authors are grateful to Dr. M. Schwarz, Organic Chemical Synthesis Lab, AR, SEA, USDA, for providing us with samples of purified AI3-36206.

The authors are also grateful to Drs. Pitt and Schindler of Research Triangle Institute for providing us with PCL tubing.

REFERENCES

1. Part I: H. Jaffe, J.A. Miller, P.A. Giang, D.K. Hayes, R.W. Miller, and C.M. Livingston, in: "Proceedings Symposium on Controlled Release of Bioactive Mat.," R.W. Baker, ed., New Orleans (1979). I.39.

2. H. Jaffe, D.K. Hayes, P. Giang, R.O. Drummond, and T.M. Whetstone, in: "Proceedings Controlled Release Pesticide Symposium," R. Goulding, ed., Corvallis 272 (1977).

3. R.E. Pfadt and T.R. Robb, Control Livestock Pests, Bull, 327R, Agricultural Experiment Station, Univ. of Wyoming, Laramie 16–20 (1966).

4. J.A. Miller, M.L. Beadles, and W.L. Gladney, in: "Proceedings Controlled Release Pesticide Symposium," R. Goulding, ed., Corvallis 253 (1977).

5. R.L. Harris, E.D. Frazar, and R.L. Younger, J. Econ. Entomol. 66:1099 (1973).

6. R.L. Harris, W.F. Chamberlain, and E.D. Frazar, J. Econ. Entomol 67:384 (1974).

7. M.L. Beadles, J.A. Miller, W.F. Chamberlain, J.L. Eschles, and R.L. Harris, J. Econ. Entomol. 68:781 (1975).

8. J.A. Miller, W.F. Chamberlain, M.L. Beadles, M.O. Pickens, and A.R. Gingrich, J. Econ. Entomol. 69:330 (1976).

9. J.L. Eschle, J.A. Miller, and C.D. Schmidt, Nature 265:325 (1977).

10. J.A. Miller, unpublished results.

11. M. Schwarz, R.W. Miller, J.E. Wright, W.F. Chamberlain, and D.E. Hopkins, J. Econ. Entomol. 67:598 (1974).

12. H. Jaffe, P.A. Giang, and J.A. Miller, in: "Proceedings Symposium on Controlled Release of Bioactive Mat.," E. Brinkman and J. Montemarano, eds., Gaithersburg, 5.5 (1978).

13. C. Pitt, Private Communication.

14. C.G. Pitt, D. Christensen, A.R. Jeffcoat, G.L. Kimmel, A. Schindler, M.E. Wall, and R.A. Zweidinger, in: "Proceedings Drug Delivery Systems," H.S. Gabelnick, ed., DHEW Publication No. (NIH) 77-1238, 141-192 (1976).

15. C.G. Pitt and A. Schindler, in: "Proceedings Symposium on Controlled Release of Bioactive Mat.," R.W. Baker, ed., New Orleans I-17 (1979).

SUSTAINED-RELEASE SYSTEMS FOR LIVESTOCK PEST CONTROL[a]

J.A. Miller, S.E. Kunz, and D.D. Oehler

U.S. Livestock Insects Laboratory
Agricultural Research
Science and Education Administration, USDA
Kerrville, Texas

INTRODUCTION

Insects, ticks, and mites cost the livestock industry an estimated $3 billion annually.[1] Two-thirds of this loss is suffered
by the beef cattle industry. Despite continued interest in alter-
nate methods of control, insecticide treatments are currently the
most widely used and most effective means of control of these pests.
It appears that pesticides will continue to be a vital part of the
producers' defense despite the inherent problems of chemical control.
Although pesticides may not be the sole control method, they are
likely to be a major tool in pest-management systems.

Progress in livestock-pest control has resulted largely from
research and development of more effective and safer compounds.
In contrast, only minimal progress has been made in the development
of methods of application and formulations of these compounds for
optimal effectiveness. Livestock are still sprayed with, dipped
in, or dusted with oils, emulsions, or powders much as they have
been for the past 25-50 years.

A part of the inefficiency in livestock-pest control is the
necessity for repeated applications of pesticides as often as every

---

[a] This paper reports the results of research only. Mention of a
pesticide in this paper does not constitute a recommendation for
use by the USDA nor does it imply registration under FIFRA as
amended. Also, mention of a commercial or proprietary product
in this paper does not constitute an endorsement by the USDA.

10-14 days. The costs in labor and pesticide and the debilitation
of cattle due to frequent applications reduce the advantage of
control and, therefore, in practice, treatments are often neglected
and the pest damage absorbed by the producer. Researchers have
long sought to prolong the effectiveness of applied pesticides.[2]
Ideally, it would be desirable to deliver the toxicant to the target
pest at a level slightly above the lethal dosage and for a prescribed
period. Advances in controlled-release technology continue to approach this ideal and thereby provide the potential for solving
many of the problems associated with chemical control.

For several years, the U.S. Livestock Insects Laboratory, Kerrville, Texas, has been investigating the potential of applying controlled-release technology to the unique problems of livestock-pest
control.[3-5] The present paper reports the continuation of this
work with the objective of developing easy-to-use, inexpensive
sustained-release systems for delivery of pest control agents to
livestock. Approaches being studied include both external and
internal applications.

EXTERNAL ATTACHMENTS

Several types of external devices for the sustained release
of pesticides are being studied at our laboratory. Thus far, ear
tags and leg bands have shown greatest promise. Both of these
devices are familiar to cattlemen and are used for identification
purposes. Therefore, they are likely to be more readily acceptable
than other control devices.

The initial research on the sustained release of pesticides
from ear tags developed from a need to control the Gulf Coast tick,
Amblyomma maculatum Koch, on cattle in south Texas.[6] These ticks
tend to congregate and feed in the ears of cattle, causing considerable damage. Infestations also make the ear more susceptible to
attack by screwworm, Cochliomyia hominivoras (Coquerel). This combination of damage from the tick and screwworm results in a condition known as "gouch ear" in which part or all of the ear may be
lost.

With the development of an ear tag that released pesticide
from a plastic matrix, ear ticks and associated screwworm infestations were controlled for seven to ten weeks, essentially the complete season.[6] In the process of this research, the ear tags were
observed to provide control of adult horn flies, Haematobia irritans
(L.), on cattle.[7,8] At present, the application of insecticide-
impregnated ear tags to the more widespread problem of horn fly
control has overshadowed the original purpose of the tag.

The 14% Rabon (2-chloro-1-(2,4,5-trichlorophenyl)vinyl dimethyl phosphate) tag originally marketed in Texas provided control of the horn fly for only eight to ten weeks and therefore required treatment of animals at least twice per season. These tags are presently marketed nationwide for control of horn flies, face flies (Musca autumalis De Geer), Gulf Coast ticks, and "spinose" ear ticks (Otobius megnini (Duges)).

The new pyrethroids are being incorporated into ear tags with promising results. Results of studies at our laboratory indicate that cattle can be protected from horn flies for up to 21 weeks with ear tags containing fenvalerate (cyano(3-phenoxyphenyl)methyl 4-chloro-α-(1-methylethyl)benzeneacetate.[9] We presently have a large-scale study in progress in New Mexico in which ca. 600 cattle on the 190,000-acre Jornada Range are being treated with tags containing fenvalerate. Early results indicate excellent horn fly control into the 16th week.

The use of insecticide-impregnated leg bands was developed at our laboratory as an alternative to the ear-tag system. These devices are attached to the hind legs of cattle just above the dew-claw. Leg bands have the advantages of being able to carry greater loads of insecticide and not requiring puncturing of the animal skin for attachment. However, they are slightly more difficult to attach than ear tags. Leg bands containing various pesticides have been shown to be equal in effectiveness to ear tags when used against the horn fly.[10]

Leg bands containing dichlorvos (2,2-dichlorvinyl dimethyl phosphate) can also protect cattle against the common cattle grub, Hypoderma lineatum (Villers).[11] It was originally speculated that the bands killed ovipositing adults, eggs, or newly hatched larvae before they penetrated the skin. However, a more recent study demonstrates that the mode of action is systemic.

In the spring of 1979, 25 Hereford yearlings were divided into five groups of five animals each. Group A was treated with ear tags containing five grams dichlorvos (DDVP). Both hind legs of each animal in Group B were treated with a leg band containing ca. five grams DDVP. Group C was treated with leg bands identical to those in Group B except for the addition of crufomate (4-tert-butyl-2-chlorophenyl methyl methylphosphoramidate) pouron at the rate of 0.3 ml/kg body weight. Group D received only the crufomate pouron at the same dosage as Group C. Finally, Group E was an untreated control group. All groups, including the untreated controls, were maintained in the same pasture to provide equal infestation pressure. The backs of the cattle were examined monthly for grubs from September 1979 through March 1980.

Results of these tests indicated that the dichlorvos ear tags
were as effective as leg bands in preventing grubs in the backs
of treated cattle (Table I). The crufomate pouron eliminates all
larave in cattle at time of treatment without preventing new infestations posttreatment. Therefore, since Group D was not infested
with grubs, we assume that there was no infestation by heel flies
posttreatment. If so, then the effect of the ear tags and leg bands
on Group A and B must have been completely systemic since all grubs
in the cattle were present prior to treatment. These results demonstrate that a sustained-release external attachment can be used
to deliver a systemically active pesticide to cattle.

The reindeer bot fly, Oedemagena tarandi L., in Alaska presents
a problem similar to that of the cattle grub in the lower United
States. Therefore, we have initiated a cooperative study with the
University of Alaska whereby the effectiveness of both sustained-
release ear tags and leg bands is being evaluated on reindeer herds.

A sustained-release formulation that could be sprayed onto
cattle would have advantages over both the ear-tag and leg-band
systems. Such a formulation might be easier to apply and perhaps
less expensive. With the objective of developing a sustained-release spray-on formulation, we incorporated permethrin (3-phenoxy-
phenyl)methyl 3-(2,2-dichloroethyenyl)-2,2-dimethylcyclopropanecar-
boxylate) in a solvent-based thermo-plastic-rubber blend. As the
volatile solvent evaporated, a thin, clear, elastic film containing
the pesticide remained. A 1% permethrin spray produced an 8% permethrin film.

TABLE I.   CONTROL OF GRUBS IN CATTLE TREATED WITH DICHLORVOS-
            IMPREGNATED EAR TAGS AND LEG BANDS

| Animal No. | Numbers of grubs in backs of animals in indicated group | | | | |
	A: Ear tags	B: Leg bands	C: Leg bands + pouron	D: Pouron	E: Untreated controls
1	2	1	0	0	30
2	2	3	0	0	43
3	0	4	0	0	27
4	17	3	0	0	37
5	7	26	0	0	32
Mean	5.6	7.4	0	0	33.8
% control[a]	83.4	78.1	100	100	--

[a] Corrected for control mortality by Abbott's formula.

We treated 12 Angus cows by spraying ca. 50 ml of a 1% permethrin formulation in a band along the backline (ca. 50 cm wide)
from the shoulder to the hip. The spray did not penetrate the hair
coat but rather appeared to remain on the outer surface. The
animals were dry and the coating nearly invisible within two to
three minutes. The number of horn flies on the treated cows and
on an untreated control herd was recorded weekly.

Table II shows the number of horn flies on the treated cattle
for eight weeks posttreatment. The results indicate excellent
control of horn flies by the sustained-release formulation for six
weeks. In previous studies, cattle sprayed with 0.05% permethrin
emulsion at a rate of 2 liters/animal were protected for only three
weeks.   Thus, the polymeric formulation more than doubled the residual life of a treatment with only half as much active ingredient.
Other such formulations are under study.

INTERNAL DEVICES

In earlier symposia, we presented the results of our research
to develop sustained-release boluses for administering insect growth
regulators to cattle for control of the horn fly and face fly.[3-5]
Boluses containing methoprene (isopropyl (E,E)-11-methoxy-3,7,11-
trimethyl-2,4-dodecadienoate), an insect juvenile hormone mimic,
and diflubenzuron (N-[[(4-chlorophenyl)amino]carbonyl]-2,6-difluoro-
benzamide), a chitin inhibitor, were shown to be effective in preventing the development of horn flies and face flies in the manure
of treated cattle for 12-32 weeks.

TABLE II.   CONTROL OF HORN FLIES WITH A SPRAY-ON
POLYMERIC FORMULATION CONTAINING PERMETHRIN

Weeks posttreatment	No. of horn flies/cow on indicated herd		
	Treated	Control	% Control[a]
0 (pretreatment)	400	400	0
1	0	600	100
2	0	1,000	100
3	5	1,000	99.5
4	5	400	99.8
5	0	300	100
6	15	150	90
7	30	150	80
8	30	125	76

[a] Corrected for control group using Abbott's formula.

The boluses are formulated from a blend of waxes with barium sulfate added to increase the specific gravity to about two. In practice, the boluses are administered orally to cattle with a standard balling gun. Because of its specific gravity, the bolus lodges and remains in the reticulum of the cow. There it slowly erodes, releasing the insect growth regulator into the digestive tract and subsequently in the manure, where immature stages of the horn fly and face fly normally develop.

During the past year, we conducted additional studies in co-operation with Philips-Roxane, Inc., a company interested in commercial production of the diflubenzuron bolus. The boluses used in these studies were manufactured according to a formulation developed at our laboratory but were compressed at the Philips-Roxane facilities on a commercial bolus press into the conventional oblong form.

Twelve Angus steers weighing 270–340 kg each were divided into three groups of four steers each. The animals in Group A were orally dosed with 10% diflubenzuron boluses at the rate of two 50-g boluses/ steer. Those in Group B were treated with two 25-g boluses from the same lot. Group C was the untreated control group.

The cattle were maintained in a common paddock on a ration of hegari hay and alfalfa cubes. Water was provided ad libitum. To collect manure samples from individual animals, we separated them into small isolation pens for 24 h. Samples of manure were collected and bioassayed against horn flies and stable flies, Stomoxys calcitrans (L.).[4]

The results of these bioassays showed that the treatments were effective against the horn fly for over 14 weeks (Table III). As expected, greater survival was observed in the stable fly bioassays than in the horn fly bioassays. Treatment with two 25-g boluses appeared insufficient for stable fly inhibition; whereas treatment with two 50-g boluses appeared to provide near minimum lethal dosages. Although the treatments were still active at 14 weeks, the test was terminated according to protocol.

The principle of using a sustained-release bolus for delivery of larvicides to control immature stages of the horn fly and face fly has been adequately demonstrated and should be applicable to a variety of new compounds that are active at low levels (< 1 mg/kg body weight). Juvenile hormone mimics, chitin inhibitors, and avermectins, a new family of potent anthelmintics, fall into this classification.

The avermectins, produced by Merck Sharp and Dohme Research Laboratories, are being studied with great interest. Not only are

TABLE III. CONTROL OF HORN FLIES AND STABLE FLIES IN THE
MANURE OF CATTLE TREATED WITH 10% DIFLUBENZURON BOLUSES

| Weeks posttreatment | % Mortality[a] of horn flies and stable flies in manure | | | |
| | Group A 2x25 g boluses | | Group B 2x50 g boluses | |
	Horn fly	Stable fly	Horn fly	Stable fly
2	100	49	100	100
4	99	0	100	75
6	100	66	100	69
8	100	0	100	63
10	73	42	97	98
12	100	83	100	97
14	90	81	91	100

[a] Corrected for control mortality by Abbott's formula.

these compounds anthelmintic, but they have shown promise as systemic
acaricides against ticks[13] and scabies and mange mites,[14] and as
larvicides against the dung-breeding diptera.[15]

Our studies indicate that a daily oral dose of < 1 μg/kg body
wt of the avermectin MK-933 provides complete inhibition of horn
flies in the manure of treated cattle. We are currently refining
a bolus formulation to deliver this dosage. Additionally, we have
found that a daily subcutaneous injection of 5 μg/kg body wt delivers
enough of the avermectin to the digestive tract to inhibit horn
fly development in the manure. This transfer from the injection
site to the digestive tract is not surprising since the compound
was developed as an injectable anthelmintic. However, this mode
of action provides an opportunity for development of an implantable
sustained-release system for control of the horn fly. Additionally,
an implantable system that would deliver ca. 10 μg/kg body wt would
be effective systemically against ticks.[13]

SUMMARY AND DISCUSSION

A variety of controlled-release systems have been developed
in recent years. The theory describing the delivery of active ingredients has been valuable to the understanding of the operation
of these systems. With that theory must come research demonstrating
the application of these systems to real world problems. The work
presented here is an attempt to apply control-release technology
to the problem of livestock-insect control. Examples are presented
which demonstrate the potential of both externally and internally
applied devices. The choice of systems is made with consideration

of the life history and behavior of the target pest. External
devices such as ear tags and leg bands would appear to be the technique of choice for control of adult horn flies on cattle. However,
such devices have been shown to be capable of delivery of systemically
active compounds as in the use of dichlorvos against the cattle
grub. Ideally, the implant appears to be a better system than tags
for delivering a systemic pesticide. The bolus form, although
capable of delivering a systemic insecticide, would be more appropriate for delivering a larvicide.

Development of new chemicals will continue to be an important
part of future progress in pesticidal control of livestock pests.
However, the development of delivery systems for more efficient
and safer use of those chemicals we now have will be equally important
to that progress.

REFERENCES

1. Anon. U.S. Dep. Agric., Agric. Res. Serv. NRP No. 20480, 1976.
2. F.W. Knapp, in: "Proceedings Controlled Release Pesticide Symposium," R. Goulding, ed., Corvallis (1977). p. 237.
3. J.A. Miller, M.L. Beadles, and W.J. Gladney, in: "Proceeding
   Controlled Release Pesticide Symposium," R. Goulding, ed.,
   Corvallis (1977). p. 253.
4. J.A. Miller and R.W. Miller, in: "Proceedings Symposium on
   Controlled Release of Bioactive Materials," E. Brinckman and
   J. Montemarano, eds., Gaithersburg (1978). p. 5.52-.61.
5. J.A. Miller, F.W. Knapp, R.W. Miller, and C.W. Pitts, Southwest. Entomol. 4(3):195 (1979).
6. W.J. Gladney, J. Econ. Entomol. 69:757 (1976).
7. E.H. Ahrens, Southwest. Entomol. 2(1):8 (1977).
8. M.L. Beadles, J.A. Miller, B.K. Shelley, and D.P. Ingenhuett,
   Southwest. Entomol. 4(1):70 (1979).
9. C.D. Schmidt and S.E. Kunz, Southwest. Entomol. in press (1980).
10. M.L. Beadles, J.A. Miller, B.K. Shelley, and R.E. Reeves, J.
    Econ. Entomol. 71(2):287 (1978).
11. L.M. Hunt, M.L. Beadles, B.K. Shelley, B.N. Gilbert, and R.O.
    Drummond, J. Econ. Entomol. 73(1):32 (1980).
12. C.D. Schmidt, J.J. Matter, J.H. Meurer, R.E. Reeves, and B.K.
    Shelley, J. Econ. Entomol. 69(4):484 (1976).
13. R.O. Drummond, T.M. Whetstone, and J.A. Miller, in manuscript.
14. W.P. Meleney, AR-SEA, USDA, Kerrville, TX, personal communica-
    tion.
15. J.A. Miller, S.E. Kunz, D.D. Oehler, and R.W. Miller, in manu-
    script.

CONTROLLED-RELEASE FEED ADDITIVES FOR RUMINANTS: I.
CELLULOSE-BASED COATING COMPOSITIONS FOR RUMEN-STABLE
NUTRIENTS

Stephen H. Wu, Clarence C. Dannelly, and
Ronald J. Komarek

Research Laboratories
Tennessee Eastman Company
Division of Eastman Kodak Company
Kingsport, Tennessee 37662

Ruminant animals such as cattle, sheep, goats, and buffalo
make a very important contribution to man's welfare by producing
both food and fiber for man's use. In addition, the dietary needs
of these animals are not largely competitive with those of man.
Thus the beef and dairy industries represent a major segment of
the U.S. economy.[1] However, ruminant animals are relatively inefficient in utilizing their diet.

A ruminant animal has a stomach compartment, the rumen, that
provides extensive pregastric microbial fermentation of ingested
feeds, which accounts for the ruminant's ability to digest cellulose.[2] The rumen is the largest of the four stomach compartments
and serves as an important location of microbial modification of
all ingested feeds. Ingested feeds are retained in the rumen for
6 to 30 hr, and longer in some instances, before entering the gastric
compartment, the abomasum. When the rumen contents pass into the
abomasum and the intestines, the microbial mass is digested by
enzymes and provides nutrients for the animal. It is particularly
difficult for labile nutrients and pharmaceuticals to survive the
effects of the rumen environment during their passage to post ruminal
absorption sites. A need existed to develop a coating with chemical
and physical properties that would not be affected by the rumen
fermentation and environment and with properties that would permit
the effective coating of a discrete particle or core. The core
would be constructed by using binders and other agents, but with
the concentration of active ingredients as high as possible.

319

In preparing nutrients and pharmaceuticals intended for administration to ruminants, it is important to protect the active ingredients from rumen microbial degradation at a pH of about 5.5 and to
provide for the controlled release of the active ingredients in
the abomasum and small intestine where they can be absorbed. The
objective of our research was to develop an efficient, controlled-
release system to protect compounds or nutrients, particularly the
essential amino acid methionine, from degradation in the rumen and
then release the compounds or nutrients postruminally in the abomasal
fluid at a pH of 3.5 or below.

This paper describes (a) coating compositions based on cellulose propionate morpholinobutyrate[3] which withstand the rumen
microbial degradation and pH conditions of 5.5 for at least 24 hours,
but release the core material upon exposure to abomasal fluid with
a pH of 3.0 after an abomasal residence of about 1 hr; (b) a coating
process that uses an air-suspension coater to apply a coating formulation that will encapsulate the pellets with a coherent and completely enveloping film; (c) the biological performance of rumen-
protected methionine in in vitro and in vivo studies; and (d) potential applications of the rumen-protective coating system.

EXPERIMENTAL

Pellet Core Preparation

The methionine pellet core consisted of 88% feed-grade DL-meth-
ionine, 10% microcrystalline cellulose, 1% methylcellulose, and
1% gum arabic. These ingredients were mixed thoroughly in a Hobart
mixer-extruder (Model N-50). Water was added slowly to wet the
dry solid mix until an extrudable dope was formed. The moisture
content of the final dope was about 16%. The dope was extruded
from the mixer-extruder through a die containing 2-mm diameter holes
with a rotating knife chopping the extruded material into small
cylindrical pellets. Other pellets containing specific nutrients,
antibiotics, hormones, growth promoters, and pharmaceuticals as
active ingredients can be made similarly. For the lysine hydrochloride, $CaCO_3$ was added to partially neutralize the hydrochloric
acid.

Polymer Composition

Cellulose propionate 3-morpholinobutyrate (CPMB) was prepared
by the addition of morpholine to the unsaturated linkage of crotonic
acid esters of cellulose.[4] The molecular weight of CPMB was about
40,000. CPMB was soluble in a variety of organic solvents such

as acetone and methylene chloride and in dilute aqueous acids below pH 5.3, but it was insoluble in water. The structure of CPMB is shown in Figure 1.

Encapsulation of Nutrient Pellets

A versatile apparatus used for spray-coating discrete particles was used for the encapsulation of dry pellet cores discussed in the previous section.[5]

Figure 2 compares the gas flows and the important design features of this spray-coating apparatus with those of conventional fluidized-bed coaters such as a Wurster coater[6] and a coater reported by Larson.[7]

In a typical coating operation, air at 250 scfm and 7 psi was admitted to the chamber to cause the methionine pellets to circulate. A coating solution composed of 6% CPMB in acetone was then pumped through the spray nozzle at a rate of 500 g/min. At the same time, 5 scfm of air at 40 psi was supplied to the nozzle to atomize the coating solution. The apparatus was operated for about 30 minutes. The product was a pellet core coated with a continuous layer of the polymer.

Other coating additives such as pigments and fatty acids and their derivatives can be dissolved or dispersed in the polymer solution and sprayed onto the pellets to modify the characteristics of the coating. A variety of pellets containing amino acids, sugar, antibiotics, growth regulators, minerals, etc. can be encapsulated successfully in a similar fashion.

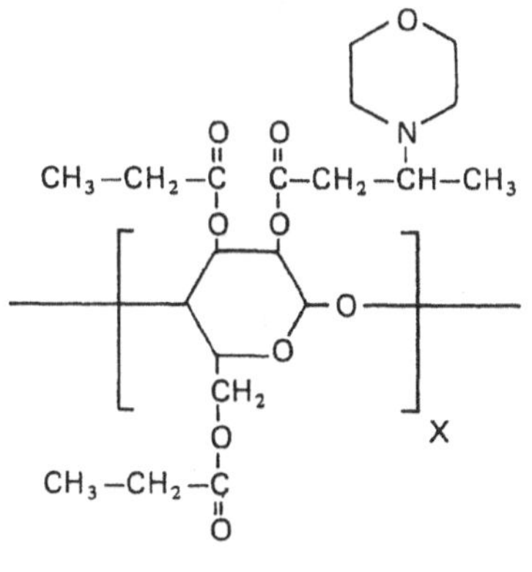

Figure 1. CPMB structure.

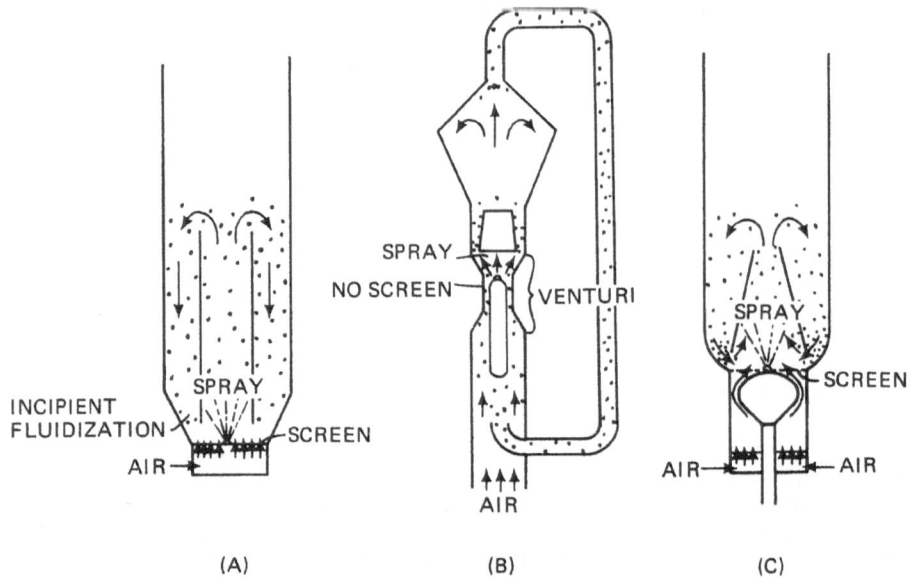

(A)   (B)   (C)

Figure 2.   Schematic diagram of air-suspension coater used at
            Eastman (C) and conventional coaters. (A) Wurster's
            coater, (B) Larson's coater (3M Co.).

Simulated Rumen Stability and Abomasal Release Tests for Coated
Pellets

     In the simulated in vitro rumen-stability test, one to two
grams of coated pellets was extracted with 50 mL of 0.1 $\underline{M}$, pH 5.4
acetate buffer for 24 hr in a shaking flask at a constant 37°C.
Similarly, in the simulated in vitro abomasal release test, a sample
of one to two grams of coated pellets was extracted with 50 mL of
0.1 $\underline{M}$, pH 3.0 glycine/NaCl/HCl buffer solution for 1 hr at 37°C.
After extraction, pellets or insoluble particles were removed,
dried, and weighed to determine the degree of amino acid protection.
The percent protection was calculated from the initial amino acid
content and the pellet weight loss. Glycine/NaCl/HCl buffer solution was used to simulate abomasal fluid; however, other pH 3.0
buffer solutions such as a citric acid/sodium phosphate solution
can also be used to extract the pellets without losing accuracy.
Amino acids in the supernatant liquid were analyzed either by an
X-ray fluorescence spectroscopic method or by a colorimetric method
with 2,4,6-trinitrobenzenesulfonic acid as a color-developing agent
in citrate buffer.[8] The percent amino acid protection data obtained
either from the gravimetric method or from the direct spectroscopic
measurements were identical within experimental error.

In Vitro and In Vivo Evaluation for Rumen Stability and Abomasal Release of CPMB-Coated Methionine Pellets

The rumen stability of CPMB-coated methionine pellets was tested in rumen fluid in vitro by incubating the pellets in freshly drawn, buffered rumen fluid for 17 hr, and tested in vivo in a nylon bag suspended in the rumen. Recovery of the CPMB-coated methionine was determined by the weight of the pellets remaining after they had been separated from the rumen fluid, washed, and dried.

Abomasal release of the pellets was tested in vitro in abomasal fluid and in vivo by administering two grams of methionine, or CPMB-coated methionine, abomasally to sheep and measuring the change of free methionine in blood plasma.

RESULTS AND DISCUSSION

To make encapsulated rumen-stable nutrient or pharmaceutical preparations by an air-suspension coating process, a number of interacting variables relative to core material and properties, coating composition and properties, and coating process were carefully considered. The important variables associated with CPMB-based rumen-stable pellets are listed in Table I.

Table II illustrates some physical properties of three amino acids: methionine, phenylalanine, and lysine.[9] Because of the relatively low water solubility of methionine and phenylalanine, excellent protection and controlled release could be achieved by merely encapsulating with a coherent, enveloping layer of CPMB. At a coating level of 10% of the finished pellet weight, the amino acid

TABLE I. VARIABLES FOR THE FORMULATION OF RUMEN-STABLE NUTRIENTS

Core Composition:	Solubility, basicity, additives (diluent, binder, disintegrant, lubricant), density, shape, size, surface.
Coating Composition:	pH sensitivity, water permeability, swelling property, solvent, polymer composition, polymer biodegradability, polymer physical properties (Tg, solubility, I.V.), polymer purity.
Coating Process:	Coater design, operating parameters (temperature, pressure, coating speed), fluid viscosity.

TABLE II.   PHYSICAL PROPERTIES OF PHENYLALANINE, METHIONINE,
AND LYSINE

Amino Acid	Mol Wt	Solubility in H$_2$O at 25°C	pK$_1$	pK$_2$	pk$_3$	PI
L-Phenylalanine	165.2	2.96	1.83	9.13	−	5.48
L-Methionine	149.2	3.8	2.28	9.21	−	5.74
L-Lysine	146.2	>70.0	2.18	o-8.95	ε-10.5	9.74

Phenylalanine: ⬡—CH$_2$-$\overset{H}{\underset{NH_2}{C}}$-C$\overset{O}{\underset{OH}{}}$

Methionine: CH$_3$SCH$_2$CH$_2$$\overset{H}{\underset{NH_2}{C}}$-C$\overset{O}{\underset{OH}{}}$

Lysine: H$_2$N-CH$_2$-CH$_2$-CH$_2$-CH$_2$-$\overset{H}{\underset{NH_2}{C}}$-C$\overset{O}{\underset{OH}{}}$

protection is 90% or greater for both of these amino acids in the
simulated rumen-stability test. Both CPMB-coated pellets readily
disintegrated within one hour in pH 3.0 buffer solution (Figure
3). The high payload of amino acids in these two preparations,
79%, is economically desirable.

Lysine monohydrochloride is the common form of feed-grade supplement lysine. Because of the high water solubility and the acidity
of the feed-grade lysine hydrochloride, pellets of lysine hydrochloride cannot be successfully rumen-protected by a simple CPMB polymeric layer. CaCO$_3$ was used as an antacid additive in the core
to partially neutralize the acid. The results are shown in Figure 4.
CaCO$_3$, in an amount equivalent to at least 10% of the HCl equivalents,
must be added to the core composition to achieve 65-70% amino acid
protection in the simulated rumen-stability test for a coating
composed of CPMB/aluminum hydroxydioleate (60/40 by weight) at the
coating level of 20% finished pellet weight.

Aluminum hydroxydioleate, [Al(OH)(Oleate)$_2$], and other hydrophobic materials such as fatty acids and waxes, were incorporated
in the polymeric coating to reduce the water permeability of the
coating and to modify the degree of swelling in water.

Figure 5 illustrates the water-swelling property of the thin
films composed of CPMB/Al(OH)(Oleate)$_2$ at different weight ratios.
The degree of swelling in water was measured by the percent increase

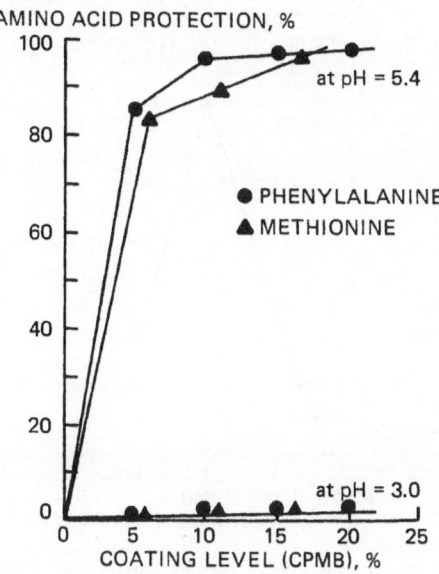

Figure 3. Simulated rumen stability and abomasal release of CPMB-encapsulated methionine and phenylalanine pellets as a function of coating weight.

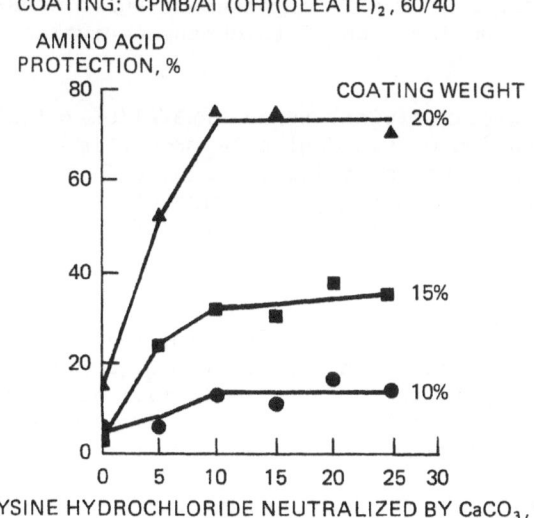

Figure 4. Effect of $CaCO_3$ as an antacid additive in the pellet core on the protection of lysine hydrochloride at pH 5.5.

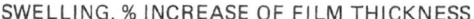

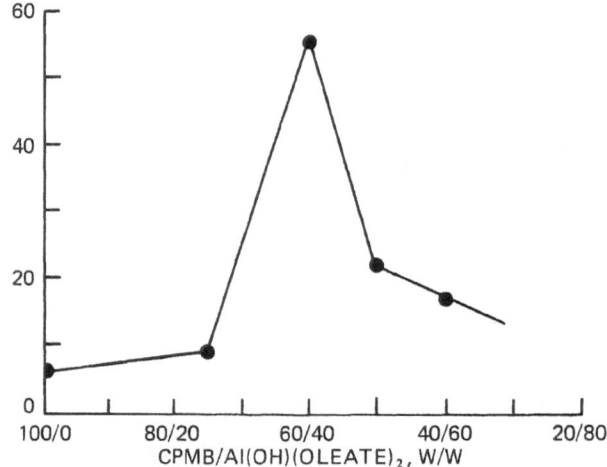

SWELLING, % INCREASE OF FILM THICKNESS

CPMB/Al(OH)(OLEATE)$_2$, W/W

Figure 5.   Degree of thin-film swelling as a function of binary
            coating composition, CPMB/Al(OH)(Oleate)$_2$; swelling
            time: 24 hr.

in the thickness of a 0.1-mm thick film immersed in pH 5.4 buffer
solution for 24 hr. The film composed of 60/40 CPMB/Al(OH)(Oleate)$_2$
exhibited a maximum increase of thickness equivalent to 55% of its
initial value.

     The coating composition, 50/50 CPMB/Al(OH)(Oleate)$_2$, provided
the best combination of all desirable properties--protection,
release, swelling, and coatability. Figure 6 illustrates the amino
acid protection as a function of varying coating compositions of
CPMB/Al(OH)(Oleate)$_2$ at four different coating levels on lysine
hydrochloride.

     Table III summarizes the results of in vitro and in vivo rumen-
stability tests of CPMB-coated methionine pellets according to the
testing methods described in the experimental section. These testing methods, in vitro and in vivo, gave virtually the same results
and, within experimental error, the data indicated nearly complete
protection of methionine in the rumen environment.

     Immersion of the CPMB-coated methionine pellets (10% coating
by weight) in freshly collected, filtered abomasal fluid taken from
an abomasally cannulated sheep resulted in the disintegration of
the coating and release of the methionine in 30 min.

PELLET CORE: LYSINE HYDROCHLORIDE 25% NEUTRALIZED WITH CaCO₃

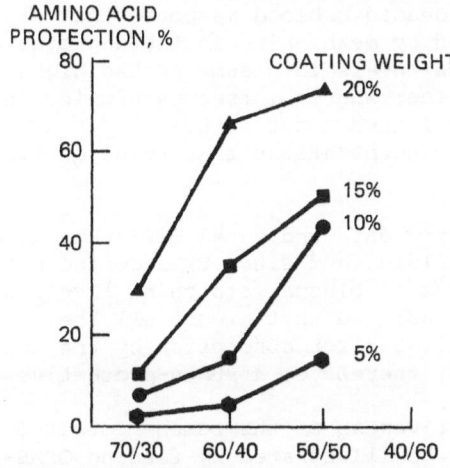

Figure 6. Protection of lysine hydrochloride at pH 5.5 as a function of binary coating composition, CPMB/Al(OH)(Oleate) ,
for 25% neutralized lysin hydrochloride pellets. Coated
at four coating levels.

     Results from the _in vitro_ and _in vivo_ rumen-stability experi-
ments and the results from the _in vitro_ abomasal-release experiment
are consistent with the data obtained from the simulated buffer-
solution tests for rumen stability at pH 5.4, and abomasal release
at pH 3.0. Thus, it was concluded that the simple simulated rumen-
stability and abomasal-release tests provide quick, reliable laboratory methods for the evaluation of these rumen-protected formulations. .

TABLE III.   IN VITRO AND IN VIVO RUMEN STABILITY
          OF CPMB-COATED METHIONINE PELLETS

	Recovery of Methionine Pellets	Range
Rumen Fluid (in vitro)	97%	92-99%
Rumen, Nylon Bag (in vivo)	95%	92-98%

The in vivo evidence of postruminal release and absorption is shown in Figure 7. Typically, abomasal administration of CPMB-coated methionine produced a blood response that was similar to the response produced by methionine in the unprotected form. Generally, free methionine levels in plasma peaked higher and somewhat earlier with methionine; whereas, free methionine levels from rumen-protected methionine peaked about an hour later and were more persistent than the blood concentrations that resulted from unprotected methionine.

Since the in vitro data indicated disintegration of the pellet coating in abomasal fluid, and since CPMB-coated methionine caused substantial elevations in plasma methionine levels when administered abomasally, it was concluded that almost all the methionine was released and was available for absorption by the animal. Indeed, the CPMB coating was, therefore, a rumen-protective coating.

The total effectiveness of the rumen-protected methionine preparation can best be illustrated by feeding CPMB-coated methionine and measuring its effect upon levels of free methionine in blood plasma.

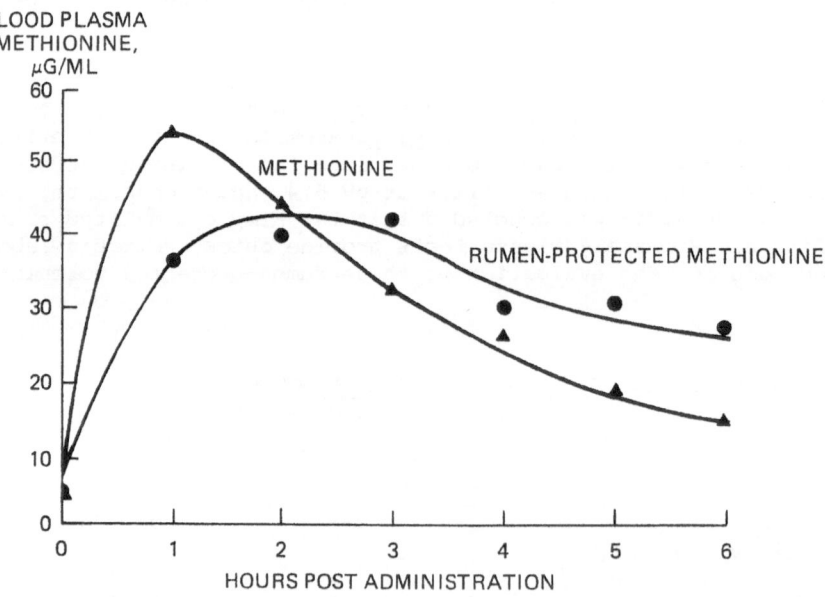

Figure 7.   Comparison of methionine concentrations in blood plasma of sheep after abomasal infusion of methionine and CPMB-coated methionine.

In one experiment, four grams of methionine (as rumen-protected methionine) was fed to sheep in their daily rations at a 0.4% level. Blood levels of methionine rose to over 200% of the control, thus illustrating that methionine had survived the rumen and had been released and absorbed. This result is shown in Table IV.

In another experiment, one group of lambs was fed a control diet; another group was fed the same diet supplemented with unprotected methionine at 4 g/day; and a third group was fed rumen-protected methionine at 4 g-equivalent/day. As shown in Figure 8, plasma methionine concentrations were not elevated with unprotected methionine after 6 days of feeding; however, rumen-protected methionine substantially elevated methionine levels.

To test the rumen-protected methionine preparation further and to investigate its utility, experiments were conducted with sheep to determine the effect of dietary rumen-protected methionine on wool growth. Rumen-protected methionine fed to lambs at the rate of 0.6% of the diet for 14 weeks increased wool production by 42%.

These results indicate that rumen-protected methionine is an effective source of postruminal methionine.

CONCLUSIONS

Cellulose propionate morpholinobutyrate, a pH-sensitive polymer, can be used to formulate controlled-release coating compositions for achieving the rumen-stability and the abomasal-release characteristics needed for labile nutrients and pharmaceuticals which are sensitive to the rumen environment and can benefit the animal through postruminal availability.

TABLE IV. FEEDING RUMEN-PROTECTED METHIONINE TO LAMBS
(0.4% RUMEN-PROTECTED METHIONINE IN DIET)

Animal	Control	Rumen-Protected Methionine	% Control
		(μg Free Methionine/ml Blood Plasma)	
1	3.5	6.8	194
2	2.6	6.2	238
3	2.4	5.1	212
$\bar{X}$	2.8	5.8	215

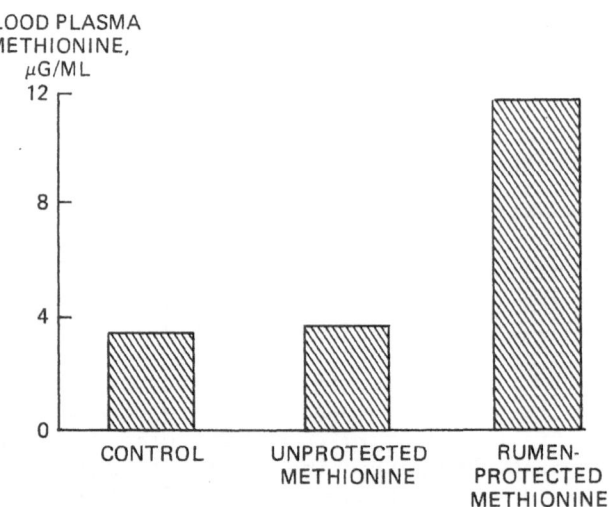

Figure 8.   Comparison of methionine concentrations in blood plasma
            for lambs fed a control diet supplemented with unprotected
            and CPMB-coated methionine.

        CPMB-based rumen-protected preparations provided an effective
and efficient way of administering essential nutrients, pharmaceuticals, and growth promoters postruminally.

        CPMB-based delivery systems also provide a useful tool for
animal nutritionists to study ruminant nutrition, an area made difficult to investigate by problems encountered in the rumen environment.

REFERENCES

1.   W. Anderson, Feedstuffs, 51(44):8 (1979).
2.   D.C. Church, in: "Digestive Physiology and Nutrition of
     Ruminants," Vol. 1, Oregon State University Book Stores, Inc.
     (1969). p. 5.
3.   P.M. Grant, B. Fulkerson, and J.W. Mench, U.S. Patent 3,562,806
     (1971).
4.   J.W. Mench and B. Fulkerson, I&EC Product & Development 7(1):2
     (1968).
5.   C.C. Dannelly and C.R. Leonard, U.S. Patent 4,117,801 (1978).
6.   H.S. Hall and T.M. Hinkes, in: "Microencapsulation Process
     and Applications," J.E. Vandegaer, ed., Plenum Press, New York
     (1974). p. 145.

7.   G.W. Larson and P.A. Mallak, U.S. Patent 3,110,626 (1963).

8.   S.L. Snyder and P.Z. Sobocinski, Anal. Bio. Chem. 64(1):284 (1975).

9.   H.R. Mahler and E.H. Cordes, in: "Biological Chemistry," Harper & Row Publishers, New York (1966). p. 8.

LIST OF CONTRIBUTORS

J.M. Anderson, Department of Macromolecular Science, Case Western
   Reserve University, Cleveland, Ohio 44106
K.W. Anderson, Department of Polymer Science, University of Southern
   Mississippi, Hattiesburg, Mississippi 39401
Lee R. Beck, Department of Obstetrics and Gynecology, University
   of Alabama in Birmingham, Birmingham, Alabama 35294
F.E. Brinckman, Chemical and Biodegradation Processes Group, Center
   for Materials Science, National Bureau of Standards, Washington,
   D.C. 20234
Nathan F. Cardarelli, Environmental Management Laboratory, The Uni-
   versity of Akron, Akron, Ohio 44325
Donald R. Cowsar, Southern Research Institute, 2000 Ninth Avenue
   South, Birmingham, Alabama 35255
Clarence C. Dannelly, Research Laboratories, Tennessee Eastman
   Company, Division of Eastman Kodak Company, Kingsport, Tennessee
   37662
Guido E. Desmarets, State University of Gent, Laboratory of Organic
   Chemistry, Krijgslaan 271 (S-4), B-9000, Gent, Belgium
Richard L. Dunn, Southern Research Institute, 2000 Ninth Avenue
   South, Birmingham, Alabama 35255
Ruben J. Ellin, Department of Chemistry, The University of Akron,
   Akron, Ohio 44325
William Evans, Environmental Management Laboratory, University of
   Akron, Akron, Ohio 44325
David J. Fink, Battelle Columbus Laboratories, 505 King Avenue,
   Columbus, Ohio 43201
P.G. Friel, International Fertility Research Program, Research
   Triangle Park, North Carolina
Gösta Gahrton, Section of Oncology and Hematology, Department of
   Medicine, Huddinge Hospital, S-141 86 Huddinge, Sweden
David L. Gardner, Battelle Columbus Laboratories, 505 King Avenue,
   Columbus, Ohio 43201
Norman L. Gauthier, Agway Inc., Syracuse, New York 13221
N.A. Ghanem, Laboratory of Polymers and Pigments, National Research
   Centre, Dokki, Cairo, Egypt
P.A. Giang, Livestock Insects Laboratory, Agricultural Research,
   Science and Education Administration, USDA, Beltsville, Maryland
   20705
Eric J. Goethals, State University of Gent, Laboratory of Organic
   Chemistry, Krijgslaan 271 (S-4), B-9000, Gent, Belgium

Craig R. Hassler, Battelle Columbus Laboratories, 505 King Avenue,
    Columbus, Ohio 43201

D.K. Hayes, Livestock Insects Laboratory, Agricultural Research,
    Science and Education Administration, USDA, Beltsville, Maryland
    20705

Dean S.T. Hsieh, Department of Nutrition and Food Science, M.I.T.,
    Cambridge, Massachusetts 02139 and the Department of Surgery,
    Children's Hospital Medical Center, Boston, Massachusetts 02114

N.E. Ikladious, Laboratory of Polymers and Pigments, National Re-
    search Centre, Dokki, Cairo, Egypt

J.C. Jackson, Department of Chemistry, The University of Akron,
    Akron, Ohio 44325

Martin Jacobson, Biologically Active Natural Products Laboratory,
    Agricultural Environmental Quality Institute, Agric. Res.,
    Science and Education Administration, Beltsville, Maryland 20705

H. Jaffe, Livestock Insects Laboratory, Agricultural Research,
    Science and Education Administration, USDA, Beltsville, Mary-
    land 20705

R.D. Jones, Departments of Pathology and Macromolecular Science,
    Case Western Reserve University, Cleveland, Ohio 44106, and
    Division of Surgical Research, St. Luke's Hospital, Cleveland,
    Ohio 44104

Irving Keiser, U.S. Department of Agriculture, Science and Education
    Administration, Tropical Fruit and Vegetable Research Laboratory,
    Honolulu, Hawaii 96804

Ronald J. Komarek, Research Laboratories, Tennessee Eastman Company,
    Division of Eastman Kodak Company, Kingsport, Tennessee 37662

S.E. Kunz, U.S. Livestock Insects Laboratory, Agricultural Research,
    Science and Education Administration, USDA, Kerrville, Texas

John W. Kusiak, Section on Macromolecules, National Institutes of
    Health, National Institute on Aging, GRC-Baltimore City Hos-
    pitals, Baltimore, Maryland 21224

Robert Langer, Department of Nutrition and Food Science, M.I.T.,
    Cambridge, Massachusetts 02139 and the Department of Surgery,
    Children's Hospital Medical Center, Boston, Massachusetts 02115.

P.I. Lee, Central Research, CIBA-GEIGY Corporation, Ardsley, New
    York 10502

Danny H. Lewis, Southern Research Institute, 2000 Ninth Avenue
    South, Birmingham, Alabama 35255

D.K. Lichatowich, Department of Polymer Science, University of
    Southern Mississippi, Hattiesburg, Mississippi 39401

Clifford S. Lofgren, USDA-SEA/AR, Gainesville, Florida 32604

C.L. McCormick, Department of Polymer Science, University of Southern
    Mississippi, Hattiesburg, Mississippi 39401

N.N. Messiha, Laboratory of Polymers and Pigments, National Research
    Centre, Dokki, Cairo, Egypt

William E. Meyers, Southern Research Institute, 2000 Ninth Avenue
    South, Birmingham, Alabama 35255

J.A. Miller, U.S. Livestock Insects Laboratory, Agricultural Re-
    search, Science and Education Administration, USDA, Kerrville,
    Texas

D.D. Oehler, U.S. Livestock Insects Laboratory, Agricultural Research, Science and Education Administration, USDA, Kerrville, Texas

L.S. Olanoff, Departments of Pathology and Macromolecular Science, Case Western Reserve University, Cleveland, Ohio 44106, and Division of Surgical Research, St. Luke's Hospital, Cleveland, Ohio 44104

E.J. Parks, Chemical and Biodegradation Processes Group, Center for Materials Science, National Bureau of Standards, Washington, D.C. 20234

Christer Paul, Section of Oncology and Hematology, Department of Medicine, Huddinge Hospital, S-141 86 Huddinge, Sweden

J.A. Pelezo, Department of Polymer Science, University of Southern Mississippi, Hattiesburg, Mississippi 39401

Curt Peterson, Department of Pharmacology, Karolinska Institute, S-104 01 Stockholm, Sweden

Josef Pitha, Section on Macromolecules, National Institutes of Health, National Institute on Aging, GRC-Baltimore City Hospitals, Baltimore, Maryland 21224

Thomas J. Quick, Environmental Management Laboratory, The University of Akron, Akron, Ohio 44325

Etienne H. Schacht, State University of Gent, Laboratory of Organic Chemistry, Krijgslaan 271 (S-4), B-9000, Gent, Belgium

A.F. Shaaban, Laboratory of Polymers and Pigments, National Research Centre, Dokki, Cairo, Egypt

Larry R. Sherman, Department of Chemistry, The University of Akron, Akron, Ohio 44325

James A. Silva, Hawaii Agricultural Experiment Station, College of Tropical Agriculture and Human Resources, University of Hawaii, Honolulu, Hawaii 96822

Daniel Smith, Department of Chemistry, University of Akron, Akron, Ohio 44325

K.N. Somasekharan, Department of Materials Science and Engineering, Washington State University, Pullman, Washington 99164

B.H. Stroud, Animal Operations Unit, Agricultural Research, Science and Education Administration, USDA, Beltsville, Maryland 20705

R.V. Subramanian, Department of Materials Science and Engineering, Washington State University, Pullman, Washington 99164

N. Tani, Department of Macromolecular Science, Case Western Reserve University, Cleveland, Ohio 44106

M. Van Dress, Department of Macromolecular Science, Case Western Reserve University, Cleveland, Ohio 44106

Robert K. Vander Meer, USDA-SEA/AR, Gainesville, Florida 32604

Nobel Wakabayashi, U.S. Department of Agriculture, Science and Education Administration, Biologically Active Natural Products Laboratory, Agricultural Environmental Quality Institute, Beltsville, Maryland 20705

R.G. Wheeler, International Fertility Research Program, Research Triangle Park, North Carolina

Stephen H. Wu, Research Laboratories, Tennessee Eastman Company, Division of Eastman Kodak Company, Kingsport, Tennessee 37662